BUSINESS REPLY CARD

FIRST CLASS   PERMIT NO. 33107   PHILADELPHIA, PA

POSTAGE WILL BE PAID BY ADDRESSEE

HANLEY & BELFUS, INC.
Medical Publishers
P.O. Box 1377
Philadelphia, PA 19105-9990

NO POSTAGE
NECESSARY
IF MAILED
IN THE
UNITED STATES

BUSINESS REPLY CARD

FIRST CLASS   PERMIT NO. 33107   PHILADELPHIA, PA

POSTAGE WILL BE PAID BY ADDRESSEE

HANLEY & BELFUS, INC.
Medical Publishers
P.O. Box 1377
Philadelphia, PA 19105-9990

Publisher: HANLEY & BELFUS, INC.
               210 South 13th Street
               Philadelphia, PA 19107
               (215) 546-7293
               Fax (215) 790-9330

CARDIAC SURGERY: State of the Art Reviews   ISSN 0887-9850
Volume 7, Number 2   ISBN 1-56053-097-9

CARDIAC SURGERY: State of the Art Reviews is published triannually (three times per year) by Hanley & Belfus, Inc., 210 South 13th Street, Philadelphia, Pennsylvania 19107.

POSTMASTER: Send address changes to CARDIAC SURGERY: State of the Art Reviews, Hanley & Belfus, Inc., 210 South 13th Street, Philadelphia, PA 19107.

This issue is Volume 7, Number 2.

The Editor of this publication is Linda C. Belfus.

CONTENTS

Use of diuretics as well as vasodilators and vasopressors with or without inotropic effects is often necessary in patients with advanced cardiac dysfunction, including congestive heart failure. This chapter examines the pharmacology of specific drugs and discusses the transition from intravenous to oral therapy.

Patient selection for mechanical circulatory support involves specific criteria for the three major clinical categories: postcardiotomy support, bridge to transplant, and acute deterioration. Refinement of the criteria should lead to expanded indications for mechanical circulatory support and to improved survival rates.

Concentration of skills and reduction of cost have necessitated the regionalization of cardiac transplant and implant centers. One result is the demand for an expedient and reliable system of transport for critically ill patients. Federal regulations as well as medical needs must be taken into account.

The Bio-Pump has undergone investigation for long-term left-heart assist since 1978. Animal experiments led to refinement of both technology and technique. Clinical trials support the long-term efficacy of the device but also indicate the need for further research into criteria for patient selection.

The thromboresistance of Duraflo II, a heparin-coating system for cardiopulmonary bypass circuits, has been demonstrated both experimentally and clinically. The system also minimizes blood trauma caused by blood-material interactions and allows optimal modification of systemic anticoagulation.

Clinical experience has been obtained with roller, centrifugal, and pulsatile pneumatic assist pumps. This chapter focuses on patient management and clinical results in treatment of postcardiotomy cardiogenic shock with the two currently available pulsatile pneumatic pumps: the Pierce-Donachy and the Abiomed.

Results of pneumatic ventricular assist devices (VADs) in patients with potentially reversible myocardial injury have been disappointing. Nonetheless, experimental data clearly demonstrate that pneumatic VADs with synchronous counterpulsation provide the ideal setting for recovery from an ischemic injury.

CONTRIBUTORS

David Abrahamson, M.D.
Assistant Clinical Professor, Department of Medicine, Division of Cardiology, University of California, Irvine, Medical Center, Orange, California

Robert M. Adamson, M.D.
Director, Heart and Lung Transplantation, Sharp Memorial Hospital, San Diego, California

Byron J. Allen, M.D.
Assistant Professor of Medicine, Division of Cardiology, University of California, Irvine, Orange, California

Thomas X. Aufiero, M.D.
Assistant Professor of Surgery, Department of Surgery, Division of Cardiothoracic Surgery, Pennsylvania State University College of Medicine, Hershey, Pennsylvania

Bradford Blakeman, M.D.
Associate Professor, Department of Thoracic and Cardiovascular Surgery, Loyola University of Chicago Stritch School of Medicine, Maywood, Illinois

Valéria Bors, M.D.
Cardiovascular Department, Groupe Hospitalier Pitié-Sapêtriere, Paris, France

Michael A. Brodsky, M.D.
Associate Professor of Medicine, Division of Cardiology, University of California, Irvine, Orange, California

A. Cabrol, M.D.
Cardiovascular Department, Groupe Hospitalier Pitié-Salpêtriere, Paris, France

David B. Calandra, M.D.
Assistant Professor, Department of Thoracic and Cardiovascular Surgery, Loyola University of Chicago Stritch School of Medicine, Maywood, Illinois

Marilyn R. Cleavinger, M.S., B.M.E.
Assistant Director, Artificial Heart Program, University of Arizona College of Medicine, Tucson, Arizona

Brian L. Cmolik, M.D.
Resident, Cardiothoracic Surgery, Allegheny General Hospital, Pittsburgh, Pennsylvania

Jack G. Copeland, M.D.
Michael Drummond Distinguished Professor of Cardiothoracic Surgery, University of Arizona College of Medicine, Tucson, Arizona

Pierre Corbi, M.D.
Cardiovascular Department, Groupe Hospitalier Pitié-Salpêtriere, Paris, France

Maria Rosa Costanzo-Nordin, M.D.
Associate Professor, Department of Thoracic and Cardiovascular Surgery, Loyola University of Chicago Stritch School of Medicine, Maywood, Illinois

Bill B. Daily, M.D., Ph.D.
Assistant Professor of Surgery, Department of Cardiovascular and Thoracic Surgery, Washington University School of Medicine, St. Louis, Missouri

Pat O. Daily, M.D.
Director, Cardiovascular and Thoracic Surgery, Sharp Memorial Hospital, San Diego, California

Walter P. Dembitsky, M.D.
Program Director, Cardiac Assist Devices, Sharp Memorial Hospital, San Diego, California

Mary Lynn Dwyer, B.S., R.N.
Baxter Healthcare Corporation, Bentley Laboratories Division, Irvine, California

Robert W. Emery, M.D.
Director, Cardiothoracic Transplantation, and Cardiovascular and Thoracic Surgeon, Minneapolis Heart Institute, Abbott Northwestern Hospital, Minneapolis, Minnesota

John Eugene, M.D.
Associate Clinical Professor of Surgery, University of California, Irvine, Orange, California

David J. Farrar, Ph.D.
Director of Research, Department of Cardiac Surgery, California Pacific Medical Center, San Francisco, California

Patria Fopiano, B.S., R.N.
Clinical Coordinator, Department of Cardiothoracic Surgery, University of California, Irvine, Medical Center, Orange, California

O.H. Frazier, M.D.
Professor of Surgery, University of Texas Medical School; Chief, Cardiopulmonary Transplantation, Texas Heart Institute, Houston, Texas

Iradj Gandjbakhch, M.D.
Professor, Cardiovascular Department, Hopital Pitié, Paris, France

Alan B. Gazzaniga, M.D.
Professor of Surgery, University of California, Irvine, Medical Center, Orange, California

Irvin F. Goldenberg, M.D.
Clinical Assistant Professor of Medicine, University of Minnesota, Minneapolis Heart Institute, Minneapolis, Minnesota

Bartley P. Griffith, M.D.
Professor of Surgery, University of Pittsburgh School of Medicine; Chief, Division of Cardiothoracic Surgery, University of Pittsburgh Medical Center, Pittsburgh, Pennsylvania

Dan E. Gutfinger, Ph.D.
Director of Artificial Heart Program, Division of Cardiothoracic Surgery, University of California, Irvine, Medical Center, Orange, California

J. Donald Hill, M.D.
Chairman, Department of Cardiac Surgery, California Pacific Medical Center, San Francisco, California

Thomas Hinkamp, M.D.
Assistant Professor, Department of Thoracic and Cardiovascular Surgery, Loyola University of Chicago Stritch School of Medicine, Maywood, Illinois

Li-Chien Hsu, Ph.D.
Senior Baxter Scientist, Bentley Division, Baxter Healthcare Corporation, Irvine, California

Timothy B. Icenogle, M.D.
Director, Inland Northwest Thoracic Organ Transplant Program, Spokane, Washington

Valluvan Jeevanandam, M.D.
Assistant Professor of Surgery, Temple University School of Medicine; Surgical Director, Heart Failure and Transplantation, Temple University Hospital, Philadelphia, Pennsylvania

Akihiko Kawai, M.D.
Research Fellow, Department of Surgery, University of Pittsburgh School of Medicine, Pittsburgh, Pennsylvania

Pratap Khanwilkar, M.S., M.B.A.
Director of Engineering, Artificial Heart Research Laboratory, University of Utah, Salt Lake City, Utah

Robert L. Kormos, M.D.
Associate Professor of Surgery; Director, Artificial Heart Program, University of Pittsburgh School of Medicine, Pittsburgh, Pennsylvania

Philippe Leger, M.D.
Cardiovascular Department, Groupe Hospitalier Pitié-Salpêtriere, Paris, France

Jean-Pierre Levasseur, M.D.
Cardiovascular Department, Groupe Hospitalier Pitié-Salpêtriere, Paris, France

Scott Lick, M.D.
Department of Cardiothoracic Surgery, University of Arizona College of Medicine, Tucson, Arizona

David H. Loffing, M.S., C.C.E.
Senior Clinical Engineer, Biomedical Engineering, University of Arizona College of Medicine, Tucson, Arizona

Vassyl Lonchyna, M.D.
Assistant Professor, Department of Thoracic and Cardiovascular Surgery, Loyola University of Chicago Stritch School of Medicine, Maywood, Illinois

George J. Magovern, Jr., M.D.
Associate Professor of Surgery, Division of Thoracic Surgery, Allegheny General Hospital, Allegheny Campus of the Medical College of Pennsylvania, Pittsburgh, Pennsylvania

James A. Magovern, M.D.
Assistant Professor of Surgery, Allegheny General Hospital, Pittsburgh, Pennsylvania

Donald J. Mahon, M.D.
Assistant Clinical Professor, Department of Medicine, Division of Cardiology, University of California, Irvine, Medical Center, Orange, California

Lawrence R. McBride, M.D.
Department of Surgery, St. Louis University School of Medicine, St. Louis, Missouri

Stephen A. Mikitish
Supervisor, Metal Trades, Facilities Management, University of Arizona Health Sciences Center, Tucson, Arizona

Timothy C. Mills, Ph.D.
Baxter L.I.S. Division, Advanced Development, Irvine, California

Alvaro Montoya, M.D.
Professor, Department of Thoracic and Cardiovascular Surgery, Loyola University of Chicago Stritch School of Medicine, Maywood, Illinois

Ricardo J. Moreno-Cabral, M.D.
Department of Cardiovascular and Thoracic Surgery, Sharp Memorial Hospital, San Diego, California

Donald B. Olsen, D.V.M.
Director for the Institute for the Artificial Heart Research Laboratory, Professor of Surgery, Research Professor of Pharmaceutics, and Research Professor of Bioengineering, University of Utah, Salt Lake City, Utah

Richard A. Ott, M.D.
Associate Professor of Surgery and Director of Cardiac Transplantation, University of California, Irvine, Medical Center, Orange, California

Lester D. Padilla, M.D.
Cardiology Fellow, Department of Medicine, Division of Cardiology, University of California, Irvine, Medical Center, Orange, California

Walter E. Pae, Jr., M.D.
Professor of Surgery, Director of Cardiac Transplantation, Division of Cardiothoracic Surgery, Department of Surgery, Pennsylvania State University College of Medicine, Hershey, Pennsylvania

Steven E. Park, M.D.
Resident, Cardiothoracic Surgery, Allegheny General Hospital, Pittsburgh, Pennsylvania

Alain Pavie, M.D.
Professor, Cardiovascular Department, Groupe Hospitalier Pitié-Salpêtriere, Paris, France

D. Glenn Pennington, M.D.
Professor of Surgery, St. Louis University School of Medicine, St. Louis, Missouri

William S. Pierce, M.D.
Evan Pugh Professor and Chief, Division of Cardiothoracic Surgery, Pennsylvania State University College of Medicine, The Milton S. Hershey Medical Center, Hershey, Pennsylvania

Roque Pifarre, M.D.
Professor and Chairman, Department of Thoracic and Cardiovascular Surgery, Loyola University of Chicago Stritch School of Medicine, Maywood, Illinois

Peer M. Portner, Ph.D.
Baxter Healthcare Corporation, Novacor Division, Oakland, California

Marc R. Pritzker, M.D.
Clinical Associate Professor of Medicine, University of Minnesota, Minneapolis Heart Institute, Abbott Northwestern Hospital, Minneapolis, Minnesota

Gregorio Rabago, M.D.
Cardiovascular Department, Hôpital Pitié, Paris, France

Narayanan Ramasamy, Ph.D.
Baxter Healthcare Corporation, Novacor Division, Oakland, California

Eric A. Rose, M.D.
Chief of Cardiothoracic Surgery, Columbia-Presbyterian Medical Center, New York, New York

David J. Sato, M.S.B.E., C.C.E.
Circulatory Assist Program, Sacred Heart Medical Center, Spokane, Washington

Bruce J. Shook, M.S.Eng.
Vice President of Clinical and Regulatory Affairs, ABIOMED, Inc., Danvers, Massachusetts

Richard G. Smith, M.S.E.E., C.C.E.
Technical Director, Artificial Heart Program, University of Arizona College of Medicine, Tucson, Arizona

Thomas L. Spray, M.D.
Professor of Surgery and Pediatrics, Department of Cardiothoracic Surgery, Washington University School of Medicine, St. Louis, Missouri

Henry J. Sullivan, M.D.
Professor and Vice-Chairman, Department of Thoracic and Cardiovascular Surgery, Loyola University of Chicago Stritch School of Medicine, Maywood, Illinois

Marc T. Swartz
Department of Surgery, St. Louis University Medical Center, St. Louis, Missouri

J. Szefner, M.D.
Cardiovascular Department, Groupe Hospitalier Pitié-Salpêtriere, Paris, France

Jonathan M. Tobis, M.D.
Professor of Medicine and Radiology, and Director of Cardiac Catheterization Laboratory, University of California, Irvine, Medical Center, Orange, California

Nina E. Topic, R.N., M.S.
Clinical Research Nurse, Department of Cardiac Surgery, California Pacific Medical Center, San Francisco, California

Eduardo A. Tovar, M.D.
Assistant Clinical Professor, Department of Surgery, University of California, Irvine, Orange, California

Elisabeth Vaissier, M.D.
Cardiovascular Department, Groupe Hospitalier Pitié-Salpêtriere, Paris, France

Milton Vana, Jr., M.D.
Assistant Clinical Professor, Department of Surgery, University of California, Irvine, Medical Center, Orange, California

Robert A. Vogel, M.D.
Herbert Berger Professor of Medicine, Division of Cardiology, Department of Medicine, University of Maryland School of Medicine; Head, Division of Cardiology, University of Maryland Hospital, Baltimore, Maryland

Jeanine M. Walenga, Ph.D.
Assistant Professor, Department of Thoracic and Cardiovascular Surgery, Loyola University of Chicago Stritch School of Medicine, Maywood, Illinois

PREFACE

We are privileged to edit this volume of **Cardiac Surgery: State of the Art Reviews** on Mechanical Cardiac Assist. This edition represents the collective effort of the leading experts in the field. We are most appreciative to the contributors who responded so enthusiastically and gave so much of their time to complete this work.

During the past three decades, an evolution of technology has provided a variety of cardiac assist systems. The objective of this issue is to present a "handbook" reference of available devices that is of value to clinicians interested in cardiovascular disease.

With new advances in technology and critical care, the prospects for mechanical support of the failing heart are more promising than ever. It seems only appropriate to review the achievements of the past and the concepts of the present with anticipation that mechanical cardiac assist will soon become conventional therapy in the future of cardiac surgery.

We extend our sincere thanks to our administrative assistant, Kay Crosser, and program consultant, Teresa Tanner, whose indispensable assistance permitted the completion of this publication. In addition, a special thanks to Robin Webb, RN, CCP and Nick Haiduc for their incomparable skill and tireless effort.

Richard A. Ott, M.D.
Dan E. Gutfinger, Ph.D.
Alan B. Gazzaniga, M.D.
GUEST EDITORS

DEDICATION

This book is dedicated to E.K.S. and the countless cardiac patients whose quiet courage give us strength and inspiration.

ALAN B. GAZZANIGA, MD

HISTORY OF EXTRACORPOREAL MEMBRANE OXYGENATION

Professor and Chief
Cardiothoracic Surgery
University of California, Irvine
Orange, California

Reprint requests to:
Alan B. Gazzaniga, MD
Professor and Chief
Cardiothoracic Surgery
University of California, Irvine
Building 53, Route 81
101 City Drive
Orange, CA 92668

The development of the bubble oxygenator did for open-heart surgery what the introduction of the membrane oxygenator did for long-term cardiopulmonary support. The father of extracorporeal circulation was John Gibbon,[1] with the assistance of Gross, Harken, Murray, and McLean after conception and of Kirklin, Lillehi, and many others after delivery. Gibbon's heart-lung machine could sustain life for 1–2 hours for intracardiac repair but beyond this time failed and in fact became lethal. Lee et al.[2] and Dobell et al.[3] identified the gas-exchange device as the source of this limitation. It was postulated that if a gas-permeable membrane could be substituted for the blood-gas interface of the bubble oxygenator, the length of extracorporeal circulation could be extended from hours to days. A membrane oxygenator had been used by Lillehi[4] with biologic preparation and cross-body circulation and by Mustard[5] with in-situ monkey lungs. Limitations of these approaches were obvious, and oxygenators continued to develop.

Kolff[6] observed oxygenation of blood through the membrane of his early dialyzers and reported gas-exchange experiments with a modified artificial kidney in 1955.[7] In 1956 Clowes[8] and coauthors designed, built, tested, and put to clinical use the first membrane oxygenator. This device used polyethylene and Teflon membranes, which were inefficient in gas transfer and required large surface areas. The cumbersome nature of the device precluded general use, but the experiments showed that construction and use of a membrane oxygenator was feasible. At the same time successful application of filming

CARDIAC SURGERY: State of the Art Reviews—Vol. 7, No. 2, 1993
Philadelphia, Hanley & Belfus, Inc.

171

oxygenators for cardiac surgery led to general acceptance and usage of the simpler devices. The bubble oxygenator, a concept described in 1966 by DeWall,[9] is now used almost universally in the operating room.

In 1957 Kammermeyer[10] reported the unique gas-transfer characteristics of a polymer of dimethylsiloxane, which came to be known as silicone rubber. Silicone polymer membranes were evaluated in blood–gas transfers by Thomas[11] and Marx.[12] In the 1960s Kolobow,[13] Crystal,[14] Bramson,[15] Pierce,[16] Lande,[17] and others designed and built membrane oxygenators with the silicone rubber membrane. Further development of the Toroidal flow oxygenator by Drinker, Bartlett, et al.[18] heightened the interest in this field. In all of the devices oxygen diffusion through blood was a limiting factor in performance in contrast with the Teflon device. The available membrane oxygenators in 1971 were the Kolobow, Bramson, and Lande oxygenators. In 1971 O'Brien and Hill[19] at Cottage Hospital in Santa Barbara, California did the first successful long-term use of the membrane oxygenator in a human. The device used was the Bramson oxygenator. Their report was followed by several other successful outcomes.[23] In 1973 Soeter et al.[20] treated a 4-year-old patient on an extracorporeal membrane oxygenator (ECMO) for 50 hours after repair of tetralogy of Fallot. In 1973 Gazzaniga successfully treated a 2-year-old patient on ECMO for 36 hours after Mustard's repair for transposition of the great vessels. The patient, later reported by Bartlett et al.,[21] made a complete recovery and at that time was the youngest survivor of long-term bypass. Several months later, the first successful use of long-term extracorporeal circulation in a neonate with persistent fetal circulation occurred at the University of California Irvine Medical Center. Following the rather dramatic result, many pediatric patients who in the past would have died were salvaged,[22] and extracorporeal circulation was used primarily for the treatment of pediatric patients because its use in adult patients with acute respiratory failure had been disappointing.[23] As the pediatric experience evolved at the University of California Irvine Medical Center and Children's Hospital of Orange County, ECMO was found to be useful in the treatment of persistent fetal circulation, meconium aspiration, retained foreign body with respiratory failure, barotrauma secondary to positive pressure ventilation, neonatal sepsis, respiratory distress syndrome, drowning, and diaphragmatic hernia. The principal investigator was Robert H. Bartlett, M.D., currently professor of surgery at the University of Michigan. Shortly after the first successful cases of neonatal ECMO, it became apparent that the criteria for selection of patients were critical. Early experience led to development of the neonatal pulmonary insufficiency index, which proved helpful in selecting patients for ECMO.[23] Similar methods of categorizing patients, such as the oxygen index, are currently in use. Although Bartlett's initial results were dramatic, they were not reproduced at other centers, and ECMO was criticized as aggressive treatment of problems that could be managed by standard methods. This criticism was put to rest when Krummel et al.[24] at the Medical College of Virginia reported 6 survivors among 8 moribund patients who were treated with ECMO. As a result of their experience, pediatric neonatal ECMO began to develop in many centers throughout the United States and around the world.

A major obstacle in the application and development of ECMO in neonates and children was vascular access. In contrast, arterial and venous access in adults was easier because the femoral artery and vein were accessible. Early experience with neonates demonstrated that the femoral vessels were too small and the jeopardy to the limb too great. Robin Jefferies, M.D., at the University of California

Irvine developed the technique of neck cannulation currently used in venoarterial bypass. His investigative techniques led to Gazzaniga's use of the right carotid artery for ECMO in 1973. Use of the right carotid artery for arterial cannulation soon raised the issue of potential neurologic damage related to the temporary or permanent interruption of right carotid artery blood flow. Although this risk was certainly of concern when neonatal ECMO was introduced, the grave nature of the patients' illness tended to override the potential hazards of using the carotid artery. Really Vasquez et al.[25] used the right carotid for arterial return in 17 moribund infants undergoing open-heart correction during the late 1970s. No neurologic deficits were noted in any of the 14 survivors. In each case of that series the carotid artery was repaired, and 8-year follow-up of survivors showed that the right carotid artery was open without evidence of narrowing. In long-term ECMO, however, the carotid artery by tradition has been simply ligated rather than repaired. Recently, several investigators have attempted to repair the artery and in some cases the vein after long-term ECMO.[27,28] Whereas on first consideration it appears desirable to restore right carotid artery flow, the complications of reopening a vessel that has been occluded for more than 24 hours are unknown. In most cases the artery has been severely damaged at the site of ligation and resection with end-to-end anastomosis is necessary. The long-term follow-up of patients who underwent ligation of the carotid artery during the initial phase of neonatal ECMO at the University of California Irvine and Children's Hospital of Orange County showed no significant neurologic deficits related to sacrifice of the carotid artery.[28]

Because of the potential problems of cannulation techniques and the possible neurologic damage from interrupting carotid flow on one side of the brain, alternate methods of ECMO have been introduced.[29] Venovenous bypass through a single cannula has proved to be feasible in some patients requiring ECMO. Figure 1 shows with the routine arterial and venous cannulas that are currently available. However, venovenous bypass has its limitations and can be used only when cardiac function is virtually normal. Figure 2A shows the venovenous bypass cannula in a patient who had been successfully treated for respiratory failure with

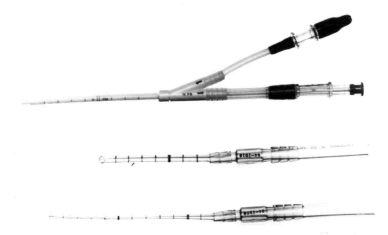

FIGURE 1.   The top cannula is used for venovenous bypass. The standard arterial and venous cannulas are shown below.

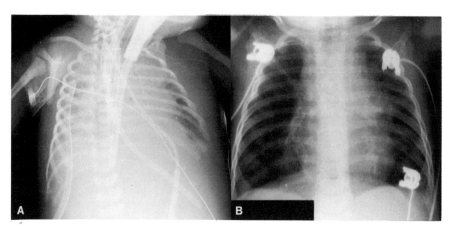

FIGURE 2. *A,* Venovenous bypass cannula is seen in the center of the chest radiograph. The patient already has been on ECMO from an earlier episode of respiratory failure. *B,* Chest radiograph of the same patient 1 month following his second time on ECMO.

standard carotid artery cannulation. Two weeks later, however, the patient again developed respiratory failure. Because the carotid vessels could not be used, an anterior thoracotomy was performed in the neonatal unit, and the patient was placed on venovenous bypass through the right atrium for 5 days, after which the cannula was successfully removed. Follow-up chest x-ray 1 month later is shown in Figure 2B. The patient has made an uneventful recovery. Venovenous bypass is practical for treatment of pulmonary failure if cardiac function is adequate. If the patient is placed on venovenous bypass and the heart become stunned,[30] then conversion to venoarterial bypass may be necessary. Nonetheless, venovenous bypass has reduced the number of patients requiring carotid arterial cannulation.

One of the more challenging applications of ECMO is for the treatment of congenital diaphragmatic hernia.[31,32] Results indicate that patients who would have died without ECMO have been successfully treated with good long-term results. Atkinson et al.[33] compared the results of patients treated for diaphragmatic hernia with and without ECMO. Their conclusions, based on the study of the oxygen index, showed that survival was 5% without ECMO versus 69% with ECMO. They concluded that ECMO significantly improves survival. The use of ECMO in the treatment of diaphragmatic hernia has raised the question of whether ECMO should be used before, during or after surgery. In any case, ECMO has greatly advanced the treatment of diaphragmatic hernia.

The use of ECMO for circulatory support after cardiac surgery in infants and children has increased in recent years. In most cases the cardiac repair may be adequate, but myocardial function is not sufficient to wean the patient from cardiopulmonary bypass. Ziomek et al.[34] reported a 75% survival rate with use of ECMO after cardiac surgery in infants and children. They concluded that ECMO has become a necessary adjunct in the treatment of congenital heart disease. At Children's Hospital of Orange County during the past 10 years, ECMO has been used in 12 children after cardiac surgery with 5 survivors. In the early experience with ECMO, postoperative bleeding was severe and uncontrollable. However, with the introduction of fibrin glue, careful heparin titration, and liberal use of coagulation components, particularly platelet transfusions, patients can be transferred from standard cardiopulmonary bypass to ECMO in the operating room. They can be maintained with the same cannula used during surgery or converted to neck cannulation. The sternum is left open, but the skin and subcutaneous tissue are closed. Patients are observed in the recovery room until they are weaned from ECMO. With wider use of ECMO in this context, difficult and complex types of defects can be treated with the hope of successful outcome.

Although the initial effort with ECMO in adults proved to be impracticable, largely because of the limitation of the diseases treated (e.g., ARDS), interest in its use among the pediatric population has been rekindled.[35] Further research and clinical trials are necessary to determine the role of ECMO in older pediatric patients as well as in adults with respiratory failure. Use of ECMO has also gained wide support for treatment of preoperative cardiac failure in patients who subsequently required a heart transplantation.[36] It also can be used as a preoperative and postoperative support for lung transplantation.[36]

Many questions need to be answered, and continued research in ECMO is crucial. The development of heparin-coated circuits by Bartlett and others shows great promise.[37,38] Other areas of interest include pulsatile perfusion, treatment of multiorgan failure and more efficient oxygenators. Recent experience with nitric oxide[39,40] indicates that alterations in pulmonary vascular resistance may even eliminate the need for ECMO in certain groups of neonatal patients. Nonetheless, in a rather short period of time the technique of extracorporeal membrane oxygenation has made tremendous strides and appears to have become an established form of treatment for certain diseases in the neonatal and pediatric populations.

REFERENCES

1. Gibbon JH Jr: Artificial maintenance of circulation during experimental occlusion of pulmonary artery. Arch Surg 34:1105, 1937.
2. Lee WH Jr, Krumhaar D, Fonkalsrud EW, et al: Denaturation of plasma proteins as a cause of morbidity and death after intracardiac operations. Surgery 50:29, 1961.
3. Dobell ARC, Mitri M, Galva R, et al: Biologic evaluation of blood after prolonged recirculation through film and membrane oxygenators. Ann Surg 161:617, 1965.
4. Lillehi CW, Cohen M, Warden HC, et al: The result of direct vision closure of ventricular septal defects in 8 patients by means of controlled cross circulation. Surg Gynecol Obstet 101:447, 1955.
5. Mustard WT: Clinical and experimental experience with hemalogous and heterologous lung perfusion. ASAIO Trans 1:94, 1955.
6. Kolff WJ, Berk HT Jr: Artificial kidney: A dialyzer with a great area. Acta Med Scand 117:121, 1944.
7. Kolff WJ, Balzer RR: Artificial coil lung. ASAIO Trans 1:39, 1955.
8. Clowes GHA Jr, Hopkins AL, Neville WE: An artificial lung dependent upon diffusion of oxygen and carbon dioxide through plastic membranes. J Thorac Surg 32:630, 1956.
9. Dewall R, Bentley DJ, Hirose M, et al: A temperature controlling (omnithermic) disposable bubble oxygenator for total body perfusion. Dis Chest 49:207, 1966.
10. Kammermeyer K: Silicone rubber as a selective barrier. Ind Eng Chem 49:1685, 1957.
11. Thomas JA: Coeur-poumon a membrane pulmonaire artificielle. CR Acad Sci (Paris) 246:1084, 1958.
12. Marx TI, Snyder WE, St. John AD, et al: Diffusion of oxygen into a film of whole blood. J Appl Physiol 15:1123, 1960.
13. Kolobow T, Bowman RL: Construction and evaluation of an alveolar membrane artificial heart lung. ASAIO Trans 9:238, 1963.
14. Day SW, Crystal DK, Wagner CL, et al: Properties of synthetic membranes in extracorporeal circuits. Am J Surg 114:214, 1967.
15. Bramson ML, Osborn JJ, Main FB, et al: A new disposable membrane oxygenator with integral heat exchanger. J Thorac Cardiovasc Surg 50:391, 1965.

16. Pierce EC II: Modification of the Clowes membrane lung. J Thorac Cardiovasc Surg 39:438, 1960.

17. Lande MR, Fallat RJ, Coeniger E, et al: Pathologic features and mechanisms of hypoxemia in adult respiratory distress syndrome. Am Rev Respir Dis 114:267, 1976.

18. Drinker PA, Bartlett RH, Bialer R, et al: Augmentation of membrane gas transfer by oscillation of a coiled tube. Surgery 66:775, 1969.

19. Hill JD, O'Brien TG, Murray JJ, et al: Prolonged extracorporeal oxygenation for acute post-traumatic respiratory failure (Shock Lung Syndrome). N Engl J Med 286:139, 1972.

20. Soeter JR, Mamiya RT, Sprague AY, et al: Prolonged extracorporeal oxygenation for cardiorespiratory failure after tetralogy correction. J Thorac Cardiovasc Surg 66:214, 1973.

21. Bartlett RH, Gazzaniga AB, Fong SW, et al: Prolonged extracorporeal cardiopulmonary support in man. J Thorac Cardiovasc Surg 68:918, 1974.

22. Bartlett RH, Gazzaniga AB, Jefferies R, et al: Extrracorporeal membrane oxygenation (ECMO) cardiopulmonary support in infancy. ASAIO Trans 22:80, 1976.

23. Bartlett RH, Gazzaniga AB: Extracorporeal circulation of cardiopulmonary failure. Curr Prob Surg 15:74, 1978.

24. Krummel TM, Lazar JG, Kirkpatrick BV, et al: Clinical use of an extracorporeal membrane oxygenator in neonatal pulmonary failure. J Pediatr Surg 17:525–531, 1982.

25. Really Vasquez F, Gazzaniga AB, Sperling DR, Bartlett RH: Use of right carotid artery for open heart surgery. In preparation.

26. Moulton SL, Lynch FP, Cornish JD, et al: Carotid artery reconstruction following neonatal extracorporeal membrane oxygenation. J Pediatr Surg 26:794–799, 1991.

27. Adolph V, Bonis S, Falterman K, Arensman R: Carotid artery repair after pediatric extracorporeal membrane oxygenation. J Pediatr Surg 25:867–869; discussion 869–870, 1990.

28. Towne BH, Lott IT, Hicks DA, et al: Long-term follow-up of infants and children treated with extracorporeal membrane oxygenation (ECMO): A preliminary report. J Pediatr Surg 20:410–414, 1985.

29. Otsu T, Merz SI, Hultquist KA, et al: Laboratory evaluation of a double lumen catheter for venovenous neonatal ECMO. ASAIO Trans 35:647–650, 1989.

30. Hirschl RB, Heiss KF, Bartlett RH: Severe myocardial dysfunction during extracorporeal membrane oxygenation. J Pediatr Surg 27:48–53, 1992.

31. Howell CG, Hatley RM, Boedy RF, et al: Recent experience with diaphragmatic hernia and ECMO. Ann Surg 211:793–797, discussion 797–798, 1990.

32. Newman KD, Anderson KD, Van Meurs K, et al: Extracorporeal membrane oxygenation and congenital diaphragmatic hernia: Should any infant be excluded? J Pediatr Surg 25:1048–1052, discussion 1052–1053, 1990.

33. Atkinson JB, Ford EG, Humphries B, et al: The impact of extracorporeal membrane support in the treatment of congenital diaphragmatic hernia. J Pediatr Surg 26:791–793, 1991.

34. Ziomek S, Harrell JE, et al: Extracorporeal membrane oxygenation for cardiac failure after congenital heart operation. Ann Thorac Surg 54:861–868, 1992.

35. Steiner RB, Adolph VR, Heaton JF, et al: Pediatric extracorporeal membrane oxygenation in posttraumatic respiratory failure. J Pediatr Surg 26:1011–1014, discussion 1014–1015, 1991.

36. Jurmann MJ, Haverich A, Demertzis S, et al: Extracorporeal membrane oxygenation (ECMO): Extended indications for artificial support of both heart and lungs. Int J Artif Organs 14:771–774, 1991.

37. Miyamoto Y, Nakano S, Kaneko M, et al: Clinical evaluation of a new synthetic protease inhibitor in open heart surgery: Effect on plasma serotonin and histamine release and blood conservation. ASAIO Trans 38:M395–M398, 1992.

38. Takano H, Nakano S, Kadoba K, Kaneko M, et al: Evaluation of the biocompatibility of a new method for heparin coating of a cardiopulmonary bypass circuit. ASAIO Trans 38:M390–M394, 1992.

39. Roberts JD, Polaner DM, Lang P, et al: Inhaled nitric oxide in persistent pulmonary hypertension of the newborn. Lancet 340:818–819, 1992.

40. Kinsella JP, Neish SR, Shaffer E, et al: Low-dose inhalational nitric oxide in persistent pulmonary hypertension of the newborn. Lancet 340:819–820, 1992.

THOMAS L. SPRAY, MD

EXTRACORPOREAL MEMBRANE OXYGENATION FOR PEDIATRIC CARDIAC SUPPORT

Professor of Surgery
Division of Cardiothoracic Surgery
Washington University School
   of Medicine
St. Louis Children's Hospital
St. Louis, Missouri

Reprint requests to:
Thomas L. Spray, MD
St. Louis Children's Hospital
400 South Kingshighway,
   Suite 5W24
St. Louis, MO 63110

Various devices have been introduced for cardiac support in adult patients, including the intraaortic balloon pump (IABP), pulsatile and nonpulsatile left ventricular and right ventricular assist devices, and the total artificial heart.[10,20] These devices have gained widespread application in postcardiotomy patients as a bridge both to recovery of natural heart function and to cardiac transplantation.

In spite of the variety of devices available for adult patients, few cardiac assist devices are applicable over the wide range of body weights of pediatric patients. The intraaortic balloon pump has been used with variable results in pediatric patients and generally has not been associated with effective improvement in myocardial performance, because ischemic disease of the myocardium is relatively infrequent after pediatric cardiac operation.[15] In addition, the rapid heart rates and relatively elastic aorta of infants and small children make effective diastolic augmentation difficult. Left ventricular assist devices have been used on rare occasions in children and infants; however, the majority of pediatric patients who require postoperative cardiac support have primarily right heart dysfunction associated with pulmonary hypertension or combined left and right heart failure.[19] For these reasons, extracorporeal membrane oxygenation (ECMO), as described by Bartlett, has been used for pediatric postcardiotomy support in the majority of reported series.[1-3,6,11,12,14,17,19,21,23,26-28] ECMO has the advantage of assisting both the right and left ventricles, although increases in afterload on the left ventricle can be a problem if the left side of the heart is not vented. ECMO does provide, however, excellent right heart support, particularly in the presence of pulmonary hypertension, which is a common indication for postoperative cardiac support in children. In addition, the ECMO circuit is adaptable to a wide range of patient sizes because pump flow can be varied according to the patient's body weight and the desired cardiac output. This chapter outlines the various types of postcardiotomy cardiac support available for use in infants and children and summarizes the reported results.

METHODS OF SUPPORT

Intraaortic Balloon Pump

The IABP is generally not effective in pediatric patients because of the difficulty in obtaining good diastolic augmentation in the face of high heart rates and aortic distensibility.[19] In addition, although many balloon sizes are currently available and modern balloon consoles can provide fast pumping rates, the balloons may be difficult to insert in the small vessels of infants without significant vascular injury. Perhaps the major reason that the IABP is generally not beneficial in pediatric cardiac support is the fact that few children after repair of congenital heart defects have isolated left ventricular failure or myocardial ischemia, for which afterload reduction and improved myocardial blood flow may result in rapid hemodynamic improvement. The IABP may not improve cardiac output significantly in the presence of primary right ventricular failure, which is more common after repair of congenital cardiac defects. A few reports of satisfactory postcardiotomy IABP support in infants and children suggest that patient selection may be the most important factor in successful use of this device.[7,19,22,25]

Ventricular Assist Devices

Adult-sized pulsatile or adult- or pediatric-sized nonpulsatile ventricular assist devices (VADs) can be used in larger children or teenagers. However, currently available VADs are too large for use in most infants and small children. Problems with thrombosis in the VAD itself or severe hemolysis due to the small cannulas required for insertion into infants and young children also limit the effectiveness of these devices. Nevertheless, Karl and associates[16] have described good results in a series of pediatric patients with the use of Bio-Medicus nonpulsatile left VADs. Twelve children, age 6 days–12 years, underwent support with left ventricular or systemic ventricular assist after cardiac operation. Nine of the children could not be weaned from cardiopulmonary bypass in the operating room. Partial anticoagulation was maintained with continuous infusion of heparin to an activated clotting time of 150 seconds. Support was continued from 38–190 hours, with a mean of 107 hours. Ten patients were weaned from the VADs, and 6 survived to leave the hospital, for an overall survival rate of 50%. The majority of the children in the series had significant ventricular dysfunction as the primary indication for support. No patient required right ventricular assistance (stable oxygenation with a right atrial pressure below 12 mmHg and lack of distention of the left or right ventricle). The major complication in this series was hemorrhage, with 5 of the 12 patients requiring mediastinal reexploration on at least one occasion. The authors note that right-to-left shunting at the atrial level can pose a problem with isolated left VAD support; thus they make a specific point of closing the atrial septal defect in all patients who undergo a biventricular repair.

Of interest, 2 patients with shunt-dependent pulmonary blood flow underwent left VAD support and were satisfactorily weaned from the device. Neither of these patients was a long-term survivor; however, the results suggest that isolated left ventricular assistance without ECMO may be associated with adequate limitation of pulmonary blood flow in the presence of a systemic-to-pulmonary shunt and in some cases may permit myocardial recovery.

Our own experience at St. Louis Children's Hospital with Bio-Medicus VADs for pediatric patients includes only 1 child who required a right VAD after homograft aortic root replacement and coronary endarterectomy for homozygous familial hypercholesterolemia and supravalvar aortic stenosis with left main coronary artery stenosis. This patient, who required postoperative cardiac support for 3 days and then was weaned successfully from ventricular assistance, is a long-term survivor 4 years postoperatively.

Extracorporeal Membrane Oxygenation

The majority of pediatric patients who have required postoperative cardiac assistance have been treated with ECMO, as described by Bartlett.[3] Advantages of ECMO include support of both the right and left ventricles and improvement in systemic oxygenation. In addition, the placement of the patient on bypass permits hemofiltration or dialysis for renal complications of low cardiac output. A major disadvantage of ECMO support is the need for continuous anticoagulation. ECMO support after cardiotomy may, be provided with either venoarterial or venovenous cannulation. Venoarterial cannulation provides the greatest cardiac support; however, studies have recently shown that venovenous bypass may improve myocardial oxygenation and decrease pulmonary vascular resistance under certain circumstances and in selected patients may thus provide adequate cardiac recovery and support primarily by improving venous oxygenation.[5,24]

Venoarterial ECMO is usually performed by cannulation via the carotid artery and jugular vein, the aorta and right atrium through the median sternotomy incision (transthoracic), or the femoral artery and vein in the groin. Cannulation of the carotid artery and jugular vein has the advantage of providing good venous drainage of the right atrium by way of a separate incision site remote from the median sternotomy wound. Carotid-jugular cannulation may best be used in patients who are weaned from cardiopulmonary bypass in the operating room and develop myocardial dysfunction and cardiogenic shock in the hours after operation. In our experience, cannulation for ECMO via the carotid artery and jugular vein in the intensive care unit is straightforward and associated with a lower incidence of bleeding from the mediastinal wound. In addition, cannulation may be performed through pursestring sutures in the vessels, and the carotid artery and jugular vein may be repaired at the time of decannulation, so that cerebral blood flow is not sacrificed. Carotid-jugular cannulation is not used if a central venous line is present in the internal jugular vein, because interruption of inotropic support through the central line during cannulation is not likely to be well tolerated. In addition, in some patients direct access from the jugular vein to the right atrium is not possible (e.g., patients with cavopulmonary Fontan connections). Direct aortic and right atrial cannulation through the median sternotomy may be preferable in these circumstances.

Transthoracic cannulation is also preferable in patients who cannot be weaned from cardiopulmonary bypass in the operating room. The standard cannulas for bypass can be converted to the ECMO circuit and the cannulas brought out through the median sternotomy incision. The sternotomy may be closed with a single stainless steel wire to aid in support of the cannulas and to permit closure of the subcutaneous tissue and skin to minimize infectious complications and bleeding. A high incidence of mediastinal hemorrhage has occurred in our patients when transthoracic cannulation is required, most commonly due to gradual erosion by cardiac motion at the cannulation sites. Because many patients who require transthoracic cannulation are not weaned from bypass in the operating room and thus never have adequate reversal of anticoagulation, an increased frequency of mediastinal hemorrhage may be expected. Disadvantages of transthoracic cannulation include the potential risks of mediastinal infection and of cannula dislodgement during patient repositioning or transport.

Femoral arteriovenous cannulation can be used in certain older pediatric patients, with placement of long intravascular catheters into the inferior vena cava or right atrium through the femoral vein and into the common femoral or iliac artery for arterial return. Generally, however, the venous drainage with such systems is not as effective as with carotid and jugular cannulation. Advantages of groin cannulation include the lack of invasion of the mediastinum and the relative security of the cannulation, which prevents dislodgement. Disadvantages include the difficulty in preventing contamination in the groin and the inability to obtain maximal blood flow.

Venovenous cannulation through the jugular and femoral veins, through both femoral veins, or with a double lumen catheter through the jugular vein positioned in the right atrium provides oxygenation support to venous blood. When myocardial dysfunction is primarily due to inadequate oxygenation or elevated pulmonary vascular resistance that can be improved by increasing saturations in venous blood, the venovenous technique may be applicable. In most circumstances venovenous ECMO does not provide adequate biventricular support; therefore, venoarterial ECMO is preferred.

The effects of ECMO on the heart include a decrease in preload, an increase in afterload, and an increase in left ventricular wall stress that may result in increased myocardial consumption of oxygen.[4,18] Although with venoarterial ECMO the right atrial and pulmonary artery pressures decrease, left atrial pressure usually remains somewhat elevated and mean arterial pressure often increases, resulting in significant afterload to the myocardium. In patients who have significant left ventricular dysfunction without the ability to unload the left ventricle through an atrial septal defect, it is therefore advisable to place a left ventricular vent to decrease the left atrial pressure and thus the wall stress and myocardial oxygen consumption of the left ventricle. This may be accomplished by connecting a vent from the left atrium or left ventricle into the venous return line of the ECMO circuit, either with gravity drainage or a small peristaltic or roller pump. An adjustable screw clamp on the vent line can modify the drainage to permit maintenance of an adequate left atrial pressure for ejection or, if necessary, to unload completely the left side of the heart.[8]

INDICATIONS FOR ECMO CARDIAC SUPPORT

Preoperative ECMO Support

Although use of ECMO for the treatment of low cardiac output syndrome after repair of congenital heart defects has been widely accepted, the preoperative use of ECMO in infants with congenital heart disease has remained controversial. Recently we reported the results of preoperative ECMO at St. Louis Children's Hospital in 8 patients, from neonates to children 16 months of age.[12] These patients had unoperated cyanotic congenital heart disease and cardiopulmonary collapse associated with hypercyanotic spells, pulmonary hypertensive crises, or sepsis. Indications for ECMO included arterial oxygen saturation <60% on maximal medical therapy, associated with hypotension and metabolic acidosis. Maximal medical therapy included hyperventilation on 100% oxygen; hemodynamic support with inotropes, vasodilators, or both; and pharmacologic paralysis and sedation. The duration of ECMO ranged from 15–840 hours (mean: 460 hours) and was associated with transient seizures in 1 patient and renal failure in another. Seven of the 8 patients underwent corrective (3 patients) or palliative (4 patients) procedures while on ECMO or within 48 hours of decannulation. One patient was bridged to double-lung transplantation after 840 hours of ECMO support. One operative and 2 late deaths occurred, for an overall survival rate of 62%. All survivors have normal growth and development. Preoperative diagnoses included tetralogy of Fallot (4 patients), total anomalous pulmonary venous return (1), Ebstein's malformation of the tricuspid valve (1), patent ductus arteriosus with systemic pulmonary vascular pressures (1), and sepsis with transposition of the great vessels (1). The results of our experience suggest that ECMO can provide effective mechanical support in cardiovascular crises that do not respond to maximal medical therapy and therefore can be used as a bridge to successful surgical repair or transplantation.[13]

Intraoperative ECMO Support

Intraoperative ECMO is used when the child cannot be weaned from cardiopulmonary bypass despite maximal inotropic therapy and optimal operative repair. The most common diagnoses for which ECMO support has been required either intraoperatively or in the immediate postoperative period are listed in Table 1. Decisions about venting of the left ventricle at the time of initiation of ECMO in the operating room depend on measurement of left atrial pressure on full ECMO support. If the left ventricle distends or left atrial pressure rises above 18 mmHg despite good flow rates, then left atrial venting is used, if technically possible. In most patients with an open atrial septal defect or a single ventricle, venting is not necessary. In the majority of patients placed on ECMO for inability to wean from cardiopulmonary bypass, ECMO is maintained via the original bypass cannulas; to improve venous return, bicaval cannulation may be converted to a two-stage, single venous cannula. The patient is then converted to a closed ECMO system with brief clamping of the cannulas and connection of new sterile lines on the operative field.

The patient with hypoplastic left heart syndrome after Norwood stage I palliative repair presents a particular problem. Use of standard venoarterial ECMO circuit is associated with overperfusion of the lungs through the

TABLE 1. Diagnoses for Which ECMO Is Most Commonly Used after Cardiac Repair

Atrioventricular septal defect	Anomalous left coronary artery from the
Truncus arteriosus	pulmonary artery
Total anomalous pulmonary venous return	Ebstein's malformation of the tricuspid valve
Tetralogy of Fallot	Pre- or post-cardiac or pulmonary transplantation

systemic-to-pulmonary shunt. This increase in pulmonary blood flow is not well tolerated by the single right ventricle and has not, in our experience, been associated with significant myocardial recovery. A recent report suggests that ECMO can be used in patients after the Norwood procedure if pulmonary blood flow is limited by temporarily occluding the systemic-to-pulmonary shunt with a vascular clip. The clip is removed before weaning from ECMO.[27] This approach may be applicable to other situations of single ventricle with shunt-dependent pulmonary blood flow.

Postoperative ECMO Support

Infants or children who require ECMO support in the postoperative period after developing progressive low cardiac output syndrome represent a uniquely favorable group. Myocardial injury is generally less severe than in patients who require intraoperative ECMO, and sufficient time for recovery of normal coagulation may decrease the incidence of major hemorrhage.[26] The indications for initiation of ECMO in such patients remain somewhat subjective. Low cardiac output syndrome, as defined by a progressive decrease in urine output to < 1 ml/kg/hr despite increasing inotropic and diuretic therapy, in association with poor peripheral perfusion, low systemic venous oxygen saturations, or progressive elevation of myocardial filling pressures, is generally considered an indication for ECMO support. In addition, refractory atrial or nodal arrhythmias resulting in or contributing to low cardiac output syndrome are also relative indications for ECMO.

Cardiac output is not readily determined in infants and small children because thermodilution catheters may not be placed and patients often have systemic-to-pulmonary shunts. Therefore, the indication for postcardiotomy ECMO must often be based on clinical judgment, according to the evidence of right or left heart failure, pulmonary hypertension, or poor peripheral perfusion and systemic acidosis. Prompt initiation of ECMO may result in a rapid return of peripheral perfusion and an increase in urine output and may obviate the need for hemodialysis or ultrafiltration in many patients who sustain a low cardiac output state after cardiac repair. No objective criteria to predict the need for ECMO support in the postoperative period have yet been determined.

Analysis of Recovery and Weaning from ECMO

Initiation of ECMO is often accompanied by rapid improvement in hemody-namics with the ability to decrease inotropic support to a minimal level. Improvement in renal function and diuresis of retained fluid is often an early sign of significant myocardial recovery. The use of 2-dimensional Doppler echocardi-ography or transesophageal echocardiography to evaluate myocardial function (left ventricular contractility) with weaning of ECMO flow rate has proved of particular value in determining myocardial recovery in patients with a single ventricle or complex anatomy. As ECMO is gradually weaned, assessment of myocardial function with a challenge infusion of inotropic agents (5 μg/kg/min of dopamine or 0.05 μg/kg/min of epinephrine) may aid in making the decision to terminate support. ECMO flows are gradually weaned to 100–200 ml/min, and if hemodynamics are good, decannulation usually can be accomplished safely. At St. Louis Children's Hospital, decannulation is usually performed in the intensive care unit to avoid the additional stress of transportation of a critically ill infant or child to the operating room.

COMPLICATIONS OF ECMO SUPPORT

The major complications of postcardiotomy ECMO in pediatric patients is hemorrhage. A large proportion of children, approaching 50%, require reexploration for hemorrhage at some point during the period of ECMO perfusion. Heparin infusion is controlled so that the activated clotting (ACT) is maintained at 150–200 seconds and platelet counts at a level above $100,000/m^3$ in an attempt to minimize the magnitude of bleeding. The primary determinant of significant hemorrhage is duration of ECMO; reexploration is unusual in the first 72 hours but is increasingly required thereafter. In our experience, once reexploration is required, additional attempts to control hemorrhage are usually necessary at decreasing intervals. Mediastinal reexploration is generally performed in the intensive care unit, while ECMO continues, to avoid the risk of cannula dislodgement or tamponade with transport to the operating room.

An additional complication of ECMO is renal insufficiency. In our experience at St. Louis Children's Hospital, however, renal insufficiency has been uncommon. If ECMO is initiated promptly on discovery of progressive low cardiac output syndrome, ultrafiltration or dialysis is rarely necessary. Initiation of ECMO prior to complete anuria has resulted in rapid improvement in renal function in our patients.

An additional risk of prolonged use of ECMO is sepsis or mediastinitis. The multiple cannulas and intravascular catheters in patients who require prolonged ECMO perfusion, in association with low cardiac output and renal insufficiency, predispose to a significant incidence of infection. Reexploration of the mediastinum, continued bleeding from mediastinal structures, and the exit of cannulas through the mediastinal wound can contribute to a significantly increased risk of mediastinal infection. Although pneumonia and intravascular sepsis have been commonly seen in our series of patients, mediastinitis requiring drainage has been infrequent.

RESULTS OF ECMO FOR PEDIATRIC CARDIAC SUPPORT

The results of the use of postcardiotomy ECMO in pediatric patients are summarized in Tables 2–5.[9,14,17,23,27,28] From July 1985 through February 1992, 48 infants and children required postoperative support with ECMO after cardiac repair at St. Louis Children's Hospital. Ten patients had tetralogy of Fallot, of whom 7 are long-term survivors (Table 6). Three patients underwent repair of truncus arteriosus, with 2 survivors. Five patients had repair of complete atrioventricular canal with postoperative pulmonary hypertension, and 4 of them survived ECMO for control of pulmonary hypertensive events. Two infants required ECMO after repair of Ebstein's malformation, with 1 survivor, and in 7 children ECMO was initiated because of hypoxemia and ventricular dysfunction after various repairs of single ventricle with shunt-dependent pulmonary blood flow. A poor survival rate was identified in this subset of patients, with late survival for only 1 of 7. The poor results emphasize the difficulty in maintaining myocardial perfusion and unloading a single ventricle in the presence of a systemic-to-pulmonary artery shunt. Six patients required ECMO for perioperative support or as a bridge to heart or lung transplantation; 2 survived. Several other types of repairs, including multiple ventricular septal defects, interrupted aortic arch, the Fontan procedure, and pulmonary atresia or stenosis, were performed in a group of 15 patients, of whom 5 survived. Of the total of 48 children, 21 survived longer than 30 days for a late survival rate of 44%. Duration of ECMO ranged

TABLE 2. Survival Rates Reported in the Registry of the Extracorporeal Life Support Organization (ELSO), October 1991

Category	Total	No. Survival	% Survival
Cardiac surgery total	435	191	44
Transplant	16	4	25
Myocarditis/cardiomyopathy	34	22	
ASD/VSD/PDA/AVSD	74	38	51
AS/MS/Coarct	17	6	35
HLHS	7	1	14
PS/PA/TA	33	12	36
Truncus/TOGV	80	25	31
TAPVR	74	38	51
TOF/Ebstein's	81	41	51
Anomalous LCA	9	5	56
Fontan	23	3	13
Other	37	22	59
OR ECMO (July, 1991)	63	17	27

ASD = atrial septal defect
VSD = ventricular septal defect
PDA = patent ductus arteriosus
AVSD = atrioventricular canal defect
AS = aortic stenosis
MS = mitral stenosis
Coarct = coarctation
HLHS = hypoplastic left heart syndrome
PS = pulmonary valve stenosis
PA = pulmonary atresia

TA = tricuspid atresia
Truncus = truncus arteriosus
TOGV = transposition of the great vessels
TAPVR = total anomalous pulmonary venous return
TOF = tetralogy of Fallot
Anom LCA = anomalous left coronary artery from
   pulmonary artery
OR ECMO = ECMO begun in operating room
Cann = cannulation for ECMO

from 7–327 hours (mean: 107 hours). These data compare favorably with the results in adult patients with various types of assist devices, including pulsatile and nonpulsatile left ventricular assist pumps.[10,20]

Table 2 summarizes the use of ECMO for cardiac perioperative assistance in the Registry of the Extracorporeal Life Support Organization (October 1991).[9] By that date, a total of 435 cases had been reported, with early survival for 191 (44%). Late survival after 1 month is not included in this summary. The best overall

TABLE 3. Results of Treatment with Extracorporeal Membrane Oxygenation, Arkansas and Detroit

Category	Total	No. Survival	% Survival
Arkansas, 1991*	24	13	54
OR ECMO	17	12	71
Detroit Children's Hospital, 1990†	36	22	61
ASD/VSD/PDA/AVSD	17	9	
Truncus/TOGV	4	4	100
TAPVR	1	1	100
TOF/Ebstein's	5	4	80
Anom LCA	2	2	10
Fontan	4	0	0
Other	3	2	75
OR ECMO	9	2	22
Cann >4 hr postoperatively	27	20	74

* From reference 27.
† From reference 17.
For abbreviations, see Table 2.

TABLE 4. Results of Extracorporeal Membrane Oxygenation, Pittsburgh, 1989

Category	Total	No. Survival	% Survival
Total	10	7	70
ASD/VSD/PDA/AVSD	4	3	75
Truncus/TOGV	1	1	100
TOF/Ebstein's	3	1	33
Fontan	1	1	100
Other	1	1	100
OR ECMO	1	0	0
ECMO 6–54 hr postoperatively	9	7	78

From reference 23.
For abbreviations, see Table 2.

TABLE 5. Results of Extracorporeal Membrane Oxygenation, St. Louis University and University of Michigan

Category	Total	No. Survival	% Survival
St. Louis Univesrity			
Cardinal Glennon (1987)*	13	6	
Transplant	1	1	100
ASD/VSD/AVSD	1	1	100
PS/PA/TA	2	1	50
Truncus/TOGV	2	0	0
TAPVR	1	1	100
TOF/Ebstein's	4	2	50
Fontan	1	0	0
Other	1	0	0
OR ECMO	1	0	0
ECMO 9–50 hr postoperatively	12	6	50
University of Michigan (1990)[†]	16	4	25
Transplant	6	2	33
ASD/VSD/AVSD	3	0	0
PS/PA/TA	1	0	0
Anom LCA	1	0	0
TOF/Ebstein's	2	0	0
Truncus/TOGV	2	1	50
Other	1	1	100

* From reference 14.
[†] From reference 28.
For abbreviations, see Table 2.

TABLE 6. Results of Extracorporeal Membrane Oxygenation, St. Louis Children's Hospital, July 1985–February 1992

Category	Total	No. Survived	% Survived
TOF	10	7	70
Truncus	3	2	67
AV canal	5	4	80
Ebstein's	2	1	50
Single ventricle	7	1	14
Heart transplant	4	1	25
Bridge	2	1	50
Other	15	5	33
Total	48	21	44

For abbreviations, see Table 2.

survival is recorded in patients with tetralogy of Fallot, truncus arteriosus, atrioventricular canal, and total anomalous pulmonary venous return, as demonstrated in the series from St. Louis Children's Hospital. The higher survival rates for patients with these conditions suggest that, as expected, a complete operative repair is associated with improved survival; more palliative operations, such as single ventricle or hypoplastic left heart syndrome with shunt-dependent pulmonary blood flow, are associated with a lower recovery rate (14%). In addition, Fontan repairs without early achievement of optimal hemodynamics are not associated with good survival (13%) despite ECMO, suggesting that in the majority of these patients ventricular function does not improve sufficiently with time or that pulmonary resistance remains elevated. A consistent finding in all reported series (Tables 2–6) is a decreased survival rate if ECMO is required to wean from bypass in the operating room, suggesting a greater level of myocardial damage in these patients.

CONCLUSIONS

Mechanical circulatory support can be effective in pediatric patients after palliative or corrective cardiac operations. Although the IABP may be used in infants and children, it has a relatively limited role. ECMO has the advantages of being applicable over a wide range of ages and weights and of providing biventricular cardiovascular and pulmonary support.

As with other mechanical circulatory assistance systems, early intervention before onset of irreversible multiple system organ failure is necessary for optimal results. In addition, adequate repair of the cardiac lesion is important to late survival. In the majority of patients who did not survive late after ECMO in the St. Louis Children's Hospital series, significant myocardial dysfunction persisted or pulmonary hypertensive events recurred after weaning from ECMO. Nevertheless, a large portion of patients who were successfully weaned from ECMO ultimately survived to leave the hospital. Of 48 patients, 27 (56%) were weaned from the device and 21 (44%) are alive. Only 6 patients died in hospital after weaning from ECMO. One patient died of sepsis after successful weaning from ECMO following repair of transposition of the great vessels. An additional patient with interrupted aortic arch was successfully weaned from ECMO but developed progressive pulmonary hypertension and died several days after discontinuation of ECMO support. One infant was successfully weaned from ECMO after repair of truncus arteriosus but developed recurrent pulmonary hypertension and died during the same hospitalization. An additional patient with single ventricle and shunt-dependent pulmonary blood flow with pulmonary hypertension was weaned from ECMO support and discharged from the hospital but developed progressive pulmonary hypertension and died several months later. One child underwent ECMO as a bridge to heart transplantation and was successfully weaned but died of progressive hypoxemia and myocardial dysfunction. A final patient was weaned from ECMO after repair of tetralogy of Fallot and a large ventricular septal defect but died of fungal sepsis.

FUTURE DIRECTIONS

Despite the relative success with ECMO for pediatric cardiac support, clearly the requirement for systemic anticoagulation makes it a suboptimal assist device. The development of bypass circuit without use of heparin may diminish the incidence of mediastinal hemorrhage in these patients. Such circuits would permit a wide range of flow rates and applicability to children of all sizes and would also permit the use of an oxygenator to improve oxygen delivery. The use of aprotinin (Trasylol) could possibly limit the coagulopathy often seen with prolonged bypass at normothermia, although no data are yet available on the use of this agent in prolonged bypass support. Which type of mechanical VAD is optimal for use with various congenital cardiac abnormalities before or after repair remains to be determined. Use of non-ECMO devices such as VADs in certain patients with shunt-dependent pulmonary blood flow may be preferable, and patients who require an increase in venous saturation to optimize pulmonary blood flow (such as after the Fontan operation) may be best served by venovenous support. Modification of adult-sized implantable or external pulsatile VADs for the pediatric patient seems to hold promise for the future. Obtaining small valves that are hemodynamically satisfactory and providing adequate support over a wide range of stroke volumes and cardiac outputs will be difficult problems in these down-sized pulsatile VADs. Until newer devices are available, ECMO is likely to provide the best range of cardiopulmonary support for postcardiotomy low cardiac output syndrome in patients after palliative or corrective repairs of congenital heart defects.

REFERENCES

1. Adolph V, Heaton J, Steiner R, et al: Extracorporeal membrane oxygenation for non-neonatal respiratory failure. J Pediatr Surg 26:326–332, 1991.
2. Anderson HL III, Attorri RJ, Custer JR, et al: Extracorporeal membrane oxygenation for pediatric cardiopulmonary failure. J Thorac Cardiovasc Surg 99:1011–1021, 1990.
3. Bartlett RH, Gazzaniga AB, Fong SW, et al: Extracorporeal membrane oxygenator support for cardiopulmonary failure: Experience in twenty-eight cases. J Thorac Cardiovasc Surg 73:375–386, 1977.
4. Bavaria JE, Ratcliff MB, Gupta KB, et al: Changes in left ventricular systolic wall stress during biventricular circulatory assistance. Ann Thorac Surg 45:526–532, 1988.
5. Cornish JD, Heiss KF, Clark RH, et al: Preferential use of venovenous ECMO for neonates with significant circulatory compromise. 8th Annual CNMC ECMO Symposium, Breckinridge, CO, February 1992 [abstract].
6. Delius RE, Zwischenberger JB, Cilley R, et al: Prolonged extracorporeal life support of pediatric and adolescent cardiac transplant patients. Ann Thorac Surg 50:791–795, 1990.
7. del Nido PJ, Swan PR, Benson LN, et al: Successful use of intra-aortic balloon pumping in a two-kilogram infant. Ann Thorac Surg 46:574–576, 1988.
8. Eugene J, Ott RA, McColgan SJ, Roohk HV: Vented cardiac assistance: ECMO versus left heart bypass for acute left ventricular failure. ASAIO Trans 32:538–541, 1986.
9. Extracorporeal Membrane Oxygenation Registry Report: Extracorporeal Life Support Organization. Ann Arbor, MI, 1991.
10. Farrar DJ, Hill D, Gray LA, et al: Heterotopic prosthetic ventricles as a bridge to cardiac transplantation: A multicenter study in twenty-nine patients. N Engl J Med 318:333, 1988.
11. Galantowicz ME, Stolar CJH: Extracorporeal membrane oxygenation for perioperative support in pediatric heart transplantation. J Thorac Cardiovasc Surg 102:148–152, 1991.
12. Hunkeler NM, Canter CE, Donze A, Spray TL: Extracorporeal life support in cyanotic congenital heart disease before cardiovascular operation. Am J Cardiol 69:790–793, 1992.
13. Jurmann MJ, Haverich A, Demertzis S, et al: Extracorporeal membrane oxygenation as a bridge to lung transplantation. Eur J Cardiothorac Surg 5:94–98, 1991.
14. Kanter KR, Pennington DG, Weber TR, et al: Extracorporeal membrane oxygenation for postoperative cardiac support in children. J Thorac Cardiovasc Surg 93:27–35, 1987.
15. Kanter KR, Pennington DG, Ruzevich SA, Swartz MT: Failure of isolated left ventricular support in children. ASAIO Trans 17:9, 1988 [abstract].
16. Karl TR, Sano S, Horton S, Mee RBB: Centrifugal pump left heart assist in pediatric cardiac operations: Indications, techniques and results. J Thorac Cardiovasc Surg 102:624–630, 1991.
17. Klein MD, Shaheen KW, Whittlesey GC, et al: Extracorporeal membrane oxygenation for the circulatory support of children after repair of congenital heart disease. J Thorac Cardiovasc Surg 100:498–505, 1990.

18. Martin GR, Short BL: Doppler echocardiographic evaluation of cardiac performance in infants on prolonged extracorporeal membrane oxygenation. Am J Cardiol 62:929–934, 1988.
19. Pennington DG, Swartz MT: Circulatory support in children. Card Surg: State Art Rev 3:381–391, 1989.
20. Pennington DG, Kanner KR, McBride LR, et al: Seven years experience with the Pierce-Donachy ventricular assist device. J Thorac Cardiovasc Surg 96:901–911, 1988.
21. Plowden JS, Kimball TR, Bensky A, et al: The use of extracorporeal membrane oxygenation in critically ill neonates with Ebstein's anomaly. Am Heart J 121:619–622, 1991.
22. Pollock JC, Charlton MC, Williams WG, et al: Intra-aortic balloon pumping in children. Ann Thorac Surg 29:522–528, 1980.
23. Rodgers AJ, Trento A, Siewers RD, et al: Extracorporeal membrane oxygenation for post-cardiotomy cardiogenic shock in children. Ann Thorac Surg 47:903–906, 1989.
24. Strieper MJ, Sharma S, Clark RH, et al: Effects of venovenous extracorporeal membrane oxygenation on cardiac performance as determined by echocardiographic measurements. 8th Annual CNMC ECMO Symposium, Breckinridge, CO, Feb 1992 [abstract].
25. Veasy LG, Webster HW, Boucek MM: Pediatric use of intra-aortic pumping. In Doyle EF, Engle MA, Gersong WM, et al (eds): Pediatric Cardiology. New York, Springer Verlag, 1986, pp 600–602.
26. Weinhaus L, Canter C, Noetzel et al: Extracorporeal membrane oxygenation for circulatory support after repair of congenital heart defects. Ann Thorac Surg 48:206–212, 1989.
27. Ziomek S, Harrell JE Jr, Fasules JW, et al: Cardiopulmonary failure after congenital heart surgery: Results of treatment with extracorporeal membrane oxygenation. Society of Thoracic Surgeons, Orlando, FL, November, 1991 [abstract].
28. Zwischenberger JB, Bartlett RH: Extracorporeal circulation for respiratory or cardiac failure. Semin Thorac Cardiovasc Surg 2:320–331, 1990.

WALTER P. DEMBITSKY, MD
RICARDO J. MORENO-CABRAL, MD
ROBERT M. ADAMSON, MD
PAT O. DAILY, MD

EMERGENCY RESUSCITATION USING PORTABLE EXTRACORPOREAL MEMBRANE OXYGENATION

From Sharp Memorial Hospital
San Diego, California

This article is reprinted, with modifications, from an article by the authors that appeared in Annals of Thoracic Surgery 55:304–309, 1993, © 1993 The American Thoracic Society, with permission.

The first experience with closed-chest methods of augmenting circulation was reported in 1878 by Boehm,[1] who worked with arrested cats. It was not until 1947 that Gurvich and Yuniev successfully performed cardioversion of experimentally induced ventricular fibrillation.[4] They found that cardioversion was not possible if arrest lasted more than 1.5 minutes. However, the interval could be extended to 8 minutes if external compressions of the chest were used. Working with this background, Kouwenhoven[7] in 1960 described the technique of applying an alternating current defibrillator to patients undergoing closed-chest cardiopulmonary resuscitation (CPR). CPR has subsequently become standard therapy for patients with cardiac arrest, whether in or out of hospital.

The physiology of extreme circulatory decompensation has been evaluated both experimentally and clinically.[2,12] During cardiac arrest with closed-chest massage, cardiac output falls to approximately 20% of normal. Systolic arterial pressure is maintained, but mean arterial pressure falls below the average level of approximately 60 mmHg because of low diastolic pressures. Venous pressure gradually rises above the normal level of 5 mmHg, as high as 20–30 mmHg. Rising venous pressure and falling mean arterial pressure gradually create an inadequate gradient of peripheral tissue perfusion, which, coupled with

CARDIAC SURGERY: State of the Art Reviews—Vol. 7, No. 2, 1993
Philadelphia, Hanley & Belfus, Inc.

189

low cardiac output, results in multiple organ failure. Because of the cumulative nature of injuries occurred during CPR, survival after experimental or clinical arrest is extremely rare if CPR lasts longer than 30 minutes.[10,18]

Abnormal circulatory dynamics can be rapidly corrected by the peripheral application of venoarterial bypass using extracorporeal membrane oxygenation (ECMO). During cardiopulmonary bypass, the central venous pressure falls to desirably low levels as mean arterial pressure and cardiac output rise. Application of peripheral bypass establishes the circulatory milieu necessary for peripheral organ sustenance and maintenance (Fig. 1). The detailed work of Levine[10] demonstrated the advantages of peripherally applied cardiopulmonary bypass for resuscitating animals after cardiac arrest (Fig. 2). After 30 minutes of cardiac arrest with standard CPR, a control group of animals was subjected to advanced cardiac life support (ACLS), including cardiotonic drugs. The test group was placed on peripheral cardiopulmonary support. All animals in the test group versus 50% in the control group were easily cardioverted. At 24 hours, 7 of 10 supported animals survived with normal central nervous system function compared with 3 of 10 animals receiving ACLS, 2 of which had normal cerebral function. Thus application of cardiopulmonary bypass to arrested animals, even after 30 minutes of CPR, can result in improved survival compared with CPR and ACLS alone. Clinical experience suggests that the same is true in humans.[9,13,16,17]

TECHNOLOGY AVAILABLE FOR PORTABLE EXTRACORPOREAL MEMBRANE OXYGENATION

Following the work of Stephen Phillips,[15] a variety of companies (Bard Cardiopulmonary Division, Tewksbury, MA; Sarnes 3M Health Care, Ann Arbor, MI; Medtronic, Inc., Minneapolis, MN) have developed commercially available portable cardiopulmonary bypass systems that can be percutaneously applied. All are relatively simple to prime; in fact, some experimental work has now been done with systems that remain permanently primed. The most encouraging recent development is the clinical use of heparin-coated peripheral bypass circuits, which offer two advantages: (1) they are minimally thrombogenic, and (2) they diminish the activation of blood components that results from surface contact. Diminished

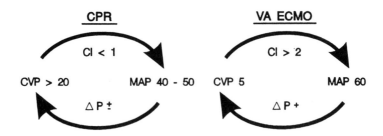

FIGURE 1. The hemodynamics produced during cardiopulmonary resuscitation are summarized on the left. The cardiac index is usually <1. The central venous pressure rises as the mean arterial pressure falls. This produces a marginal tissue perfusion gradient (delta P). Introduction of peripherally applied venoarterial ECMO (right) immediately creates a satisfactory cardiac index and improves the peripheral tissue perfusion gradient. (From Dembitsky WP, et al: Ann Thorac Surg 55:304–309, 1993, with permission.)

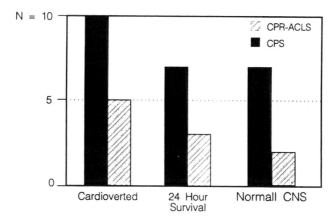

EXPERIMENTAL RESUSCITATION WITH ECMO FOLLOWING 30 MIN. ARREST WITH CPR

FIGURE 2. Experimental evidence demonstrating improved survival after 30 minutes of cardiac arrest with CPR in animals supported by peripherally applied ECMO and venoarterial bypass compared with animals receiving continued CPR and ACLS. (From Levine R, et al: Ann Emerg Med 16:620–627, 1987, with permission.)

activation of the complement cascade, preserved platelet levels, and normal prothrombin, partial thromboplastin, and bleeding times have permitted their use in situations in which hemorrhage is either an active or a potentially active problem. They have successfully supported patients with multiple trauma and patients requiring major surgery. An unproved possible advantage of coated circuits for emergency cardiopulmonary bypass, in which the usual precoating of a circuit with albumin is impractical, is that the more biocompatible surfaces may reduce the incidence of multiple-systems injury.

SURGICAL TECHNIQUES

Venous Cannulation

Because the portable systems do not use a reservoir and therefore aspirate blood directly from the heart, higher flows through relatively small-bore cannulas can be achieved. In contrast, conventional cardiopulmonary bypass uses relatively large-bore venous cannulas in a gravity drainage system to fill a reservoir. No. 20 Fr venous cannulas can be percutaneously positioned in the right atrium, through either the femoral vein or the right internal jugular vein. In 1 of our patients, emergency percutaneous femoral cannulation resulted in retroperitoneal venous disruption that required circulatory arrest for repair and survival. Retroperitoneal perforation can be avoided by use of internal jugular vein as a percutaneous site for right atrial access. Repair is simpler in the rare patient with internal jugular vein injury. Furthermore, venous flows are apt to be higher because of the shorter catheters required for more direct right atrial access.

Arterial Cannulation

Arterial blood is returned to the femoral artery. Because cardiac arrest is generally due to cardiac rather than pulmonary dysfunction, it is not necessary to direct the arterial blood flow back to the supravalvular region. The cannulas can be placed percutaneously using a Seldinger technique with progressive dilatation of the artery or, especially in arrested patients, by cutdown, usually combined with the modified Seldinger technique. Rapid peripheral arterial access may not be possible in patients with aortoiliac occlusive disease. Even with cannulation, obstructive disease in some patients does not permit adequate retrograde perfusion. In occasional patients the small, high-flow jet from the arterial cannula can dislodge atheromatous excrescences and produce systemic arterial embolization. Rarely peripheral cannulation can result in aortic dissection. In cases that require prolonged perfusion, it may occasionally be necessary to cannulate the peripheral femoral artery and vein to prevent leg ischemia and venous stasis.

Oxygenators

Currently the most commonly used oxygenators for emergency cardiopulmonary bypass have "hollow-fiber" membranes. Because the microporous fibers are not true membranes, they tend to exude plasma progressively after 12–36 hours of use. In the future, diminishing pore size as well as the potential addition of a silicone coat to one side of the fiber may eliminate plasma leakage. Available oxygenators with heparin-coated fibers are minimally thrombogenic; however, all are currently constructed in biologically improbable ways that create thrombosis in areas of stasis. This problem makes the use of some circulating heparin desirable.

Pumps

Two types of pumps are used in emergency CPR with portable bypass units. Currently the most widely applied are the nonocclusive, pressure-limited centrifugal pumps, which include (in order of frequency of use) the Biomedicus, the Sarnes, and the St. Jude pumps. All three are minimally hemolytic, although over long-term use, they appear to be mildly thrombogenic. Their advantage for emergency cardiopulmonary bypass is that the centrifugal pumps are pressure-limited; therefore, any abrupt occlusions of inflow and outflow cannulas are unlikely to result in either aspiration of air or disruption of lines. Use in long-term support is less desirable because of thrombogenicity.

The second type of pump used for peripheral resuscitating bypass units is the common roller pump, which is not pressure-limited and consequently can develop extremely high venous inflow and arterial outflow pressures. This potential can make its use in emergencies somewhat cumbersome if patient mobility is important. For support lasting more than 1 or 2 days, the roller pump becomes more advantageous.

The Conduct of Emergency Cardiopulmonary Bypass

After vascular access has been established, cardiopulmonary bypass is conducted in the usual way, with a few exceptions. Because peripherally applied cardiopulmonary bypass usually does not capture all venous return to the heart, some blood may continue to flow through the lungs, into the left ventricle, and subsequently, into the coronary arteries and cerebral circulation. Thus, continued high endotracheal oxygen insufflation is necessary to prevent the left ventricle from ejecting desaturated blood. Distention due to varying amounts of aortic insufficiency and bronchial flow into the arrested left heart can be minimized by prompt cardiac defibrillation. Cardioversion is made easier by collapsing the engaged left ventricle with simple sternal compression. Experimental left ventricular decompression during peripheral cardiopulmonary bypass in animals with ventricular fibrillation has been achieved by placing a helical coil across the pulmonary valve to render it incompetent and to permit left ventricular decompression.[6] Clinical use of this technique has not been reported. In our experience, left ventricular distention is infrequent. It can be monitored with transthoracic or transesophageal echocardiography or with a catheter that monitors pulmonary artery pressure (pulmonary artery pressure during ventricular fibrillation is equal to left intraventricular pressure). After initiation of full cardiopulmonary bypass, arrested patients may suddenly awaken and become combative; in this situation, immediate sedation or muscle paralysis is required.

Because emergency cardiopulmonary bypass is often established in patients who are not fully monitored, the adequacy of perfusion must initially be determined by clinical examination. Temperature of the upper extremities is assessed. The arterial pressure is determined initially by a Doppler apparatus with pressure cuffs and later by arterial monitoring lines. The arterial and venous access lines are examined to determine roughly the arterial venous oxygen difference. If both arterial and venous catheters are desaturated, oxygen flow to the oxygenator is insufficient. If both are fully saturated, venovenous bypass must be ruled out. Alternatively, in some patients after cardiac arrest with prolonged CPR, peripheral oxygen extraction may be so low that arteriovenous oxygen difference, even with low flows, is minimal. This usually denotes peripheral organ death and a poor prognosis.

During cardiopulmonary bypass in patients with cardiac arrest due to acute coronary occlusion, it is theoretically advantageous to reduce the systemic temperature to prolong the safe ischemic time for the injured heart. Some commercially available emergency cardiopulmonary bypass units have cooling as well as heating units incorporated into their circuits.

CURRENT RESULTS OF CLINICAL TRIALS USING PORTABLE EMERGENCY CARDIOPULMONARY BYPASS SYSTEMS

On the thirty-first anniversary of the discovery and clinical application of CPR,[8] reported results have been less encouraging than the initial experience seemed to project. Two recent studies have reviewed the current results of CPR in in-hospital patients.[3,11,14,18] Approximately 50% of patients can be resuscitated initially, but only 10% ultimately leave the hospital. At Sharp Memorial Hospital in San Diego, the discharge rate has been somewhat higher. Over a 1-year period, approximately 65% (91) of 140 arrested patients were resuscitated. Twenty-six percent (23 patients) were discharged. The average duration of CPR was approximately 22 minutes. Many have questioned how widely CPR should be applied in the hospital setting. The procedure is expensive, and in patients with little hope of long-term survival, it may be undesirable and even inhumane. Each institution must address patient selection individually. Our results with in-hospital CPR have improved primarily because of more judicious use of the technique.

Based on the experimental evidence available, one expects enhanced survival in patients if, after CPR, they are supported early by judiciously applied peripheral extracorporeal bypass circuits. Control studies evaluating the technique are unlikely to be created in the near future. The only evidence available is anecdotal clinical reports now appearing in the literature. Data from the 1991 National Cardiopulmonary Support Registry for emergency applications have been recently reported.[5] The registry collected information from 17 different institutions treating 187 patients with emergency cardiopulmonary bypass. Forty of 187 patients ultimately survived for an overall survival rate of 21%. Diagnostic and therapeutic interventions were performed on 75% (140) of the 187 patients while on cardiopulmonary bypass. These procedures included pulmonary embolectomy, pulmonary artery bypass grafting, and pulmonary and arterial angiography as well as angioplasty. Approximately 77% (31/40) of survivors underwent therapeutic intervention during support, compared with only half (73/147) of nonsurvivors. This suggests that cardiopulmonary bypass allows the patient to be transferred to more advanced forms of diagnostic and therapeutic intervention that may enhance survival. Figure 3 shows the results of witnessed arrests in 116 patients reported in the registry. Although differences among the three groups of arrest times are not statistically significant, survival, even after 221 minutes of cardiac arrest, is clearly possible with peripherally applied ECMO.

Because registry data represent the broad application of a technology in multiple institutions, some insight can be gained by examining the experience of single institutions. At the 37th Annual ASAIO Meeting, Dr. Charles Moore reported his experience with 67 patients, including a 30-day survival rate of 31%.[13a] In 11 patients undergoing emergency cardiopulmonary bypass, Mooney[13] reported a 64% (7) survival rate. When we analyzed data from our initial series and divided patients into early and late experience, the long-term survival rate of our most recent cohort was approximately 30% (7/20) compared with a long-term survival rate of only 10% (2/20) in our earlier cohort. Improved survival is the result of better patient selection as well as an emphasis on early institution of emergency ECMO.

We have created an emergency ECMO team consisting of informed physicians, nurses, and practitioners. Training for the team includes an initial didactic session describing the physiology of the technology as it is applied to the patient as well as potential complications. Direct, hands-on, "wet lab" experience is also provided

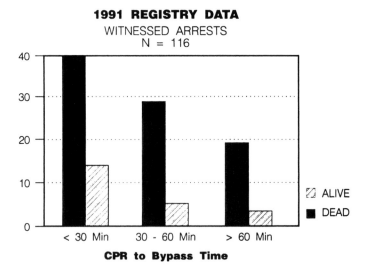

1991 REGISTRY DATA
WITNESSED ARRESTS
N = 116

FIGURE 3. Summary of 1991 registry data, including 116 patients with witnessed arrests. Even with cardiopulmonary resuscitation lasting > 30 minutes, prolonged survival is possible. (From Hill J, Bruhn P, Cohen S, et al: Emergent applications of cardiopulmonary support: A multi-institutional experience. Ann Thorac Surg, in press, with permission.)

during the initial training session. After introductory training, designated nurses with beepers are readily available to bring resuscitative units to the bedside of arrested patients, to prime the pump, and to begin cardiopulmonary bypass. These nurses, who participate in laboratory training every 2 months, are able to prime the pump and begin cardiopulmonary bypass within 10 minutes of notification.

Careful attention must be paid to the hospital deployment plan for this potentially lifesaving technology. The plan must begin at bedside with the physician attending the arrested patient. The physician must decide almost immediately if the arrested patient is a good candidate for long-term survival. Once that decision is made, the physician issues a call for the cardiopulmonary bypass unit, which ultimately may or may not be used. In our hospital, perfusionist and cardiothoracic surgeon are notified at the same time as the nurse who brings the unit to the bedside. Cannulas are placed at the bedside by the physician in attendance. Physicians capable of placing percutaneous catheters for use as dialysis access conduits are also capable of placing cannulas for extracorporeal circulation. In precarious patients, it is prudent to place percutaneous access lines in the femoral artery, internal jugular vein, or common femoral vein before cardiac arrest. This facilitates the later use of larger-bore cannulas after cardiopulmonary arrest, when finding an arterial pulse can be difficult. Cannulas are placed, and the patient is attached to the perfusion unit, which is activated by the nurses. Ultimate disposition is decided by the physician in attendance.

COMPLICATIONS

Complications unique to emergency peripherally applied cardiopulmonary bypass are largely related to vascular access sites. In our reported experience, vascular access was not possible in approximately 10% (2/38) of patients.[17] In Moore's experience, 2/53 could not be cannulated (reported at the 37th Annual ASAIO Meeting). In the Multi-Institutional Experience, 14% (26/187) of patients experienced technical problems with cannulations (Table 1). Of the 135 patients who died, the major organ dysfunctions contributing to death are summarized in Table 2. It is not possible to determine whether these maladies preceded or resulted from emergency cardiopulmonary bypass. Probably some resulted from delayed institution of cardiopulmonary bypass after prolonged CPR. Moreover, the introduction of emergency hemodilutional cardiopulmonary bypass into patients undergoing prolonged CPR may predispose these patients in some way to

TABLE 1.   Complications Related to Bypass

Complication	Number	Percent
None	161	86.1
Technical perfusion problem—cannulas	6	3.2
Poor venous drainage	5	2.7
Bleeding at groin	2	1.1
Technical perfusion problem—circuit	2	1.1
Arterial injury	1	0.5
Equipment failure	1	0.5
Perforated vena cava	1	0.5
Other	2	1.1
Unknown	7	3.7

From Hill J, Bruhn P, Cohen S, et al: Emergent application of cardiopulmonary support: A multi-institutional experience. Ann Thorac Surg, in press, with permission.

TABLE 2. Factors Contributing to Death (n = 135)

Factor	Number	Percent
Cardiac	101	74.8
Pulmonary	30	22.2
Central nervous system	37	27.4
Bleeding	35	25.9
Renal	1	0.7
Other	22	16.2

From Hill J, Bruhn P, Cohen S, et al: Emergent application of cardiopulmonary suppot: A multi-institutional experience. Ann Thorac Surg, in press, with permission.

multiple organ failure. The Elective Supported Angioplasty Register reported its multicenter experience with the first 100 cases undergoing supported angioplasty. This experience represents a best-case scenario for introduction of peripheral percutaneous cardiopulmonary bypass in the relatively controlled environment of the cardiac catheterization laboratory.[19] Table 3 shows the reported morbidity. Understandably, local cannulation problems are less frequent, and multisystem organ failure does not appear. A few cases may result from retrograde embolization (cerebrovascular accident, renal failure, small bowel infarction), thus reflecting the incidence of this problem in a large population of patients likely to receive emergency resuscitative cardiopulmonary bypass.

CONCLUSION

Early, judicious use of emergency cardiopulmonary bypass in properly selected patients in cardiac arrest appears to offer a survival advantage. Devices

TABLE 3. Morbidity in 105 Patients

Vessel cannulation	
Femoral artery repair (required)	4
Femoral artery occlusion	1
Femoral artery pseudoaneurysm	3
Large hematoma	4
Thrombophlebitis	5
Cannula site infection/necrosis	8
Femoral nerve injury (transient)	2
Embolism	
Superior mesenteric artery embolus/thrombus	1
Cerebrovascular accident	1
Transient cerebral ischemia	1
Angioplasty	
Left ventricular dysfunction requiring balloon pump	1
Post-PTCA myocardial ischemia	5
Post-PTCA myocardial infarction	7
Cardiac arrest	1
Other	
Gastrointestinal bleeding	2
Diabetic ketoacidosis (bowel ischemia)	1
Acute renal failure	1

PTCA = percutaneous transluminal coronary angioplasty.
From Vogel RA, Shawl F, Tommaso C, et al: Initial report of the National Registry of Elective Cardiopulmonary Bypass Supported Coronary Angioplasty. J Am Coll Cardiol 15:23–29, 1990, with permission.

should be used only in patients with witnessed arrests, with the possible exception of arrested victims suffering from hypothermia. Technology to miniaturize the circuitry, thus making it more biocompatible and less expensive, is available. Whether or not the technology is distributed to those using and needing it depends on the economic pressures of supply and demand. In the meantime, readily available equipment can be successfully used for patient care only when combined with an organized, carefully considered team approach.

REFERENCES

1. Boehm RV: Arbeiten aus dem pharmakologischen Institute der Universitat Dorpat: 13. Ueber Wiederbelebung nach Vergiftungen und Asphyxie. Arch Esper Pathol Pharmakol 8:68–101, 1878.
2. Cobb LA, Werner JA, Trobaugh GB: Sudden cardiac death. I: Experience with out-of-hospital resuscitation. II: Outcome of resuscitation, management, and future directions. Mod Concepts Cardiovasc Dis 49:31, 1980.
3. Fox M, Lipton HL: The decision to perform cardiopulmonary resuscitation. N Engl J Med 309:607–608, 1983.
4. Gurvich HL, Yuniev GS: Restoration of heart rhythm during fibrillation by condenser discharge. Am Rev Soviet Med 4:252–256, 1947.
5. Hill J, Bruhn P, Cohen S, et al: Emergent application of cardiopulmonary support: A multi-institutional experience. Ann Thorac Surg [in press].
6. Kolebow T, Rossi F, Borelli M, Foti G: Long-term closed chest partial and total cardiopulmonary bypass by peripheral cannulation for severe right and/or left ventricular failure, including ventricular fibrillation. ASAIO Trans 34:485–489, 1988.
7. Kouwenhoven WB, Jude JR, Knickerbocker GG: Closed chest cardiac massage. JAMA 173:1064–1067, 1960.
8. Kyff J, Puri VK, Raheja R, Ireland T: Cardiopulmonary resuscitation in hospitalized patients: Continuing problems of decision-making. Crit Care Med 15:41–43, 1987.
9. Laub GW, Banaszak D, Kupferschmid J, et al: Percutaneous cardiopulmonary bypass for the treatment of hypothermic circulatory collapse. Ann Thorac Surg 47:608–611, 1989.
10. Levine R, Gorayeb M, Safar P, et al: Cardiopulmonary bypass after cardiac arrest and prolonged closed-chest CPR in dogs. Ann Emerg Med 16:620–627, 1987.
11. Longstreth WT, Cobb LA, Fahrenbruch CE, Copass MK: Does age affect outcomes of out-of-hospital cardiopulmonary resuscitation? JAMA 264:2109–2110, 1990.
12. Maier GW, Tyson GS Jr, Olsen CO, et al: The physiology of manual external cardiac massage: High impulse cardiopulmonary resuscitation. Circulation 70:86, 1984.
13. Mooney MR, Arom KV, Joyce LD, et al: Emergency cardiopulmonary bypass support in patients with cardiac arrest. J Thorac Cardiovasc Surg 101:450–454, 1991.
13a. Moore CH, Dailey JW, Canon S, Rubin MO: Non-pulsatile circulatory support in 90 cases. ASAIO J 38:627–630, 1992.
14. Peterson MW, Geist LJ, Schwartz DA, et al: Outcome after cardiopulmonary resuscitation in a medical intensive care unit. Chest 100:168–174, 1991.
15. Phillips SJ, Ballentine B, Slonine D, et al: Percutaneous initiation of cardiopulmonary bypass. Ann Thorac Surg 36:223–224, 1983.
16. Phillips SJ, Zeff RH, Kongtahworn C: Percutaneous cardiopulmonary bypass: Application and indication for use. Ann Thorac Surg 47:121–123, 1989.
17. Reichman RT, Joyo CO, Dembitsky WP, et al: Improved patient survival after cardiac arrest using a cardiopulmonary support system. Ann Thorac Surg 49:101–105, 1990.
18. Taffet GE, Teasdale TA, Luchi RJ: In-hospital cardiopulmonary resuscitation. JAMA 260:2069–2072, 1988.
19. Vogel RA, Shawl F, Tommaso C, et al: Initial report of the National Registry of Elective Cardiopulmonary Bypass Supported Coronary Angioplasty. J Am Coll Cardiol 15:23–29, 1990.

MARC T. SWARTZ
D. GLENN PENNINGTON, MD

DEVELOPMENT OF A CIRCULATORY SUPPORT TEAM

From the Department of Surgery
St. Louis University Medical
  Center
St. Louis, Missouri

Reprint requests to:
Marc T. Swartz
Department of Surgery
St. Louis University Medical
  Center
3635 Vista Ave. at Grand Blvd.
P.O. Box 15250
St. Louis, MO 63110-0250

The past decade has brought substantial improvements in the clinical application of mechanical circulatory support devices,[7] which are now used not only for treatment of postcardiotomy shock but also as a bridge to cardiac transplantation and as support after acute hemodynamic deterioration.[2,3,8–11,13] Expanded application is due to improved survival and decreased morbidity as well as development of more reliable devices. During the same time period, a multidisciplinary approach to the management of critically ill patients has proved advantageous. For this reason we developed a team with expertise to aid in the clinical evaluation of mechanical circulatory support devices.

Host/device interactions are now recognized to be extremely complicated and multisystemic in nature.[7] Therefore, clinical care and research must be a cooperative effort among physicians, engineers, perfusionists, and nurses. Because the annual number of patients who require circulatory support devices is usually small at any given institution, a core group should be developed to provide consistent care. For these reasons, we developed a circulatory support team with the goal of increasing survival, decreasing morbidity, reducing cost, and identifying areas in need of further investigation.

EVOLUTION OF A TEAM

The popularity of cardiac transplantation, along with the promising results among early patients bridged to cardiac transplantation, led to a dramatic expansion of mechanical circulatory

CARDIAC SURGERY: State of the Art Reviews—Vol. 7, No. 2, 1993
Philadelphia, Hanley & Belfus, Inc.

199

support. A significant percentage of cardiac transplant centers now have active programs for bridge to transplantation. Many of these institutions initially assigned a heart transplant coordinator to supervise the newly formed programs. Other institutions place technical responsibilities under the auspices of the perfusion staff and clinical care under the management of the heart transplant team. Because a majority of centers involved in bridging to transplantation usually perform 2–5 procedures per year, it is difficult to justify personnel who are responsible solely for an assist device program.

At St. Louis University we have developed a program that uses a family of devices to treat cardiac failure, including extracorporeal membrane oxygenation (ECMO), centrifugal pumps, external pneumatic ventricular assist devices (VADs), electrical implantable left ventricular assist systems (LVASs), and pneumatic total artificial hearts (TAHs). These devices have been used as support for patients pending myocardial recovery or as a bridge to cardiac transplantation. Some can be used in children, and all can be used in adults. Because our program involves children and adults at three different hospitals, technical and clinical support is the responsibility of several distinct groups. Our circulatory support team, which coordinates investigational device studies, is separate from the perfusion, nursing, and heart transplant staffs. Because investigational devices are more complex than commercially available pumps and because the durations of support at St. Louis University have significantly increased over the last decade (Fig. 1), we need a group of experts who can dedicate their time solely to patients with assist devices.

Initially (1978) we used the Medtronic centrifugal pump, with technical support from laboratory personnel who had also performed animal experiments.[6] In 1981 we received a contract from the National Heart, Lung, and Blood Institute (NHLBI) to evaluate temporary VADs. For this contract, we selected the Pierce-Donachy Thoratec VAD.[5] The NHLBI provided salary support for one technical position. From 1981–1985, technical support and data collection were performed by a research technician. In 1985 St. Louis University acquired the Novacor left ventricular assist system (LVAS).[3] The sponsor of the study required readily available biomedical engineering support at each clinical site. We therefore added a biomedical engineer to our staff. This was a logical step in the evolution of our team because devices were becoming more complex. Over the next year our program continued to grow, with the durations of support increasing. In 1986 we purchased the Symbion Jarvik-7 TAH and also added a clinical nurse specialist to the circulatory support team. At this time, nursing support was essential because patients were supported for longer periods and some patients were transferred to the step-down floor.[12] Researchers, biomedical engineers, and perfusionists are not familiar with the care of patients or protocols in the intensive care unit (ICU). Although nonnursing personnel can collect and evaluate data and provide technical support, they are often not educated in infection control or treatment, nutrition, drug interrelationships, or other areas of patient management. A second nursing position was added in 1988 to assist with long-term management of patients.

Concurrent with the development of the adult circulatory support team, we also developed programs for pediatric and adult ECMO. The pediatric ECMO program was modeled after the University of Michigan's program, in which perfusionists supervise specially trained intensive care nurses. This system has worked well in neonatal and pediatric patients suffering cardiac and/or respiratory

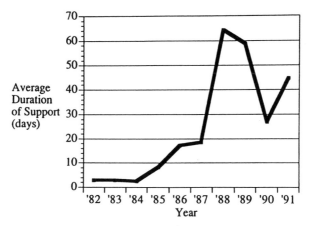

FIGURE 1. Average duration of mechanical circulatory support per year at St. Louis University.

failure. The perfusion staff is responsible for technical aspects of the adult ECMO program; research as well as clinical and engineering support are supplied by the investigational circulatory support team as needed. Because the duration of most adult ECMO perfusions at St. Louis University is usually < 3 days and most often ≤ 24 hours,[11] the perfusion staff has been able to manage the program with little or no detrimental effects on their routine case work.

We have found the combination of researcher, engineer, and nurses to be effective. The nature of the studies requires that protocols be under constant change; methods of treatment need to undergo prospective and retrospective analysis. Engineering support ensures device readiness and safety as well as professional education. Nursing support is critical, especially in the management of patients supported for longer durations. Of necessity, job responsibilities overlap to some degree; however, primary functions should be well defined and maintained within a reasonable set of limits.

TEAM RESPONSIBILITIES

The circulatory support team should be responsible for much more than technical considerations. Once stabilized, the patient can be managed by this team (under physician supervision), whose decisions are guided by specific protocols. As a group, the circulatory support team should perform the following functions:

1. Maintain device readiness.
2. Assist with the evaluation of potential candidates for mechanical circulatory support.
3. Provide technical support during device implantation.
4. Provide technical and clinical support during interval of perfusion.
5. Provide information to the family and patient.
6. Act as liaison between consulting services, house officers, nursing staff, and investigators.
7. Report data to clinical investigators and regulatory bodies.
8. Evaluate data and suggest areas for further research.
9. Suggest changes in protocol.

10. Provide ongoing education to staff.
11. Perform animal experimentation when necessary.
12. Disseminate information through publications and scientific meetings.
13. Maintain a database for long-term follow-up and evaluation of results.

Responsibilities of individual team members are described in the following paragraphs.

A team member with background in medical research is responsible for the collection and initial evaluation of data. In addition, he or she may be responsible for regulatory affairs and coordinate interdepartmental and multicenter studies. Animal implantations are often necessary for team readiness or for evaluating the effectiveness of a device. This person may be responsible for animal experiments and for collection of associated data. Under optimal conditions, he or she should possess a degree in nursing or perfusion technology to provide clinical/technical support if necessary.

The biomedical engineer is responsible for the readiness of the device at all times and the function of the device while it is implanted. Duties include the maintenance and calibration of consoles, along with ensuring an adequate supply of available implantable devices. In addition, the engineer is involved in the evaluation of different control modes and the identification of optimal parameters. Because these are clinical investigations, the biomedical engineer should take an active role in the development and modification of all system components. He or she may also assist with data collection as well as ambulation, exercise, and transport of the patient. Once the patient is stable, the engineer may be used to monitor the device if 24-hour technical coverage is necessary.

Clinical nurse specialists should have previous experience in a cardiovascular ICU. Familiarity with assist devices is encouraged because their primary role is to coordinate the care of supported patients. Clinical nurse specialists are also responsible for developing, maintaining, and updating nursing protocols. Their most critical role, however, is to act as a liaison among nursing staff, house officers, and attending physicians. They are responsible for educating the housestaff and nurses who care for patients. Other departments that interact directly with the patient—such as physical therapy, social service, nutritional support, and cardiac rehabilitation—are given individual educational sessions that provide an overview of clinical protocols and device function.

Clinical nurse specialists assist in the evaluation of potential candidates and in the operating room with preparation of the device before insertion; they also assist with transport of the patient. As the patient progresses, the nurse specialist can assist with equipment when the patient ambulates. Additional responsibilities include collection of data and patient follow-up.

Of necessity, each team member should be cross-trained and capable of covering for an absentee member. Additional responsibilities, including call, are divided among the team members. The team is responsible to the principal investigator, who coordinates its activities. One of the team's most important responsibilities is to evaluate clinical data and to identify areas that require further investigation. An objective evaluation of the total program needs to be performed periodically to target patient- and device-related complications that influence survival.

CONSULTING SERVICES

Cardiologists play a vital role in any assist device program. They are responsible for the initial evaluation and referral of many transplant candidates as well as other potential candidates for circulatory support. In conjunction with cardiac surgeons, they follow the patients throughout their hospital course and are often responsible for long-term management after discharge.

One of the most common complications associated with assist device support is infection.[4] Thus, communication with the infectious disease division is essential. Members of this division should be familiar with the type of mechanical devices used and with host/device interactions.[1] Bleeding is another significant complication. The severity of bleeding depends on many factors. For decades hematologists have studied the effects on blood when it comes in contact with an artificial surface. This research continues. However, the best method to avoid and/or to treat bleeding has yet to be determined. At the same time, anticoagulation protocols have been dramatically improved, and thromboembolic-free perfusions of >30 days are now commonplace.[15]

ANCILLARY SERVICES

A physical therapist sees the patient initially within 24 hours of device insertion. The physical therapist follows the patient throughout his or her hospital course, providing instruction to facilitate the return to near-normal activity by the time of hospital discharge. We have two physical therapists who assist with all patients receiving mechanical circulatory support.

We have a social worker exclusively for patients with cardiac transplants and assist devices. The social worker assists with financial, medical, and social arrangements as well as individual and family counseling. The social worker often acts as a liaison between the patient and the insurer and as a resource person for referral to community agencies.

DISCUSSION

The team described above results from more than 10 years of clinical and experimental work. We do not believe that such a team is the only possible organizational structure capable of providing adequate survival and meaningful research. Many institutions use employees who serve other functions when no patient is on a mechanical assist device. This arrangement, however, distracts the employees (generally perfusionists or transplant coordinators) from their normal duties whenever an assist device is inserted. Our group has two major objectives: (1) to improve the survival of patients currently supported with temporary assist devices, and (2) to collect data that will be useful in managing current patients on temporary support as well as future patients on permanent assist device systems and artificial hearts. At present, the temporary systems are limited to a small patient population, but their use will increase dramatically if it can be demonstrated that temporary ventricular assistance is beneficial to patients with acute myocardial infarction shock. This technology, however, will become most useful when permanent systems are available.

Most institutions are unable to assign four people exclusively for circulatory support. But the financial burden may ease if this capability increases patient referrals. In addition, salaries of personnel and cost of devices can be partially recovered by billing for the devices and the care related to their use.[14] We believe our assist device program is an investment in the future. The dividends of this investment will become obvious when permanent devices are available.

The above description of team members is the result of an evolutionary process. Formal education of team members and division of responsibilities are not the major factors that determine success or failure. Strict definition of the team's responsibility and its goals is the most important factor in success. Although the ideal team should contain nursing and engineering personnel, this make-up is not essential. Any combination of researchers, perfusionists, nurses, or engineers can be successful.

REFERENCES

1. Didisheim P, Olsen DB, Farrar DJ, et al: Infections and thromboembolism with implantable cardiovascular devices. ASAIO Trans 35:54, 1989.
2. Farrar DJ, Lawson JH, Litwak P, Cederwall G: Thoratec VAD system as a bridge to heart transplantation. J Heart Transplant 9:415, 1990.
3. Kanter KR, McBride LR, Pennington DG, et al: Bridging to cardiac transplantation with pulsatile ventricular assist devices. Ann Thorac Surg 46:134, 1988.
4. McBride LR, Ruzevich SA, Pennington DG, et al: Infectious complications associated with ventricular assist device support. ASAIO Trans 33:201, 1987.
5. Pennington DG, Kanter KR, McBride LR, et al: Seven years' experience with the Pierce-Donachy ventricular assist device. J Thorac Cardiovasc Surg 96:901, 1988.
6. Pennington DG, Merjavy JP, Swartz MT, Willman VL: Clinical experience with a centrifugal pump ventricular assist device. ASAIO Trans 28:93, 1982.
7. Pennington DG, Swartz MT: Assisted circulation and the mechanical heart. In Braunwald E (ed): Heart Disease: A Textbook of Cardiovascular Medicine, 4th ed. Philadelphia, W.B. Saunders, 1992, pp 535–550.
8. Pennington DG, Swartz MT: Temporary circulatory support in patients with postcardiotomy cardiogenic shock. In Spence PA, Chitwood WR (eds): Card Surg: State Art Rev 5:373–392, 1991.
9. Phillips SJ, Zeff RH, Kongtahworn C, et al: Percutaneous cardiopulmonary bypass: Application and indication for use. Ann Thorac Surg 47:121, 1989.
10. Portner PM, Oyer PE, Pennington DG, et al: Implantable electrical ventricular assist system: Bridge-to-transplantation and the future. Ann Thorac Surg 47:142, 1989.
11. Raithel SC, Swartz MT, Braun PR, et al: Experience with an emergency resuscitation system. ASAIO Trans 35:475, 1989.
12. Reedy JE, Ruzevich SA, Swartz MT, et al: Nursing care of a patient requiring prolonged mechanical circulatory support. Prog Cardiovasc Nurs 4:1–9, 1989.
13. Reichman RT, Joyo CI, Dembitsky WP, et al: Improved patient survival after cardiac arrest using a cardiopulmonary support system. Ann Thorac Surg 49:101, 1990.
14. Swartz MT, Reedy JE, Lohman DP, et al: Cost and reimbursement rates for investigational circulatory support. ASAIO Trans 37:549, 1991.
15. Szukalski E, Reedy JE, Pennington DG, et al: Oral anticoagulation in patients with ventricular assist devices. ASAIO Trans 36:700, 1990.

D.J. MAHON, MD, L.D. PADILLA, MD
D. ABRAHAMSON, MD, D.E. GUTFINGER, MD
M.L. DWYER, MD,* J.M. TOBIS, MD

CORONARY ANGIOPLASTY SUPPORTED BY EXTRACORPOREAL MEMBRANE OXYGENATION

From the Department of Medicine
Division of Cardiology
University of California, Irvine
Orange, California

* Baxter Healthcare Corporation
Bentley Laboratories Division
Irvine, California

Reprint requests to:
D.J. Mahon, MD
Department of Medicine
Division of Cardiology
University of California, Irvine
    Medical Center
101 The City Drive
Orange, CA 92668

Although the use of extracorporeal membrane oxygenation (ECMO) for cardiopulmonary failure has been well documented,[1,3,10,13] a portable cardiopulmonary bypass (CPB) system that could be rapidly instituted was not available until 1986.[6] The system initially was used in a variety of settings in patients with cardiac arrest.[11] Since then, its main emergent use has been in the cardiac catheterization laboratory.[8]

With the availability of a portable ECMO system that can be rapidly instituted,[6] the application of percutaneous transluminal angioplasty (PTCA) has been expanded to patients with severe ventricular dysfunction who otherwise would not be suitable candidates. Prophylactic use of ECMO during high-risk PTCA has been termed supported angioplasty.[12]

The effectiveness of supported angioplasty in high-risk patients has been well documented,[12,15,16] along with the indications for use.[2] In 1990 the National Registry of Elective Cardiopulmonary Bypass Supported Angioplasty reported 105 high-risk patients who underwent supported angioplasty. The procedural success rate was 95%, and the overall in-hospital mortality rate was 7.6%.[17]

ECMO during PTCA permits maintenance of adequate systemic perfusion, regardless of underlying cardiac function. The data show that patients undergoing supported angioplasty rarely have hypotension, chest pain, or ST-segment changes during balloon inflation.[15] Also, some data show that the use of ECMO during PTCA

CARDIAC SURGERY: State of the Art Reviews—Vol. 7, No. 2, 1993
Philadelphia, Hanley & Belfus, Inc.

205

can potentially reduce ischemia by decreasing myocardial oxygen consumption,[9] which may subsequently affect infarct size in the event of myocardial infarction.[4] Finally, supported angioplasty allows longer balloon inflation (5 min) as well as mixed procedures (e.g., PTCA and valvuloplasty) in high-risk patients.

The use of supported angioplasty will continue to play a role in sophisticated cardiac catheterization laboratories accustomed to high-risk patients who require PTCA.[2] In 1988 supported angioplasty was clinically introduced in the cardiac catheterization laboratory at the University of California Irvine Medical Center (UCIMC).[7] This chapter describes the results of our experience with ECMO-supported angioplasty.

MATERIALS AND METHODS

The ECMO system consists of the Bard H-4300 Cardiopulmonary Support System (CPS), as described by Tommaso.[15] The perfusion circuit is a compact, preassembled CPB system with a non-occlusive blood pump (BioMedicus 540, Irvine, CA), heat exchanger, oxygenator, and interconnecting tubing. The circuit also includes arterial and venous blood-sampling ports, recirculation loop, rapid infusion mechanism, and tubing clamps that expedite institution of CPB.

Set-up and priming can be accomplished within minutes. The prime consists of 1,500 cc of plasmalite A (Travenol Labs, Inc., Deerfield, IL) and 5,000 units of heparin. Arterial and venous access is obtained percutaneously with the Seldinger technique and standard cannulas developed specifically for the system (C.R. Bard Company, Inc., Billerica, MA), as described by Shawl.[12] Cannulation can be rapidly achieved, provided appropriate arteriograms are performed to assess the suitability of the femoral and iliac vessels.

Heparin is infused at 300 units/kg and adjusted so that the activated clotting time (ACT) is between 400 and 500 seconds. Prophylactic antibiotic coverage with 1.5 g of cefuroxime is administered before instituting bypass at the operator's discretion.

PATIENT SELECTION

Three modes under which ECMO is instituted have been identified: elective, standby, and emergent. In the elective mode, the patient is placed on ECMO before initiation of PTCA. The criteria for patient selection in the elective mode consist of either or both of the following conditions:

- Unstable angina with poor left ventricular function (ejection fraction <25%)
- Dilation of a vessel that supplies >50% of the remaining viable myocardium

Because of the risks of bleeding and vascular complications at the cannulation site, standby mode has sometimes been favored over elective mode. In the standby mode, arteriographic evaluation of the iliac and femoral vessels, placement of 5-Fr sheaths, and ECMO priming are performed before initiation of PTCA.[8] These measures permit rapid institution of ECMO in the event of hemodynamic collapse. This approach decreases the additional risk of ECMO support but increases the cost of the PTCA because of priming.

The optimal criteria for patient selection in the standby mode are uncertain. Tommaso,[15] however, provides separate selection criteria for the elective and standby procedures, using the elective mode in patients undergoing dilation of a single patent vessel or demonstrating hemodynamic instability. On the other hand, standby is used in patients either with impaired left ventricular function (ejection fraction <25%) or with greater than 50% of the viable myocardium supplied by the target vessel. For ECMO standby, Tommaso reports a set-up time of 4–6 minutes before partial bypass is initiated.

In the emergent mode, ECMO is instituted in response to failed PTCA with hemodynamic collapse. The presence of the sheaths and the availability of fluoroscopy expedite cannulation of the femoral vessels. However, priming of the ECMO and rapid initiation of bypass depend on training and expertise. Experience with emergency use of ECMO shows that survival rates are higher when rapid institution is possible (i.e., within 5–7 minutes).[8] Conversely, delays in instituting ECMO have been associated with an unfavorable outcome.

Patients may undergo supported angioplasty even if they are not surgical candidates because of poor surgical anatomy, severely depressed left ventricular function, multiple previous procedures for surgical revascularization, or secondary systemic conditions.

For transplant candidates with ischemic cardiomyopathy and unstable angina, supported angioplasty can relieve symptoms and function as a bridge to transplantation. This approach effectively reduces the cost of medical care and the increased morbidity associated with prolonged pretransplant hospitalization.

Absolute exclusion criteria include target vessel(s) not technically suited for PTCA, severe iliofemoral disease, or history of a significant bleeding diathesis.[12]

RESULTS

Between February 1989 and September 1992, 14 patients underwent PTCA with ECMO at the UCIMC. The patient population consisted of 11 men and 3 women with a mean age of 58 years. Nine of 14 patients had left ventricular ejection fractions ranging from 14–30% (mean: 20%). Four patients had normal ejection fractions (50–70%) but during PTCA developed hypotension that led to use of ECMO. ECMO was initiated with PTCA either electively or emergently (Table 1). In 7 patients, prophylactic supported PTCA was selected based on poor left ventricular function and associated unstable angina. One of the patients with aortic stenosis (no. 13) had elective ECMO. Emergent ECMO was applied to 1 patient (no. 3) who developed angioplasty-associated dissection of the proximal left anterior descending (LAD) artery with cardiopulmonary arrest and to 1 patient (no. 11) undergoing PTCA and aortic valvuloplasty when he developed hypotension with the initial coronary angiogram. Bypass times ranged from 26–200 minutes, with a mean of 116 minutes at a mean flow of 2.7 L/min (Table 2).

All patients had one or more coronary vessels with >50% luminal stenosis (Table 3), and two patients (nos. 11 and 13) had severe aortic stenosis with three-vessel coronary artery disease. Thirteen of 14 patients underwent successful PTCA of 33 of 39 lesions. Successful balloon aortic valvuloplasty was performed on 2 patients. Four patients (nos. 1, 4, 6, and 11) required additional intraaortic balloon pumping. Two patients (nos. 3 and 5) died during or immediately after the procedure. Patient no. 3 developed cardiopulmonary arrest after LAD dissection and could not be resuscitated despite emergent ECMO. In the other mortality, patient no. 5 developed hypotension during surgical removal of arterial and venous cannulas after weaning from ECMO. One other patient (no. 1) developed pulmonary edema and respiratory arrest after PTCA, which were felt to be secondary to cardiomyopathy and poor cardiac reserve. This patient subsequently underwent orthotopic cardiac transplantation 2 days after PTCA. No apparent episodes of significant chest pain or hemodynamic instability occurred in the remaining 11 patients during angioplasty with ECMO.

TABLE 1.   Supported Angioplasty at the University of California Irvine Medical Center

Patient No.	Age (yrs)	Sex	EF (%)	Cardiac Disease	ECMO, Indication
1	62	M	15	USA, ischemic	Elective, cardiomyopathy
2	59	M	53	USA	Elective, secondary to hypotension with initial inflation
3	66	M	54	s/p MI	Emergent, cardiopulmonary arrest with dissection of proximal LAD
4	54	M	15	Ischemic cardiomyopathy	Elective
5	47	M	30	Acute MI, CHF	Elective
6	64	M	25	USA, Hx CABG, CHF	Elective
7	51	M	14	USA, ischemic cardio-myopathy	Elective
8	41	M	25	USA, Hx MI	Elective, hypotension with initial inflation
9	68	F	70	Postinfarct angina	Elective, hypotension with PTCA of LAD
10	48	M	23	USA, Hx CABG	Elective
11	65	M		Aortic stenosis, CAD	Emergent, hypotension with coronary angiogram
12	50	F	50	Postinfarct angina	Elective, hypotension with inflation
13	91	F		Aortic stenosis, CAD	Elective
14	54	M	15	Ischemic cardiomyopathy	Elective, hypotension with inflation

EF = ejection fraction, USA = unstable angina, MI = myocardial infarction, CHF = congestive heart failure, Hx = history, CABG = coronary artery bypass grafting, LAD = left anterior descending artery, CAD = coronary artery disease.

Complications of ECMO angioplasty (Table 4) included blood transfusions (6 patients), a large groin hematoma (2 patients), and arterial insufficiency requiring thrombectomy (2 patients). Bleeding was the most common complication, with a mean of 2 units of packed red blood cells transfused per patient (Table 3). One patient (no. 12) experienced all of these complications except blood transfusion. She eventually developed a large left groin lymphocele, which required surgical drainage 2 months after the procedure. Cannulas were removed surgically in 5 patients on an elective basis; this procedure was not considered a complication.

Follow-up (Table 4) was available for 6 of the patients, ranging from 2 months to 2 years. Patients nos. 12 and 2 had no recurrent ischemia at 2 months and 24 months, respectively. At 8 months patient no. 14 developed recurrent restenosis and subsequently underwent PTCA without ECMO. Patient no. 4 had recurrent

TABLE 2.   Data Related to Extracorporeal Membrane Oxygenation

Patient No.	Bypass Time (min)	Flow Rate (L/min)	Transfusions (units PRBC)	Patient No.	Bypass Time (min)	Flow Rate (L/min)	Transfusions (units PRBC)
1	85	2.8	0	8	26	2.8	
2	90	3.0	0	9	80	2.8	2
3		2.0		10			
4		4.0		11			
5	200	2.3	3	12	150	3.0	3
6	150	1.8	2	13	150	2.4	3
7	60	3.0		14	170	2.2	1

PRBC = packed red blood cells.

TABLE 3. Data Related to Percutaneous Transluminal Coronary Angioplasty

Patient No.	Vessels Dilated	Stenosis, Pre- and Post-dilation (%)	Maximal Inflation Time (sec)
1	Proximal LAD	90/60	60
	Proximal LAD	75/30	60
	Mid LAD	70/40	60
2	Mid RCA	85/40	270
3	Proximal LAD	80/dissection	80
4	Proximal LAD	90/40	90
	Mid LAD	70/0	90
	Distal LAD	80/30	150
	Proximal RCA	95/40	120
	Mid RCA	70/0	50
	Distal RCA	70/40	40
5	Proximal LAD	80/40	50
	First septal portion	70/50	
6	Svg, Cx	95/0	60
	LAD	100/100	60
7	Proximal LAD	95/0	
	Mid Cx	100/0	
	RCA	80/0	
8	Mid Cx	95/30	60
	Proximal RCA	60/30	
9	Proximal LAD	95/0	
	Mid LAD	95/50	
	Distal LAD	95/0	
10	Proximal Cx	95/30	
	Distal Cx	80/30	
11	Distal Cx	90/	70
	Diagonal	95/	60
	LAD	60/	60
12	Mid RCA	85/35	50
	Mid LAD	70/20	60
13	Proximal LAD	85/25	60
	Mid LAD	80/25	105
	Mid RCA	70/15	60
	Distal RCA	75/75	60
	Aortic valve	120/20 mmHg	
14	Proximal RCA	100/30	70
	Mid RCA	100/30	30
	Distal RCA	100/30	125
	Proximal LAD	100/30	30
	Mid LAD	100/100	60

LAD = left anterior descending artery, RCA = right coronary artery, Cx = circumflex artery.

ischemia at 1 year and underwent successful two-vessel coronary bypass grafting. Orthotopic cardiac transplantation was performed in patient no. 1 two days after supported angioplasty. At 1-year follow-up, patient no. 4 had expired from recurrent congestive heart failure and ventricular arrhythmias.

DISCUSSION

Our initial experience with ECMO-assisted PTCA supports the belief that partial bypass decreases the risks in patients with severe left ventricular dysfunction. The reduction of physiologic work provided by ECMO allows complex PTCA as well as mixed procedures in patients whose conditions would otherwise prohibit

TABLE 4.   Complications and Follow-up of Supported Angioplasty

Patient No.	Complication
1	Postprocedural hypotension, pulmonary edema, and respiratory arrest requiring IABP and intubation/mechanical ventilation Subsequent orthotopic cardiac transplant 2 days after ECMO angioplasty At 21-month follow-up, patient doing well
2	Surgical removal of cannulas Transfusion of 1 unit PRBC with surgery At 24-month follow-up, no recurrent ischemia
3	Proximal LAD dissection with persistent hypotension, requiring continued ECMO and institution of IABP; ultimate death despite resuscitative measures
4	Groin hematoma At 12-month follow-up, death from from recurrent CHF and ventricular arrhythmias
5	Hypotension after weaning from ECMO, requiring placement of IABP and reinstitution of ECMO; ultimate death despite prolonged resuscitation Surgical removal of cannulas
6	Surgical removal of cannulas Postsurgical agitation with intubation/mechanical ventilation secondary to CO_2 retention; extubated successfully
7	No significant complications
8	No significant complications
9	Left femoral artery occlusion (ECMO site), with thrombectomy performed 2 days after the procedure At 2-month follow-up, patient was without recurrent cardiac ischemia but had left lower extremity claudication
10	No significant complications
11	IABP inserted after ECMO
12	Left lower extremity ischemia requiring urgent surgical removal of cannulas Subsequent large left groin hematoma, complicated by deep venous thrombosis At 2 months after procedure, surgical drainage of large left groin lymphocele At 1 year after procedure, underwent successful two-vessel CABG
13	No significant complications
14	Left lower extremity ischemia requiring urgent surgical removal of cannulas and embolectomy procedure At 6-month follow-up, EF improved by MUGA to 25%; clinically doing well At 8-month follow-up, catheterization revealed restenosis; patient underwent successful PTCA without ECMO

IABP = intraaortic balloon pumping, PRBC = packed red blood cells, LAD = left anterior descending artery, CHF = congestive heart failure, CABG = coronary artery bypass grafting, EF = ejection fraction, MUGA = multiple gated acquisition.

intervention. ECMO also served well in PTCA cases in which irreversible hemodynamic deterioration was not initially expected.

The UCIMC experience is comparable to results obtained in the initial report from the National Registry of Elective Supported Angioplasty.[18] However, the small numbers in our experience, including 12 elective and 2 emergent ECMO cases, preclude meaningful statistical comparison. Successful balloon dilation occurred in 83% (29/35) of lesions in our elective group vs. 95% (173/182) in the initial registry experience. The average number of attempted lesions per patient was higher in our elective group (2.9 vs. 1.7). Complications occurred frequently in both the registry group (39%) and in our elective population (58%). The overall hospital mortality rate in our elective population was 8.3% vs. 7.6% reported by the registry. A significant proportion of the deaths in the registry experience occurred in patients older than 75 years or with significant left main disease.[18]

Emergent use of ECMO during PTCA could not be compared with prophylactic use from our limited patient data. The standard approach for standby ECMO includes the placement of 5-Fr sheaths in the contralateral femoral artery and vein, arteriography of the iliofemoral system, and priming of the ECMO pump. Priming of the pump adds significant cost to the PTCA. With these measures, we have found that emergent institution of ECMO can be accomplished within several minutes. Tierstein et al.[14] reported the results of prophylactic vs. standby ECMO in high-risk PTCA from the registry data, which included 258 patients with prophylactic and 98 patients with standby ECMO. The two groups had similar rates of procedural success, need for emergent bypass grafting, and mortality. The difference was greater morbidity in the prophylactic group, specifically a trend toward more complications at the femoral site and a significant increase in required blood transfusions (47% vs. 17%).[14] In a subgroup analysis, patients with an ejection fraction <20% had a significantly lower procedural mortality (4.8% vs. 18.8%) with prophylactic ECMO compared with standby ECMO.[14]

As with our experience, the complications of supported angioplasty have been principally bleeding and vascular complications at the cannulation site.[8,12,15,17] Vogel[17] reported that 52% of the complications involved arterial, venous, or nerve injury at the cannulation site. However, fewer problems were encountered when the newer 18-Fr cannluas (possible flow of 4–5 L/min) were used instead of the 20-Fr cannulas (possible flow of 5–6 L/min).[17] Shawl[12] reported that the most common complication appears to be the need for blood transfusions, which he associated with the large amount of administered heparin, loss of blood during exchange of catheters, and hemodilution. He reported that more recently he has reduced the complication rate by modifying the procedure for removal of cannulas. Instead of removing the cannulas in the catheterization laboratory, he removes them 6 hours later. This method reduces the clamp compresssion time to <4 hours (vs. 8–16 hours), and no complications or blood transfusions were encountered in his most recent 20 patients.[12] The introduction of heparin-bonded tubing and pump[5] may be another approach for reducing the need for anticoagulation and hence the risk of complications. This approach is expected to reduce bleeding but is unproved clinically.

Other practical considerations may reduce complications with supported PTCA. In a center at which ECMO use is infrequent, routine maintenance of the system is essential. Our experience includes 1 case of CPS pump failure during attempted emergent ECMO in a patient with dissection of the left main coronary artery. One possible preventive measure is scheduled test priming of the pump; this measure, however, adds considerable expense. We recommend the use of auxillary clamps for the arterial/venous lines in addition to the clamps provided by the manufacturer. Clamp failure for even a brief moment may lead to significant blood loss.

Despite the risk of complications, our results confirm the efficacy of supported angioplasty in a variety of high-risk patients. Investigators have used the technique in patients with severe ischemic cardiomyopathy, associated critical valvular disease, significant left main disease, single patent artery, and poor surgical risk. Ultimately, the probable key to high-risk angioplasty is the expediency with which the task is accomplished. The belief that patency rates may be improved with prolonged inflations is a factor that may favor prophylactic ECMO. We believe, however, that most high-risk PTCA cases can be managed with standby ECMO instead. Prophylactic use has not improved success but has been associated with increased complications. Moreover, the success of other percutaneous techniques in high-risk angioplasty (such as intraaortic balloon counterpulsation or anterograde transcatheter coronary perfusion) provides alternatives to prophylactic ECMO. Data from the registry experience[14] suggest that patients with a severely depressed ejection fraction (<20%) would benefit from prophylactic ECMO; further investigation, however, is required to define the appropriate use of prophylactic ECMO in high-risk angioplasty.

CONCLUSION

ECMO-supported coronary angioplasty represents yet another valuable tool for the interventional cardiologist. Supported coronary angioplasty offers a viable therapeutic option for patients otherwise unsuitable for cardiac surgery or conventional interventional procedures. In addition, supported angioplasty may provide a unique modality for patients with ischemic cardiomyopathy and unstable angina, either as primary therapy or as a bridge to transplantation.

Critical to the effective management of high-risk patients are careful patient selection and knowledge of the pathophysiology of cardiopulmonary bypass.

Finally, with particular attention to the potential for complications at the femoral site and transfusion requirements, patients with an ejection fraction >20% are likely to benefit as much from standby as from prophylactic ECMO-supported coronary angioplasty.

REFERENCES

1. Bartlett RH, Gazzaniga AB, Fong SW, et al: Extracorporeal membrane oxygenator support for cardiopulmonary failure: Experience in 28 cases. J Thorac Cardiovasc Surg 73:375–386, 1977.
2. Ellis SG, Myler RK, Spencer BK III, et al: Causes and correlates of death after unsupported coronary angioplasty: Implications for use of angioplasty and advanced support techniques in high-risk settings. Am J Cardiol 68:1447–1451, 1991.
3. Hill JD, DeLeval MR, Fallat RJ, et al: Acute respiratory insufficiency: Treatment with prolonged extracorporeal oxygenation. J Thorac Cardiovasc Surg 64:551–562, 1972.
4. Laks H, Ott RA, Standever J, et al: Servo-controlled cardiac assistance. Effect of left ventricular-to-aortic and left atrial-to-aortic assistance on infarct size. Am J Cardiol 42:244–250, 1978.
5. Larm O, Arrader L, Olsson P: Influence of blood flow and the effect of protamine on the thrombo resistant properties of a covalently bonded heparin surface. J Biomed Mater Res 859–868, 1988.
6. Litzie AK, Roberts CP: Emergency femoral-femoral cardiopulmonary bypass. Proc Am Acad CV Perfus 8:60–65, 1987.
7. Ott RA, Mills TC, Tobis JM, et al: ECMO assisted angioplasty for cardiomyopathy patients with unstable angina. ASAIO Trans 36:483–485, 1990.
8. Overlie PA: Emergency use of portable cardiopulmomary bypass. Cathet Cardiovasc Diag 20:27–31, 1990.
9. Pavlides GS, Hauser AM, Stack RK, et al: Effect of peripheral cardiopulmonary bypass on left ventricular size, afterload and myocardial function during elective supported coronary angioplasty. J Am Coll Cardiol 18:499–505, 1991.
10. Pennington DG, Merjavy JP, Codd JE, et al: Extracorporeal membrane oxygenation for patients with cardiogenic shock. Circ Cardiovasc Surg 70(Suppl I):130–137, 1984.
11. Reichman RT, Daily PO, Overlie PA, et al: Improved patient survival after cardiac arrest using a cardiopulmonary support system. Ann Thorac Surg 5230:599, 1990.
12. Shawl FA, Domanski MJ, Punja S, Hernandez TJ: Percutaneous cardiopulmonary bypass support in high-risk patients undergoing percutaneous transluminal coronary angioplasty. Am J Cardiol 64:1258–1263, 1989.
13. Swartz MT, Pennington DG, McBride LR, et al: Temporary mechanical support: Clinical experience with 148 patients. In Unger F (ed): Assisted Circulation 3. Berlin, Springer Verlag, 1989, pp 132–151.
14. Teirstein PS, Vogel RA, Dorros G, et al: Prophylactic versus standby cardiopulmonary support for high risk percutaneous transluminal coronary angioplasty. J Am Coll Cardiol 21:590–596, 1993.
15. Tommaso CL: Use of percutaneously inserted cardiopulmonary bypass in the cardiac catheterization laboratory. Cathet Cardiovasc Diag 20:32–38, 1990.
16. Vogel RA: The Maryland experience: Angioplasty and valvuloplasty using percutaneous cardiopulmonary support. Cardiology 62:11K, 1988.
17. Vogel RA, Tommaso CL: Special feature: Cardiopulmonary support. Elective supported angioplasty: Initial report of the National Registry. Cathet Cardiovasc Diag 20:22–26, 1990.
18. Vogel RA, Shawl F, Tommaso C, et al: Initial report of the National Registry of Elective Cardiopulmonary Bypass Supported Coronary Angioplasty. J Am Coll Cardiol 15:23–31, 1990.

ROBERT A. VOGEL, MD

FEMOROFEMORAL CARDIOPULMONARY BYPASS ASSISTED CORONARY ANGIOPLASTY

Robert A. Vogel, MD
Herbert Berger Professor
  of Medicine
Head, Division of Cardiology
University of Maryland School
  of Medicine
Baltimore, Maryland

Reprint requests to:
Robert A. Vogel, MD
University of Maryland Hospital
22 S. Greene Street, Suite N3W77
Baltimore, MD 21201

Although coronary angioplasty was originally employed predominantly in patients with single-vessel coronary artery disease, stable angina, and good left ventricular function, it has been increasingly used in those with more extensive coronary disease, severe and acute chest pain syndromes, and poor ventricular function.[3,4,8,23] Technical advances in guidewires and balloon catheters, new interventional devices, increased operator experience, improved imaging equipment, and use of circulatory support systems have facilitated the widespread application of coronary angioplasty. Three techniques for circulatory support have been used: the intra-aortic balloon pump,[1,6,7,12] autoperfusion catheters,[21,28] and femorofemoral cardiopulmonary bypass.[13,16–19,24,25,34] Intra-aortic balloon pumping and cardiopulmonary bypass primarily support the systemic circulation, whereas the autoperfusion catheter augments coronary blood flow during balloon inflation. The use of autoperfusion catheters deviates least from standard angioplasty technique, but provides limited increases in coronary blood flow in circumstances of profound shock or cardiac arrest. The intra-aortic balloon pump augments systemic circulation about 30% in circumstances of mild hypotension, but is of little value in arrested patients. In contrast, cardiopulmonary bypass provides the greatest degree of systemic circulatory augmentation, but is the most complex and invasive to implement. Each of the three systems for circulatory support can be used prophylactically, held in standby, or applied emergently during angioplasty complications. This review summarizes the experience of a multicenter registry of cardiopulmonary bypass use in patients undergoing high-risk angioplasty, and identifies those circumstances in whom prophylactic, standby, and emergency support have been found helpful.

SUPPORTED ANGIOPLASTY TECHNIQUE

The cardiopulmonary bypass system employed was originally designed for emergency femorofemoral bypass support.[16] As seen in Figure 1, it contains in series a centrifugal pump, heat exchanger, and membrane oxygenator. It provides 4–6 L/min of nonpulsatile flow through 17–20-Fr cannulas inserted into the femoral artery and vein.[16,19,34] The system differs from standard, intraoperative passive drainage bypass systems by placement of the centrifugal pump directly in line with the venous afferent cannula. This allows active aspiration of venous blood, thus reducing the required diameter of the venous cannula. Contrary to use of the intra-aortic balloon pump, full systemic circulatory support is provided irrespective of intrinsic cardiac output or rhythm.[15,20] Myocardial ischemia distal to balloon occlusion is not reduced, however, and myocardial lactate production has been shown to increase upon institution of bypass support. Because left ventricular pumping is not employed, it is important to maintain sinus rhythm to preclude progressive left ventricular dilatation and irreversible myocardial injury.

Procedures are performed in the catheterization laboratory by an interventional cardiologist, perfusionist, and technician team using mild sedation and local anesthesia.[16,19,34] Coagulation, blood gases, and electrolytes are routinely monitored in the catheterization laboratory. Although femoral cannulation was initially performed

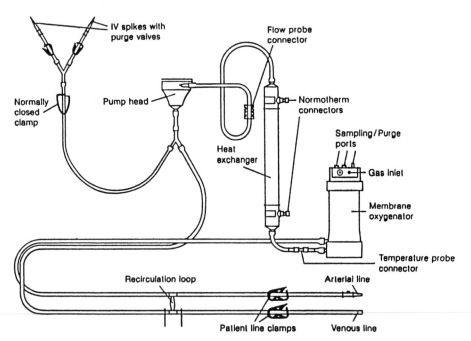

FIGURE 1. The cardiopulmonary bypass circuit employed in conjunction with high-risk angioplasty.

using surgical cutdown, the more recently developed percutaneous technique of Shawl et al.[18,19] is associated with lesser morbidity and allows for standby support.[25] Iliofemoral angiography is routinely performed prior to cannulation to ensure vessel adequacy. Occasionally, femoral angioplasty has been required to obtain an adequate lumen. The percutaneous technique uses placement of flexible, followed by stiff guidewires over which progressive vessel dilatation (10, 14 Fr) is accomplished. Under fluoroscopic guidance, the 18–20 Fr-venous cannula is positioned at the right atrial–inferior vena caval junction, and the 17–19-Fr arterial cannula positioned in the distal aorta. Comparison of this percutaneous approach with traditional cutdown cannulation has consistently demonstrated lower morbidity and mortality for both electively and emergently supported patients. Activated clotting times are maintained at greater than 400 and 300 seconds for standard and heparin-bonded oxygenator systems, respectively.

Coronary angioplasty is performed after the initiation of circulatory support. Pump flow is adjusted to reduce pulmonary artery wedge pressure to less than 5 mmHg and maintain mean blood pressure above 70 mmHg (usually 2–3 L/min). As with intraoperative cardiopulmonary bypass, fluid administration is frequently found necessary to maintain adequate venous return. If left ventricular tachycardia or fibrillation occurs, cardioversion/defibrillation is promptly instituted to prevent ventricular dilatation. If sinus rhythm cannot be maintained, left ventricular aspiration with 10-Fr pigtail catheters has been employed. Patients suffering hemodynamic collapse associated with angioplasty complications have been found to undergo successful defibrillation more easily when placed on bypass support.

Once the patient is on bypass support, coronary angioplasty is undertaken. Prolonged dilatations can be performed without fear of circulatory collapse. The circulatory stability allows for optimal dilatation and more complete revascularization. The minority of patients undergoing dilatation on bypass support experience angina and/or EKG changes, perhaps due to reductions in preload. Despite this, the myocardium distal to the balloon occluded segment clearly becomes ischemic and overall ventricular function declines. Transesophageal echocardiography has shown that patients with very poor ventricular function cease left ventricular blood ejection during angioplasty. Following successful angioplasty, pump flow is gradually decreased over a few minutes. Cannula removal is accomplished either immediately using surgical closure or percutaneously 4–6 hours later following decrease in the activated clotting time to about 240 seconds. In the latter instance, a mechanical groin clamp is used to achieve hemostasis following cannula removal. Progressively, lesser clamp pressure is employed over a period of 2–6 hours. In approximately 10% of cases, hemostasis cannot be maintained and surgical closure is performed. Other centers prefer to perform direct surgical closure immediately following the procedure, even if cannulas were placed percutaneously, which allows continued use of heparin in situations of unstable angina or less than optimum dilatation results. Packed red cells are retrieved from the bypass circuit and returned to the patient.

Standby support has been increasingly employed for high-risk, but not critical, individuals.[25] Standby support requires the same teamwork, perfusion expertise, and bypass system availability as does prophylactic support. Iliac angiography is performed, followed by placement of 5-Fr sheaths in the artery and vein contralateral to the guiding catheter sheath. Pump priming is performed in about half of standby cases, especially if it appears likely that circulatory support will be necessary. If hemodynamic instability or vessel closure occurs, cannulation and initiation of cardiopulmonary bypass can be accomplished in less than 5 minutes in at least 90% of instances. In general, the standby approach can be used successfully only in those laboratories that have considerable elective cannulation experience, cardiopulmonary technician support, and maintenance of the system in the catheterization laboratory. Laboratories performing standby supported angioplasty have found that only 5–10% of high-risk patients require circulatory support, although it is difficult to select those who will require it in advance. Although patients with extensive coronary artery disease and/or severe left ventricular dysfunction are most likely to encounter circulatory collapse following a complication of dilatation, the latter is associated more with lesion complexity and dilatation technique.

Emergency initiation of cardiopulmonary support following unexpected protracted circulatory collapse or cardiac arrest has also been employed in centers with the technical expertise.[13,18] The greatest success has been achieved when circulatory support is encountered in the catheterization laboratory or coronary care unit. Initiation of bypass support in under 20 minutes is associated with an approximate 50% long-term survival in contrast to an 10–20% survival if support is not initiated within that period. Although approximately 80% of individuals can be resuscitated with emergency bypass support, only approximately 35% survive hospitalization. Follow-up of these latter individuals, however, reveals that 2-year survival is about 90%.

The majority of patients sustaining vessel closure during supported angioplasty have not required emergency bypass surgery due to the circulatory stability, which allows time for correction of the coronary occlusion. The same has been found for patients undergoing emergency bypass initiation. More than half of this latter group can undergo completion of their angioplasty without need for emergency bypass surgery. Patients requiring surgical bypass can be taken to the operating room on support. Because cardiopulmonary bypass does not augment perfusion, autoperfusion catheters have been found additionally helpful following sustained vessel closure. As left ventricular venting is generally not employed, it is also important to maintain sinus rhythm to prevent ventricular dilatation.

NATIONAL REGISTRY EXPERIENCE

The multicenter experience of 25 institutions performing elective and emergency supported angioplasty have been collected in a national registry since March, 1988.[22,26,30,32,33] Through March 1992, the data on 801 elective procedures have been collated. Patients were considered candidates for prophylactic or standby support if they had severe or unstable angina, a lesion judged by the interventionalist to be appropriate for angioplasty, and a target vessel supplying more than one-half the residual viable myocardium and/or a left ventricular ejection fraction <25%. Of the 801 patients, 76% were male, their mean age was 65 years, and 85% had either class III or IV angina. Multivessel coronary disease was present in 90%, left main coronary disease was present in 15%, and dilatation of the only patent coronary vessel including bypass graft was undertaken in 21%.[5,12,22] Using local criteria, 20% of patients were deemed bypass surgery inoperable. The mean left ventricular ejection fraction was 30%, and 28% of patients had an ejection fraction ≤20%.

Prophylactic and standby support were undertaken in 73% and 27% of patients, respectively.[27] The characteristics of these two groups of patients were the same except for a higher ejection fraction in the patients undergoing standby support (32.8 vs. 28.4%, p <0.01). Angioplasty was undertaken at 1.9 vessel sites

TABLE 1. National Registry of Elective Supported Angioplasty:
Mortality by Subgroup

	Mortality	Patients
Women	7.7%	195
Age >70	12.0%	248
Left main stenosis	12.0%	116
Only patent vessel	7.1%	169
Inoperable	5.1%	158
Ejection fraction ≤20%	8.8%	226
Standby	6.5%	217
Prophylactic	7.0%	584
Total	6.9%	801

per patient with a primary success rate of 93% (final diameter stenosis <50%). Acute myocardial infarction occurred in 0.87%, emergency bypass surgery was required in 2.6%, and the overall hospital mortality rate for the entire group was 6.9%. Hospital mortality is categorized in Table 1. Only the presence of age >70 years and left main coronary disease were associated with increased mortality. Unexpectedly, patients with ejection fraction ≤20%, surgical inoperability, and those undergoing dilatation of their only patent vessel did not experience significantly higher mortality than the group mean.

Table 2 lists morbidity and mortality according to the use of percutaneous or cutdown prophylactic support or standby support. In general, the fewest vascular complications and need for transfusions occurred in the standby supported group, and the most in the cutdown cannulation-prophylactic supported group. Hospital mortality was least for percutaneous cannulation-prophylactic support and standby support, trending higher for cutdown cannulation-prophylactic support. These data raise the question of whether any specific subgroup benefited from prophylactic support. Those with left ventricular ejection fraction <20% had significantly less hospital mortality when prophylactic support was employed compared with standby support (Table 3). An opposite trend was observed for those with ejection fraction >20%. Although patients older than 70 years trended in favor of prophylactic support, no other subgroup clearly benefited from predilatation initiation.

Of the 217 patients undergoing standby support, 91% underwent successful coronary dilatation without protracted hypotension or cardiopulmonary arrest

TABLE 2. National Registry of Elective Supported Angioplasty:
Morbidity and Mortality by Technique

	Prophylactic Support (Cutdown) (n = 108)	Prophylactic Support (Percutaneous) (n = 476)	Standby Support (n = 219)
Transfused	69.0%	31.0%	14.0%
Vascular complications	19.0%	15.0%	6.1%
Acute myocardial infarction	1.9%	0.6%	0.9%
Emergency bypass surgery	1.9%	2.5%	3.2%
Death	11.0%	6.3%	6.0%

TABLE 3.   National Registry of Elective Supported Angioplasty:
Mortality by Ejection Fraction (EF)

	EF ≤20%	EF >20%
Standby support	7/39 (18%)	7/178 (3.9%)
Prophylactic support	13/187 (7%)	28/397 (7.1%)
	P <0.05	P = NS

(Fig. 2).[22] This finding underscores the lack of need of circulatory support for most high-risk patients undergoing coronary angioplasty. Three patients (1.4%) underwent emergency bypass support following unsuccessful dilatations unassociated with circulatory collapse. Sixteen patients (7.4%) on standby required emergency initiation of bypass support, predominantly due to protracted cardiac arrest. Of these, support was initiated successfully in 15 cases in less than 5 minutes. One patient required 10 minutes for initiation of support with resulting irreversible neurological damage. The majority (75%) of patients requiring circulatory support underwent successful angioplasty without need for bypass surgery, and 7 survived long-term hospitalization. Four patients required emergency bypass surgery following initiation of circulatory support, and two survived long-term hospitalization. These findings suggest that standby support reduces the need for emergency bypass surgery by about two-thirds and reduces the mortality of high-risk angioplasty by about one-half.

Although five standby supported patients underwent angioplasty on intra-aortic balloon support, the registry did not attempt to compare or randomize these therapies. Good experience in high-risk patients with use of intra-aortic balloon support has been reported, but these studies also have not directly compared support therapies.[7,9,27] Moreover, the registry's experience suggests that only patients with very poor ventricular function appear to benefit from prophylactic support of any type.

Long-term follow-up of 527 prophylactic and standby supported patients was reported, although this was not an initial goal of the registry.[29,31] At follow-up,

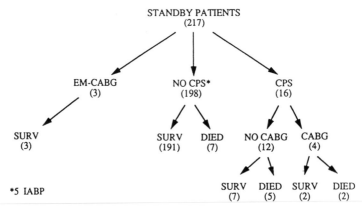

FIGURE 2.   Outcome of 217 patients in the national registry who underwent standby use of cardiopulmonary bypass support (CABG = bypass surgery, CPS = cardiopulmonary bypass support, EM = emergency, SURV = survived).

90% had class I or II angina, and the mean ejection fraction had risen from 27.3% to 35.7% (p <0.05). An even more substantial increase in left ventricular ejection fraction was experienced in those with initial ejection fractions ≤20% (17.5–28.0%). Improvement in ventricular function is more likely in those with residual viable but hibernating myocardium. Additional procedures were required as follows: unsupported angioplasty: 36; supported angioplasty: 22; bypass surgery: 34; AICD placement: 5; and cardiac transplantation: 4. The survival including original hospital mortality at 1, 2, and 3 years was 82%, 80% and 77%, respectively. Even those with initial left ventricular ejection fractions ≤20% experienced a 77% 2-year survival.

EMERGENCY CARDIOPULMONARY BYPASS SUPPORT

Percutaneous cardiopulmonary bypass was originally envisioned as an emergency technique to support patients with hemodynamic collapse or profound hypotherapy.[18] It has continued to be employed in this fashion, generally occurring in the catheterization laboratory, coronary care unit, or emergency room. Overlie et al. collated the national registry experience of the last 4 years, now totaling 210 patients.[13,14] The most frequent clinical situations requiring emergency support have been angioplasty complicated by vessel occlusion, acute myocardial infarction associated with shock, and post–cardiac surgery hemodynamic collapse.[18] The registry's experience underscores the need for prompt initiation of support, as noted above.

CONCLUSION

Percutaneous cardiopulmonary bypass support, initiated prophylactically, in standby fashion or emergently, can be employed in conjunction with high-risk angioplasty. Multicenter experience suggests that only patients with ejection fraction ≤20% clearly benefit from prophylatic support. Lesser morbidity and equally good outcomes are experienced in patients with ejection fractions >20% using standby support. Only 5–10% of the standby patients appear to require any form of circulatory support, although these patients are difficult to predict in advance. With experience, cardiopulmonary bypass can be initiated in the standby situation promptly in almost all cases. The ability to initiate bypass support in the standby circumstance reduces the need for emergency bypass surgery by about two-thirds and procedural mortality by about one-half. Emergency use of bypass support is most successful when initiated in under 20 minutes. The experience to date suggests that high-risk patients are appropriate candidates for coronary angioplasty as they undergo intervention with acceptable morbidity and mortality, improvement in anginal status and ventricular function, and good long-term survival.

REFERENCES

1. Alcan KE, Stertzer SH, Walsh JE, et al: The role of intraaortic balloon counterpulsation in patients undergoing percutaneous transluminal coronary angioplasty. Am Heart J 105:527–530, 1983.
2. Anderson HV, Leimgruber PP, Roubin GS, Gruentzig AR: Distal coronary artery perfusion during percutaneous transluminal coronary angioplasty. Am Heart J 110:720–726, 1985.
3. Bentivoglio LG, Van Raden MJ, Kelsey SF, Detre KM: Percutaneous transluminal coronary angioplasty (PTCA) in patients with relative contraindications: Results of the National Heart, Lung and Blood Institute PTCA Registry. Am J Cardiol 53:82C–88C, 1984.
4. Ellis SG, Topol EJ: Results of percutaneous transluminal angioplasty of high-risk angulated stenosis. Am J Cardiol 66:932–937, 1990.
5. Freedman RJ, Wrenn RC, Gudley ML, et al: Complex multiple percutaneous transluminal coronary angioplasty with vortex hospital setting. Cathet Cardiovasc Diagn 17:237–242, 1989.

6. Hartzler GO, Rutherford BD, McConahay DR, et al: "High-risk" percutaneous transluminal coronary angioplasty. Am J Cardiol 61:33G–36G, 1988.

7. Kahn JK, Rutherford BD, McConahay DR, et al: Supported "high-risk" coronary angioplasty using intraaortic balloon pump counterpulsation. J Am Coll Cardiol 15:1151–1155, 1990.

8. Kohli RS, DiSciascio G, Cowley MJ, et al: Coronary angioplasty in patients with severe ventricular dysfunction. J Am Coll Cardiol 16:807–811, 1990.

9. Lincoff AM, Popma JJ, Ellis SE, et al: Percutaneous support devices for high-risk or complicated coronary angioplasty. J Am Coll Cardiol 17:770–780, 1991.

10. Margolis JR: The role of percutaneous intraaortic balloon in emergency situation following percutaneous transluminal coronary angioplasty. In Kaltenbach M, Gruentzig A, Rentrop P, Bassman W-D (eds): Transluminal Coronary Angioplasty and Intracoronary Thrombolysis. Berlin, Springer-Verlag, 1982, pp 145–150.

11. Morrison DA, Barbierre C, Cohan A, et al: Percutaneous transluminal coronary angioplasty for rest angina pectoris requiring intravenous nitroglycerin and intraaortic balloon counterpulsation. Am J Cardiol 66:168–171, 1990.

12. Muller DWM, Ellis SG, Topol EJ: Atherectomy of the left main coronary artery with percutaneous cardiopulmonary bypass support. Am J Cardiol 64:114–116, 1989.

13. Overlie PA: Emergency use of portable cardiopulmonary bypass. Cathet Cardiovasc Diagn 20:27–31, 1990.

14. Overlie PA, Vogel RA, Shawl FA, et al: Initial and long-term followup in patients treated with emergency cardiopulmonary bypass: The National Registry Experience [abstract]. J Am Coll Cardiol 21:139A, 1993.

15. Pavlides GS, Hauser AM, Stack RK, et al: Effect of peripheral cardiopulmonary bypass on left ventricular size, afterload and myocardial function during elective supported coronary angioplasty. J Am Coll Cardiol 18:499–505, 1991.

16. Phillips SJ, Ballentine B, Slonine D, et al: Percutaneous initiation of cardiopulmonary bypass. Ann Thorac Surg 36:223–225, 1983.

17. Reichman RT, Joyo CI, Dembitsky WP, et al: Improved patient survival after cardiac arrest using a cardiopulmonary support system. Ann Thorac Surg 49:101–105, 1990.

18. Shawl FA, Domanski MJ, Hernandez SP: Emergency percutaneous cardiopulmonary support in cardiogenic shock from acute myocardial infarction. Am J Cardiol 64:967–970, 1989.

19. Shawl FA, Domanski MJ, Wish MH, Davis M: Percutaneous cardiopulmonary bypass support in the catheterization laboratory: Technique and complications. Am Heart J 120:195–203, 1990.

20. Stack RK, Pavlides GS, Miller R, et al: Hemodynamic and metabolic effects of venoarterial cardiopulmonary support in coronary artery disease. Am J Cardiol 67:1344–1348, 1991.

21. Stack RS, Quigley PJ, Collins G, Phillips HR: Perfusion balloon catheter. Am J Cardiol 61:776–806, 1988.

22. Teirstein PS, Vogel RA, Dorros G, et al: Prophylactic versus standby support for high-risk percutaneous transluminal coronary angioplasty. J Am Coll Cardiol 21:590–596, 1993.

23. Tommaso CL: Management of high-risk coronary angioplasty. Am J Cardiol 64:33E–37E, 1989.

24. Tommaso CL: Use of percutaneously inserted cardiopulmonary bypass in the cardiac catheterization laboratory. Cathet Cardiovasc Diagn 20:32–38, 1990.

25. Tommaso CL, Johnson RA, Stafford JL, et al: Supported coronary angioplasty and standby supported coronary angioplasty for high-risk coronary artery disease. Am J Cardiol 66:1255–1257, 1990.

26. Tommaso CL, Vogel JHK, Vogel RA: Coronary angioplasty in high-risk patients with left main coronary stenosis: Results from the National Registry of Elective Supported angioplasty. Cathet Cardiovasc Diagn 25:169–173, 1992.

27. Topol EJ: Emerging strategies for foiled percutaneous transluminal coronary angioplasty. Am J Cardiol 63:249–250, 1989.

28. Turi ZG, Campbell CA, Gottimukkala MV, Kloner RA: Preservation of distal coronary perfusion during prolonged balloon inflation with an autoperfusion angioplasty catheter. Circulation 75:1273–1280, 1987.

29. Vogel RA: Elective supported angioplasty registry: Benefit of prophylactic bypass support in low ejection fraction patients [abstract]. Circulation 86(Suppl I):1–787, 1992.

30. Vogel JHK, Ruiz CE, Jahnke EJ, et al: Percutaneous (nonsurgical) supported angioplasty in unprotected left main disease and severe ventricular dysfunction. Clin Cardiol 12:297–300, 1989.

31. Vogel RA, Shawl F: Long-term followup of patients undergoing cardiopulmonary supported coronary angioplasty: Registry results [abstract]. Circulation 84(Suppl II):II-132, 1991.

32. Vogel RA, Shawl F, Tommaso C, et al: Initial report of the national registry of elective cardiopulmonary bypass supported coronary angioplasty. J Am Coll Cardiol 15:23–29, 1990.

33. Vogel RA, Tommaso CL: Elective supported angioplasty: Initial report of the national registry. Cathet Cardiovasc Diagn 20:22–26, 1990.

34. Vogel R, Tommaso CL, Gundry S: Initial experience with angioplasty and aortic valvuloplasty using elective semipercutaneous cardiopulmonary support. Am J Cardiol 62:811–813, 1988.

BYRON J. ALLEN, MD
MICHAEL A. BRODSKY, MD

MEDICAL MANAGEMENT OF SEVERE CONGESTIVE HEART FAILURE

From the Division of Cardiology
University of California, Irvine
Orange, California

Reprint requests to:
Byron J. Allen, MD
Division of Cardiology
University of California, Irvine
101 The City Drive South
Orange, CA 92668

This chapter focuses on pharmacologic interventions to support the failing heart. Heart failure has been defined traditionally as the inability of the heart to supply blood to peripheral tissues at a level that meets metabolic demands. This discussion assumes that patients have advanced states of cardiac dysfunction and require additional support beyond the usual therapy with oral agents such as digoxin, diuretics, and vasodilators.

APPROACH TO THE PATIENT

The physical examination has long been used in estimating the severity of congestive heart failure. Elevated jugular venous pressure, pulmonary rales, a third heart sound, and peripheral edema often indicate heart failure. The limitation of this approach was recently demonstrated, especially in patients with chronic left ventricular dysfunction. Pulmonary rales, edema, and elevated jugular venous pressure were insensitive predictors of an elevated pulmonary capillary wedge pressure. The sensitivity of all three combined signs was only 58%. However, proportional pulse pressure (systolic-diastolic/systolic pressure) correlated well with cardiac index. A proportional pulse pressure <25% predicted a cardiac index <2.2 L/min/m² with 91% sensitivity and 83% specificity.[19] Subtle signs of inadequate cardiac output, such as cold vasoconstricted extremities, lethargy, confusion, unexplained nausea, and anorexia, should not be ignored. Deterioration in renal function with prerenal azotemia may signal progression to endstage congestive heart failure.

CARDIAC SURGERY: State of the Art Reviews—Vol. 7, No. 2, 1993
Philadelphia, Hanley & Belfus, Inc.

221

Acutely ill patients suspected of having a low cardiac output should have invasive cardiac monitoring with a pulmonary artery catheter. Because patients with severe congestive heart failure often have moderate-to-severe tricuspid insufficiency that leads to inaccurate thermodilution measurements of cardiac output, an alternative method of estimating cardiac output is often useful. Catheters equipped with a fiberoptic port allow continuous measurement of mixed venous oxygen saturation, which correlates well with changes in cardiac output. This technique can be used in evaluating the effectiveness of pharmacologic interventions.

Once the patient is properly instrumented, pharmacologic interventions can be instituted to maximize cardiac output. It is useful to establish hemodynamic goals to tailor medical therapy for the patient with heart failure. Although individualization of therapy is necessary, general guidelines have been proposed to aid in the initial management of congestive heart failure. A pulmonary capillary wedge pressure <15 mmHg, a systemic vascular resistance <1200 dynes/sec/cm^5, and right atrial pressure <8 mmHg, with maintenance of a systolic blood pressure >80 mmHg, have been advocated.[18] The optimal left ventricular filling (pulmonary capillary wedge) pressure must be determined; it cannot be assumed that abnormally high filling pressures will help to maintain cardiac output in patients with heart failure. This may be the case in some patients with acute ischemic syndromes. However, patients with chronic heart failure and a dilated heart often achieve optimal cardiac performance at normal or minimally elevated filling pressures.[20]

Medical therapy of advanced heart failure involves the use of one or a combination of drugs. These can be broadly divided into diuretics, inotropic agents, and vasodilators. Some drugs overlap in the latter two categories. The predominant symptom complex should determine the order and extent of therapy.

PHARMACOLOGY

Diuretics

Table 1 lists the diuretics commonly used to relieve volume overload and congestion in the treatment of congestive heart failure. In general, the most useful agents are the so-called loop diuretics, which act primarily to inhibit an enzyme responsible for pumping chloride across the lining cells of the ascending limb of the loop of Henle. The consequences are excretion of sodium, chloride, potassium, hydrogen, and water. Furosemide is often the drug of choice because it acts rapidly and remains effective despite low glomerular filtration rates. In addition, furosemide promotes venodilation and preload reduction.[2] Ethacrynic acid and bumetanide are also loop diuretics with similar modes of action. Ethacrynic acid requires a larger volume of injectate than furosemide when given intravenously, and no compelling evidence supports anecdotal claims that it is effective in instances in which furosemide fails. Bumetanide is much more potent milligram per milligram than furosemide[1] but has not been shown to be clearly superior. The various loop diuretics share similar metabolic side effects, including hypokalemia, hyponatremia, hypomagnesemia, hypochloremia, and alkalosis.[13] Hyperuricemia may also develop, especially in patients prone to gout.

Combining the various loop diuretics does not achieve greater diuresis.[10] The effectiveness of loop diuretics, however, can be enhanced by the addition of thiazide or thiazidelike diuretics that act in the early distal tubule. Metolazone,

TABLE 1. Diuretics

Agent	Site of Action	Peak Action IV	Peak Action PO	Duration IV	Duration PO	Dose IV	Dose PO
Furosemide	Ascending limb loop of Henle	20–30 min	2 hr	3–4 hr	6 hr	20–320 mg	20–320 mg/day
Ethacrynic acid	Ascending limb loop of Henle	5–30 min	2 hr	3–4 hr	8 hr	25–100 mg	25–200 mg/day
Bumetanide	Ascending limb loop of Henle	20–30 min	1.5 hr	3–4 hr	6 hr	1–4 mg	1–10 mg/day
Metolazone	Early distal tubule		1.5–3 hr		12–24 hr		2.5–10 mg/day
Spironolactone	Late distal tubule		2–4 hr		8–12 hr		50–100 mg/day
Triamterene	Late distal tubule		2–4 hr		8–12 hr		25–200 mg/day

IV = intravenously; PO = orally.

which has been used extensively for this purpose, is the current agent of choice because it maintains its effect even in patients with reduced renal function.[6]

Hypokalemia is a frequent and potentially severe side effect of loop diuretics, especially in combination with metolazone. High doses of potassium supplement may be required; however, high-dose potassium is often poorly tolerated. An alternative is to administer a potassium-sparing diuretic. Triamterene, spironolactone, and amiloride are the commonly used drugs in this category. Triamterene has minimal side effects and is generally well tolerated. However, danger of developing hyperkalemia in patients with very low cardiac outputs is significant, especially when the drugs are given concomitantly with angiotensin-converting enzyme inhibitors; in this setting, the patient's serum potassium must be monitored compulsively.

Vasodilators

Primary vasodilators may be useful in patients with low cardiac output and high systemic vascular resistance (Table 2). Intravenous nitrates are the most commonly used drugs in this category. Nitroprusside is often effective in providing rapid, easily titratable vasodilatation.[14] It affects primarily the systemic arterioles, providing a profound reduction in systemic vascular resistance. Nitroprusside also has a lesser effect on venodilation and thus lowers left ventricular filling pressures. However, nitroprusside may worsen regional myocardial ischemia because it primarily affects vessels with small resistance. This effect may lead to a fall in perfusion pressure in ischemic zones and thus to reduced perfusion.[3] Nitroprusside should be used cautiously, therefore, in patients with uncorrected ischemia.

Nitroprusside should be instituted at low doses in patients with low systemic blood pressure (<110 mmHg). Its use is limited by the potential for cyanide toxicity that may manifest as lactic acidosis. Nitroprusside is converted to cyanmethemoglobin and cyanide. The cyanide is metabolized to thiocyanate by the liver and excreted by the kidneys. The problem can be assessed by monitoring blood levels of thiocyanate, but this is often impractical. Toxicity can best be avoided by limiting the duration of therapy to <72 hours.

Nitroglycerin is predominantly a venodilator. Its ability to dilate epicardial coronary arteries may ameliorate coronary ischemia. It also dilates coronary

TABLE 2. Intravenous Vasodilators and Inotropes

Drug	Concentration	Dose	Predominant Effect
Nitroglycerin	50 mg/250 cc	0.5–7 μg/kg/min	Venodilatation
Nitroprusside	50 mg/250 cc	0.5–7 μg/kg/min	Arterial dilatation
Dobutamine	500 mg/500 cc	2.5–20 μg/kg/min	Positive inotrope
Amrinone	500 mg/500 cc	5–15 μg/kg/min	Positive inotrope
Dopamine	400 mg/500 cc	2–4 μg/kg/min	Increased renal blood flow
		4–6 μg/kg/min	Beta agonist
		>10 μg/kg/min	Alpha agonist
Epinephrine	4 mg/250 cc	2–20 μg/min	Positive inotrope
Norepinephrine	4 mg/250 cc	2–20 μg/min	Vasoconstrictor

collateral vessels and improves regional myocardial ischemia. Nitroglycerin may be preferable to nitroprusside, or added to it, in cases with a significant ischemic component to cardiac dysfunction. Because it is a potent venodilator, it can rapidly lower left ventricular filling pressure in patients who are acutely decompensated. Because nitroglycerin is a less potent and less effective peripheral vasodilator than nitroprusside, it is often ineffective as solitary therapy in patients with severe hypertension, but it can be combined with other vasodilators. Nitroglycerin is poorly tolerated in patients with hypotension or borderline hypotension. Its use is generally inadvisable in the presence of a systolic blood pressure <90 mmHg.

Vasodilators/Inotropes (Table 2)

Dobutamine. Dobutamine is a synthetic catecholamine that directly stimulates beta-1, beta-2, and alpha receptors. It has direct inotropic effects that do not require the release of myocardial norepinephrine. Its effects are maintained in the catecholamine-depleted heart, and dobutamine also produces vasodilatation that reduces systemic vascular resistance and filling pressures. It has modest positive chronotropic properties and a small potential to increase arrhythmias.[17,22] In modest doses (2.5–5.0 μg/kg/min) it is generally well tolerated without increasing ischemia or arrhythmias. Dobutamine may be effective in patients who are not candidates for nitrate therapy because of hypotension or marginal blood pressure. It often has an adjunctive effect in patients already receiving nitrates. On occasion, high doses (up to 40 μg/kg/min) are required to achieve the desired effects on cardiac output and filling pressures. High-dose dobutamine often causes significant tachycardia and may increase myocardial oxygen demand out of proportion to supply, thus worsening ischemia and arrhythmias. In these instances, it is preferable to lower the dose of dobutamine and use combination therapy with an agent such as amrinone.[7,21]

Amrinone. Amrinone, a phosphodiesterase inhibitor with vasodilatory and inotropic properties, is well suited for use in congestive heart failure.[11] However, it has a relatively long half-life that makes it difficult to titrate. When side effects occur, their duration may be extensive compared with short-acting agents such as dobutamine. As a result, dobutamine is more commonly used than amrinone. Despite these reservations, amrinone is useful in patients with severe congestive heart failure. It lowers systemic and pulmonary vascular resistance and pulmonary capillary wedge pressure as well as increases cardiac output through a vasodilatory effect and a direct inotropic effect. The major side effects are thrombocytopenia and exacerbation of arrhythmias. Thrombocytopenia is rare with <72 hours of therapy. In our experience, however, it is common with prolonged infusions.

Thrombocytopenia is generally mild and reversible if amrinone therapy is terminated. Amrinone has been shown to have additive effects when combined with dobutamine and may be used most effectively when the doses of both drugs can be titrated downward in combination as opposed to solitary therapy.

Vasopressors/Inotropes (Table 2)

Dopamine. Dopamine, a catecholaminelike drug, is the immediate precursor to norepinephrine and causes release of norepinephrine from cardiac stores. Dopamine exerts its effects by stimulation of dopaminergic, beta-adrenergic, and alpha-adrenergic receptors. Ultimately it exerts its positive effect in congestive heart failure by stimulation of adenylate cyclase activity, thus elevating levels of cyclic adenosine monophosphate and leading to increased inotropy and vasodilatation. Dopamine also modulates release of norepinephrine by stimulation of dopamine receptors.

Dopamine's effects are dose-dependent.[8] In low doses (2–4 µg/kg/min) the predominant effect is stimulation of dopamine receptors in the renal and mesenteric beds, which leads to increased renal blood flow and a net fall in systemic vascular resistance. In increasing doses the predominant clinical effect is mediated by stimulation of beta receptors; an increase in heart rate and inotropic state leads to increased cardiac output and often an increase in blood pressure. Alpha-receptor effects occur at high doses and predominate at infusion rates ≥20 µg/kg/min. Significant increases in blood pressure can be obtained at high infusion rates, but often at the expense of constriction of the renal vascular bed and a fall in renal blood flow and urine output.

Epinephrine. Epinephrine is a potent stimulator of alpha- and beta-adrenergic receptors. It increases heart rate and blood pressure as well as pulmonary and systemic vascular resistance. It may worsen arrhythmias and ischemia and markedly diminish renal blood flow and urine output. Its use in congestive heart failure should be reserved for patients refractory to other agents. Duration of therapy should be limited to the minimal time necessary for stabilization.

Vasopressor Agents (Table 2)

Norepinephrine. Norepinephrine, a naturally occurring catecholamine, is the principal neurotransmitter released from sympathetic nerve endings. The predominant clinical effect of intravenous norepinephrine is to stimulate alpha-adrenergic receptors to promote peripheral vasoconstriction. To a lesser degree it is a beta-1 agonist, producing both a positive inotropic and a positive chronotropic effect. It causes an increase in blood pressure that may lead to reflex changes in vagal tone and thus mitigate the positive chronotropic effect of beta-1 stimulation. The adverse consequences of vasoconstriction (increased afterload) can be overcome by concomitant administration of phentolamine, an alpha-receptor antagonist. This combination has been used in patients with low-output states associated with low systemic vascular resistance after cardiopulmonary bypass.[9,12] Low-dose dopamine (4 µg/kg/min) has also been shown to preserve renal blood flow and renal function during therapy with norepinephrine.[16]

TRANSITION FROM INTRAVENOUS TO ORAL THERAPY

Institution of long-term oral therapy generally begins as patients are weaned from intravenous drugs. Digoxin should be administered to patients with depressed systolic function, and diuretic therapy should be adjusted to maintain optimal filling pressures. Oral vasodilators should be initiated in low doses and titrated upward to tolerance. In severely ill patients this process may require several days to several weeks.

Current data suggest that long-term survival of patients with severe heart failure can be enhanced by drug regimens using vasodilator therapy. These studies have been conducted in patients generally receiving diuretic and digoxin therapy. The first study demonstrating an unequivocal increase in survival of patients with severe heart failure was the Veterans Cooperative Study, which combined hydralazine and isosorbide dinitrate. This therapy resulted in a 38%, 25%, and 23% reduction in 1-, 2-, and 3-year mortality rates, respectively.[4]

However, the incidence of intolerance to this combination is relatively high. Consequently, angiotensin-converting enzyme inhibitors are currently the drugs of choice for afterload reduction and oral vasodilator therapy. These drugs increase cardiac output and decrease pulmonary and systemic vascular resistance with only a modest decrease in systemic arterial pressure. Controlled trials have shown that therapy with angiotensin-converting enzyme inhibitors improves survival of patients with heart failure. The Cooperative North Scandinavian Enalapril Survival Study (CONSENSUS) reported a decrease of 31% in 1-year mortality for patients with congestive failure.[5] Captopril has also been shown to reduce the mortality of patients with varying degrees of heart failure. In another trial, captopril-treated patients had a better survival rate than patients treated with hydralazine (without nitrates) as vasodilator therapy.[15]

REFERENCES

1. Asbury MJ, Gatenby PBB, O'Sullivan S, Bourke E: Bumetanide: Potent new "loop" diuretic. BMJ 1:211–213, 1972.
2. Biddle TL, Yu PN: Effect of furosemide on hemodynamics and lung water in acute pulmonary edema secondary to myocardial infarction. Am J Cardiol 43:86–90, 1979.
3. Chiariello M, Gold HK, Leinbach RC, et al: Comparison between the effects of nitroprusside and nitroglycerin on ischemic injury during acute myocardial infarction. Circulation 54:766–733, 1976.
4. Cohn JN, Archibald DG, Ziesche S, et al: Effect of vasodilator therapy on mortality in chronic congestive heart failure: Results of a Veterans Administration Cooperative Study. N Engl J Med 314:1547–1552, 1986.
5. CONSENSUS Trial Study Group: Effects of enalapril on mortality in severe congestive heart failure. Results of the Cooperative North Scandinavian Enalapril Survival Study (CONSENSUS). N Engl J Med 316:1429–1435, 1987.
6. Dargie HJ, Allison MEM, Kennedy AC, Gray MJB: High dosage metolazone in chronic renal failure. BMJ 4:196–198, 1972.
7. Gage J, Rutman H, Lucido D, LeJemtel TH: Additive effect of dobutamine and amrinone on myocardial contractility and ventricular performance in patients with severe heart failure. Circulation 74:367–373, 1986.
8. Goldberg LI, Rajfer SI: Dopamine receptors: Applications in clinical cardiology. Circulation 72:245–248, 1985.
9. Gray R, Shah PK, Singh B, et al: Low cardiac output states after open heart surgery. Chest 80:16–22, 1981.
10. Hook JB, Williamson HE: Addition of the saluretic action of furosemide to the saluretic action of certain other agents. J Pharmacol Exp Ther 148:88–93, 1965.
11. LeJemtel TH, Keung E, Sonnenblick EH, et al: Amrinone: A new nonglycosidic, nonadrenergic cardiotonic agent effective in the treatment of intractable myocardial failure in man. Circulation 59:1098–1104, 1979.
12. Lemmer JH, Botham MJ, McKenney P, et al: Norepinephrine plus phentolamine improves regional blood flow during experimental low cardaic output syndrome. Ann Thorac Surg 38:108–116, 1984.

13. Lowe J, Gray J, Henry DA, Lawson DH: Adverse reactions to furosemide in hospital patients. BMJ 2:360–362, 1979.
14. Miller RR, Vismara LA, Zelis R, et al: Clinical use of sodium nitroprusside in chronic ischemic heart disease: Effects on peripheral vascular resistance and venous tone and on ventricular volume, pump and mechanical performance. Circulation 50:328–336, 1975.
15. Newman TJ, Maskin CS, Dennick LG, et al: Effects of captopril on survival in patients with heart failure. Am J Med 84(Suppl 3A):140–144, 1988.   .
16. Schaer GL, Fink MP, Pqarrillo JE: Norepinephrine alone versus norepinephrine plus low-dose dopamine: Enhanced renal blood flow with combination pressor therapy. Crit Care Med 13:492–496, 1985.
17. Sonnenblick EH, Frishman WH, LeJemtel TH: Dobutamine: A new synthetic cardioactive sympathetic amine. N Engl J Med 300:17–22, 1979.
18. Stevenson LW, Dracup KA, Tillisch JH: Efficacy of medical therapy tailored for severe congestive heart failure in patients transferred for urgent cardiac transplantation. Am J Cardiol 3:461–464, 1989.
19. Stevenson LW, Perloff JK: The limited reliability of physical signs for estimating hemodynamics in chronic heart failure. JAMA 261:884–888, 1989.
20. Stevenson LW, Tillisch JH: Maintenance of cardiac output with normal filling pressures in dilated heart failure. Circulation 74:1303–1308, 1986.
21. Sundram P, Reddy HK, McElroy P, et al: Myocardial energetics and efficiency in patients with idiopathic cardiomyopathy: Response to dobutamine and amrinone. Am Heart J 119:891–898, 1990.
22. Vatner SF, McRitchie RJ, Braunwald E: Effects of dobutamine on left ventricular performance, coronary dynamics, and distribution of cardiac output in conscious dogs. J Clin Invest 53:1265–1273, 1974.

D. GLENN PENNINGTON, MD
MARC T. SWARTZ

PATIENT SELECTION FOR MECHANICAL CIRCULATORY SUPPORT

From the Department of Surgery
St. Louis University Medical
　Center
St. Louis, Missouri

Reprint requests to:
D. Glenn Pennington, MD
Department of Surgery
St. Louis University Medical
　Center
3635 Vista Ave. at Grand Blvd.
P.O. Box 15250
St. Louis, MO 63110-0250

Over the last decade, considerable progress has been made in mechanical circulatory support,[26,27] with significant advances in device technology as well as patient management. Concurrently, criteria for patient selection have been refined. However, identification of the ideal patient group continues to elude clinicians. Although some predictors of survival have been identified before device placement, patient populations have been small and selection protocols have not been tightly controlled. Investigational protocols and historical criteria have been used as guidelines, but in most instances the decision to initiate mechanical circulatory support has been based on limited objective criteria and clinical impressions. The clinician's decision to initiate mechanical circulatory support has been hampered by several factors, including the inability to determine whether irreversible major organ damage has occurred, the uncertainty of whether mechanical circulatory support is superior to conventional therapy, and the necessity to commit a large amount of resources with no assurance of a favorable outcome. Clearly, some rapidly deteriorating patients have the potential to benefit from mechanical circulatory support. However, a larger group of patients with marginal hemodynamics in spite of what appears to be optimal conventional therapy present the clinician with the most difficult decisions.

This chapter discusses criteria for patient selection in each of the major patient groups: postcardiotomy support, bridge to transplant,

CARDIAC SURGERY: State of the Art Reviews—Vol. 7, No. 2, 1993
Philadelphia, Hanley & Belfus, Inc.

229

and acute deterioration. Information in this chapter was derived from our clinical experience, a literature review, device manufacturers, and data from the Combined Registry of the American Society of Artificial Internal Organs (ASAIO)–International Society of Heart and Lung Transplantation (ISHLT) for the clinical use of mechanical ventricular assist devices (VAD) and total artificial hearts (TAH) maintained at Pennsylvania State University.

POSTCARDIOTOMY SUPPORT

Despite improvements in surgical techniques, technology, and myocardial preservation, postoperative cardiogenic shock requiring intraaortic balloon pump (IABP) support continues to occur in 1–10% of patients undergoing cardiac surgical procedures.[1,2,5,15,17] Published survival rates in these IABP patients range from 45–65%.[1,2,5,15,17] The reported incidence of postoperative patients requiring VAD support is 0.1–0.8%, with survival rates ranging from 29–50% in the larger series,[6,7,19,21] but the overall survival rate of the VAD population is 23%.[11] Most patients who develop postcardiotomy cardiogenic shock are treated only with conventional therapy, including drugs and IABP, and the survival rates of 45–65% in patients receiving operative or postoperative IABP support have improved little over the last decade. Thus one might conclude that postoperative VAD support should be pursued more vigorously.

The hemodynamic criteria used to evaluate a patient's candidacy for postcardiotomy VAD support are derived from the studies of Norman and associates.[17] These criteria include a cardiac index <1.8 L/min/m^2, systemic vascular resistance $>2,100$ dynes/sec/cm^5, systolic arterial blood pressure <90 mmHg, left and/or right atrial pressures >20 mmHg, and urine output <20 ml/hr, despite the use of maximal pharmacologic and IABP support. Although these criteria are more than 15 years old, they are in many ways still applicable for postcardiotomy patients. However, these exact hemodynamic criteria should not be rigidly applied and should not be the only factors determining VAD placement. Other factors to be considered are the previous medical history, the amount of pharmacologic support necessary to wean from cardiopulmonary bypass (CPB), and factors such as those listed in Table 1. Some of the risk factors in Table 1 have been shown to influence survival in retrospective studies; others have been traditionally held to be true.[11,18,20,23]

In some patients, the intended cardiac procedure may have been unsuccessful. Patients with unsuccessful operations who cannot be weaned from CPB should be excluded from temporary VAD support unless they are candidates for cardiac transplantation. Patients suffering acute myocardial infarctions within 24–48 hours of operation have a reduced chance of cardiac recovery.[18,20] Intraoperative myocardial infarction is difficult to diagnose in the operating room, but it is often diagnosed preoperatively.

TABLE 1. Risk Factors to Evaluate Before VAD Insertion (After CPB)

Unsuccessful operation
Preoperative or intraoperative myocardial infarction
Biventricular failure
Multiple previous infarctions or history of congestive heart failure
Physiologic age
Uncontrollable bleeding while on cardiopulmonary bypass
Cardiac surgical procedure within 10 days

In some cases, it may be possible to determine whether left, right, or biventricular failure is present before placement of the assist device. This can be accomplished by visual inspection of the heart and measurements of the left and right atrial pressures. With CPB temporarily discontinued, the atrium with the highest pressure usually indicates the ventricle with the worst failure. If both the left and right atrial pressures are elevated, biventricular failure is usually present. This determination is important because biventricular failure decreases the opportunity for myocardial recovery.[18,23] Many patients who initially appear to have univentricular failure develop biventricular failure after placement of a single device. If biventricular failure is present, biventricular support may improve the patient's chances for survival; however, in the registry, the survival rate for patients requiring biventricular assist devices (BVAD) is lower than that for patients with right ventricular assist devices (RVAD) or left ventricular assist devices (LVAD) (Table 2). These differences in survival rates are related to the degree and extent of ventricular damage rather than to technical problems associated with biventricular support.[24]

Another important predevice risk factor is age. Advanced age is probably the most common criterion used to exclude patients from mechanical circulatory support. From the registry data, the overall survival rate for patients less than 59 years of age requiring postoperative VAD support was 34%, whereas patients older than 70 years had a survival rate of only 10%.[11] A recent report suggests that if patients are carefully selected, age over 65 years may not be such a critical predictor of survival.[34] From these data, one might conclude that physiologic age is more important than chronologic age. Physiologic age is an extremely important factor to evaluate because the mean age of patients undergoing cardiac surgical procedures has increased significantly over the last decade.[16]

Traditionally it has been thought that intraoperative bleeding so intense that adequate systemic perfusion cannot be maintained on CPB is a relative contraindication to VAD placement. Placement of some devices, especially those in which the heparin can be reversed, may lead to less bleeding. However, patients continue to die in the operating room from bleeding complications associated with coagulopathies or technical problems related to VAD implantation.

A recent review of 68 patients who received Thoratec VADs (Thoratec Laboratories Corporation, Berkeley, CA) at St. Louis University showed that 10 of 68 died in the operating room, 8 from a combination of bleeding and biventricular failure and 2 from bleeding from left atrial tears. Eight of these operating room deaths occurred in our first 2 years of using the Thoratec VAD, whereas only 2 occurred in our last 8 years. Analysis of the remaining 58 patients showed that 30/58 (52%) had significant bleeding (>1500 cc/m^2 chest drainage during the first 24 postoperative hours and/or reoperation). However, there was no difference in

TABLE 2. Postcardiotomy Results Based on Type of Support*

Type of Support	No. of Patients	Weaned	Discharged
LVAD	349	167 (47.9%)	95 (27.2%)
RVAD	86	33 (38.4%)	20 (23.3%)
BVAD	226	82 (36.3%)	37 (16.4%)[†]
Total	661	282 (42.7%)	152 (23.0%)

* ASAIO-ISHLT Registry.
[†] p = 0.003 by chi-square on discharge; BVAD vs. LVAD
LVAD = left ventricular assist device, RVAD = right ventricular assist device, BVAD = biventricular assist device.

TABLE 3. Incidence of Complications versus Survival in Postcardiotomy Patients*

Complication	Survived (%) (n = 152)	Died (%) (n = 509)	Level of Significance[†]
Bleeding	43	40	NS
Renal failure	14	38	p < 0.0001
Biventricular failure	12	31	p < 0.0001
Respiratory failure	12	21	p < 0.0156
Infection	16	12	NS
Neurologic	7	13	NS
Thrombosis/embolus	9	13	NS

* ASAIO-ISHLT Registry.
[†] Chi square.
NS = not significant.

chest tube drainage, number of units of packed red blood cells or units of fresh frozen plasma transfused between survivors and nonsurvivors. These data suggest that bleeding remains a major complication, but its effect on overall survival is less than previously thought. When analyzing subpopulations of patients, bleeding is a determinant of survival in the bridge-to-transplantation group, but not in the postcardiotomy group. This is true for the St. Louis University experience and for data from the ASAIO-ISHLT Registry (Tables 3 and 4).

In patients who cannot be weaned from CPB with conventional therapy, the decision of whether or not to insert the VAD is not so problematic. If a VAD is not used, the patient will die in the operating room. If supported, most patients can be returned to the intensive care unit and have a 20–45% chance of survival. In these cases, the clinician must evaluate the risk/benefit ratio for reach particular patient. Factors such as the likelihood of long-term survival and the degree of functional status have to be evaluated. Some thought must be given as to whether or not the patient would wish the therapy to be undertaken. Concerned family members usually choose any opportunity for survival versus death, no matter what the cost. The way the physician presents the options to the patient and/or family can greatly influence their decision. At St. Louis University we have tried to be as objective as possible when talking with patients and families. In fact, we often emphasize the negative aspects in discussing the decision to initiate mechanical circulatory support and in describing potential complications. Despite this approach, only 1 of more than 130 adult patients or families at St. Louis University refused to participate.

The decision to place a VAD is less clear in patients who can be weaned from CPB but require large amounts of pharmacologic support and an IABP. Many of

TABLE 4. Complications of Bridge to Transplantation* (n = 216)

Complication	Survivors (n = 106)	Nonsurvivors (n = 110)	Level of Significance[†]
Bleeding	29 (27%)	61 (55%)	p < 0.0001
Renal failure	3 (3%)	42 (38%)	p < 0.0001
Infection	15 (14%)	32 (29%)	p < 0.05
Thrombosis/embolus	8 (8%)	11 (10%)	NS

* ASAIO-ISHLT Registry.
[†] Chi square.
NS = not significant.

these patients are returned to the intensive care unit only to detriorate later. Many develop multiorgan failure and die several days or weeks after operation. At our institution, the survival rate in patients who could not be weaned from CPB and had VADs inserted at the time of operation is 44%. This contrasts with the 14% survival rate of patients who required VADs within 6 hours to 10 days of the initial operation. Delays in the decision to provide adequate support often lead to longer periods of hypoperfusion and multiorgan failure.

Other factors have been traditionally thought to influence survival. Intraoperative ventricular arrhythmias are negative prognostic indicators if a stable rhythm cannot be maintained. However, intermittent episodes of ventricular tachycardia or fibrillation before device insertion do not influence survival.[14] Patients with controlled bacterial endocarditis (sterile blood cultures) preoperatively should be considered reasonable candidates for mechanical circulatory support. Patients in both the postcardiotomy and bridge-to-transplant populations have been successfully supported during and after episodes of bacteremia,[10,21] particularly if the duration of support is short. Historically patients having reoperations have been thought to have a decreased chance of survival, and in some clinical trials, patients undergoing cardiac reoperations were excluded from VAD implantation. The most reliable information on reoperative patients requiring postcardiotomy VAD support comes from the Thoratec clinical trials. These data show that 16 of 79 (20.2%) patients survived VAD support after their first cardiac operation, whereas 5 of 23 (21.7%) reoperative patients survived. At St. Louis University we have inserted VADs in 5 postcardiotomy patients after reoperation, with 1 survivor. From these small groups, reoperation does not appear to be a contraindication to VAD support.

The exclusion criteria developed for the 1981 clinical trial of the National Heart, Lung and Blood Institute to evaluate temporary VADs are listed in Table 5. Because most cardiac surgical procedures are performed electively, it is unlikely that many of the potential VAD patients would suffer from any of these disorders. Some patients undergoing emergency cardiac procedures have developed renal or hepatic dysfunction, coagulopathy, or severe infectious complications preoperatively. In these cases, the cardiac procedure is rescue therapy. If these patients cannot be weaned from CPB or if they deteriorate shortly after arrival in the intensive care unit, placement of a mechanical circulatory support device may reverse the acute hemodynamic deterioration. However, the reversal of major organ dysfunction is highly unlikely, and their survival rate is expected to be very low.

A large study describing a multivariate analysis of preoperative risk factors in postcardiotomy patients has yet to be performed. Such a study might answer some of the questions presently facing clinicians. Unless more usable risk factors can be

---

TABLE 5.   Traditional Exclusion Criteria for Mechanical Circulatory Support

Renal failure (BUN > 100 mg/dl, creatinine > 5)
Severe peripheral vascular disease
Symptomatic cerebrovascular disease
Cancer with metastasis
Severe hepatic disease
Coagulopathy
Severe infections resistant to therapy
History of congestive heart failure or multiple myocardial infarctions
   (unless transplant candidate)

identified, overall survival rates are unlikely to improve. In this scenario, post-operative mechanical circulatory support will continue to be used only in times of desperation and will never achieve the status of a reasonable therapeutic option.

BRIDGE TO TRANSPLANTATION

The selection criteria to determine candidates for bridging to transplantation are quite different from the criteria used in evaluating postcardiotomy and acute deterioration patients. Many bridge-to-transplant candidates are reasonably stable and not undergoing CPB at the time the decision to implement prolonged circulatory support is made. Because the adverse effects of CPB are not a consideration, a rapid decision is not mandatory (as is so often the case in postcardiotomy patients.) Many bridge-to-transplant candidates can be stabilized with IABP and pharmacologic support. Although some may progressively deteriorate, their condition is usually stable enough to allow a thorough evaluation. Patients who have been previously evaluated and accepted for cardiac transplantation are often the best candidates. In this group, the medical and psychosocial histories are well known to the physicians caring for the patient as well as to those evaluating the candidate for mechanical circulatory support. The hemodynamic criteria to determine candidacy for device insertion in postcardiotomy patients were developed during the mid 1970s[17] for patients with cardiogenic shock immediately after or within 24 hours of cardiac surgery. Device manufacturers and clinicians used these same criteria in preparing protocols for the bridge-to-transplant studies, but the criteria have not been uniformly appropriate. Since the initial protocols were developed, a great deal has been learned concerning patient selection for bridge to transplantation. Because myocardial recovery is not the issue, the question becomes how long the patient can be effectively maintained with conventional therapy while waiting for a donor heart. Cardiac transplantation continues to increase in popularity, and the time required to locate donor hearts is also increasing. Waiting periods of weeks or months are now the general rule, even for patients in the most urgent category. Therefore the crucial decision of when to implant circulatory support devices is confounded by many unknowns: How long will it take to locate a donor heart? Is the organ dysfunction already present reversible? Is mechanical circulatory support superior to conventional therapy in this patient? Determination of when a donor heart will become available for a particular patient is impossible. The reversibility of major organ dysfunction requires further investigation; however, limits of reversibility are beginning to be defined. A recent study from St. Louis University showed that bridging to cardiac transplantation with VADs is superior to conventional therapy in status 1 (urgent need) patients.[30]

In our experience at St. Louis University, some patients initially rejected as candidates for bridging to transplantation because they were hemodynamically stable later developed complications that excluded them from mechanical circulatory support or cardiac transplantation.[31] Based on these results, we concluded that hemodynamic stability alone should not exclude patients from mechanical assistance. The amount of pharmacologic, respiratory, and IABP support necessary to maintain stability must be considered. If these supportive measures cannot be reduced within 24–48 hours, mechanical support with a more sophisticated device should be considered. Patients have been successfully supported with IABPs and drugs for several weeks prior to transplantation. Today, however, this may not be an adequate length of time to locate a donor heart. It is our preference to insert a more sophisticated device that provides adequate cardiac output without the need for inotropic support. In this case, patients may have all intravenous lines removed, take oral medications, and begin regular ambulation and exercises.

Some bridge-to-transplant candidates are so unstable that they require immediate implantation of an assist device. These patients may be at a higher risk of developing complications than the hemodynamically stable patient in whom device implantation can be performed under more controlled conditions. Several criteria exclude patients from mechanical circulatory support prior to cardiac transplantation: (1) unresolved pulmonary emboli; (2) renal failure requiring dialysis; (3) recent unresolved cerebrovascular accident; (4) unacceptable psychosocial history; and (5) severe bleeding. At the time of device insertion, it is not absolutely essential that patients meet all the transplantation criteria. Complications such as acute renal insufficiency, infection, and hypoxia can sometimes be better treated if the patients receive circulatory support, with the hope of converting the patient from a nontransplant to a transplant candidate. Unfortunately, in some patients, the complications worsen after support is initiated.

Most of the patients at St. Louis University who were refused mechanical support prior to cardiac transplantation were rejected on the basis of infection or renal failure. Infection is a major concern because placement of a large amount of prosthetic material may worsen the infectious process.[4] In addition, the immuno-suppressive drugs used after transplantation may reactivate or accentuate the infection. The potential need for invasive monitoring lines over a prolonged period may also play a role in the development of infection. However, some patients with predevice infectious complications have responded well to antibiotics after VAD placement and restoration of adequate perfusion. Patients with superficial infections, urinary tract infections, or mild pneumonia with low-grade fever and minimal elevation in white blood cell count should be considered as reasonable candidates for mechanical circulatory support. However, patients who have a combination of renal and infectious complications before device insertion are at increased risk. Those with uncontrolled sepsis or symptomatic bacteremia should be excluded.

Predevice renal insufficiency is the single most important exclusion criterion at St. Louis University.[8] In our experience, a predevice serum creatinine ≥ 2.5 mg/dl is highly predictive of postdevice renal failure and death. For this reason, we exclude patients who have an acute increase in creatinine above 2.5 mg/dl with a decrease in urine output and increased resistance to diuretic therapy. Patients who have had multiple episodes of renal insufficiency manifested by elevated creatinines that return to normal should be considered. Unfortunately, in many instances renal failure worsens after VAD implantation. CPB, bleeding, and infectious complications can influence the reversibility of predevice renal insufficiency.

Some centers have avoided the use of VADs as bridges to transplantation in patients who have had previous cardiac surgery because of the increased risk of infection, the fear of additional myocardial damage due to injury to a patent bypass graft, and the potential development of circulating antibodies. Our experience has shown that a history of previous transfusions may lead to the development of circulating antibodies. However, if clinicians and patients are willing to commit to a long duration of support (3 months–1 year), it may be possible to find a compatible heart. At St. Louis University, we have not noted higher infection rates in patients who have previously undergone cardiac surgery and have not encountered a problem with injury to bypass grafts at the time of VAD insertion.[9]

Other factors that can be evaluated before device placement, such as the number of days hospitalized, number of days requiring inotropic support, and whether or not an IABP is necessary, have not been shown to be useful. Similarly, predevice hemodynamic parameters, such as cardiac index, right atrial pressure, and pulmonary capillary wedge pressure, are not predictors of survival in our experience.[31]

The most commonly reported complications of patients receiving devices as bridges to transplant are shown in Table 4.[12] The presence of biventricular failure is not as important a predictor of survival in the bridge-to-transplant population as it is in post-CPB patients as long as biventricular support is supplied, because myocardial recovery is not necessary for survival. If the type of ventricular failure is correctly supported, the result in the bridge-to-transplant population should be similar, whether the patient has univentricular or biventricular failure. Renal failure requiring dialysis has been highly predictive of nonsurvival in assist device populations at St. Louis University and in the ASAIO/ISHLT Registry. Pretransplant infections must be carefully evaluated to determine their potential to affect outcome. If all of these factors, bleeding, renal failure, and infection are evaluated thoroughly before device placement, many implant complications that preclude patients from cardiac transplantation could be avoided by limiting the entry criteria.

In most series, at least 50% of patients have been successfully stabilized with mechanical circulatory support and have undergone subsequently successful transplantation. The remainder of patients in whom bridging was attempted have deteriorated after device placement or have initially improved and then suffered multiple complications that precluded transplantation. Almost all of these patients have died. The scarcity of donor hearts makes it imperative that only the best candidates for mechanical circulatory support be selected in order to optimize the distribution of a limited resource and to avoid the unpleasant task of denying high-risk patients cardiac transplantation.

ACUTE DETERIORATION

Patients who develop acute cardiogenic shock or cardiac arrest may benefit from temporary circulatory support. These patients may already be in the hospital or may arrive in the emergency department, intensive care unit, or cardiac catheterization laboratory with acute myocardial injuries and cardiogenic shock. Many such patients have not had a previous evaluation of cardiac function and present in varying states of deterioration in which conventional resuscitative techniques, such as pharmacologic therapy and IABPs, are ineffective. These patients may be resuscitated by placement of femorofemoral extracorporeal membrane oxygenation (ECMO). Once stabilized, cardiac catheterization, echocardiograms, and nuclear multigated acquisition scans can be obtained while the patient continues on circulatory support. Although registry information is being compiled, few pre-ECMO predictors of survival have been identified. The past medical history may or may not be available. Only patients with witnessed cardiac arrest who have been effectively perfused during the period of resuscitation should be considered for ECMO. Certainly patients who have had multiple myocardial infarctions and/or a history of congestive heart failure are considered at high risk unless they are candidates for cardiac transplantation. Advanced age is an additional risk factor. Long periods of conventional resuscitation or preexisting complications such as infection, renal failure, or coagulopathy also limit survival. In this group, it is critically important that the patients be supported as soon as possible. Thus a rapid decision must be made concerning eligibility. Patients undergoing elective procedures such as coronary angioplasty or cardiac catheterization should be supported. Patients who have undergone elective cardiac surgical repair and deteriorate in the intensive care unit should also be supported. Patients receiving this therapy include those with postcardiotomy cardiogenic shock while in the intensive care unit, failed percutaneous transluminal coronary angioplasty (PTCA), myocardial infarction and cardiogenic shock, massive pulmonary embolus, deterioration after cardiac transplantation, cardiomyopathy and acute shock, aortic stenosis, hypothermia, traumatic injury, and refractory ventricular fibrillation.[13,28,29,32] The survival rate is best in those who have failed PTCAs and undergo surgical revascularization after a brief period of stabilization with ECMO. Patients who have suffered large myocardial insults and are not candidates for cardiac transplant and patients who undergo conventional cardiopulmonary resuscitation for extended periods have the least chance of survival.

DISCUSSION

Objective guidelines for choosing the optimal candidate for mechanical circulatory support are not well developed. The clinician is frequently confronted with the difficult decisions of whether the potential recipient may still respond favorably to conventional therapy and therefore "is not ill enough to require the device" or whether the patient is so far advanced that irreversible organ dysfunction precludes a good result and is "too ill to receive the device." In general, clinical investigators have erred on the side of using devices in patients in the latter category, particularly in the postcardiotomy group. Much of the difficulty in this group of patients centers on the difficult determination of reversibility of organ dysfunction. Pulmonary, renal, hepatic, and cerebral insufficiency must be carefully assessed and decisions made as to whether each organ can regain normal function if adequate blood flow is reestablished. Moreover, the question of the potential for myocardial recovery is a challenge in the postcardiotomy group, particularly if the patient is a possible transplant candidate. If the patient is supported with a device that can provide extended perfusion (beyond 1 month), myocardial recovery can be evaluated over a period of several weeks; if recovery is not apparent, transplantation may be the only option. Approximately 50% of postcardiotomy patients supported with VADs recover myocardial function sufficiently to be weaned from the device. However, of the 50% who become device-dependent, only a small percentage would be likely candidates for transplantation, because they often have suffered other organ damage or developed infections. In our experience at St. Louis University it has been rare for a postcardiotomy patient who required VAD support to become a successful transplant candidate. On the other hand, prolonged mechanical support for more than 1 week has allowed the recovery of a small group of patients with acute myocarditis or postpartal cardiomyopathy without the need for transplantation.

Successful perfusions of more than 1 month are now commonplace for patients bridged to transplantation, and survival rates are generally excellent in patients who receive a transplant. Over the last 8 years, when bridge to transplantation was performed with greater frequency, many centers have reported their individual experiences. These retrospective reviews have identified some risk factors that aid in patient selection. A prospective randomized multicenter study of the various risk factors may be able to provide the needed information. Although such studies are highly desirable, they are unlikely because of the lack of funding for clinical research of this type.

Perhaps a more important aspect of bridging to transplantation has been the opportunity to observe patients from periods of months to longer than 1 year with support devices in place. Such information is invaluable in planning future studies of permanently placed, totally implanted devices. Criteria for patient selection for these devices will be of necessity more restrictive than those for temporary support.

Another major factor in determining whether to offer temporary circulatory support is the amount of resources each case may absorb. At St. Louis University, the average charges for patients receiving VADs after cardiac surgery are approximately $70,000 higher than for patients undergoing routine cardiac surgery without the need for postoperative VAD support. In the bridge-to-transplant group, status I patients supported with conventional techniques (drugs and IABP) before transplantation had an average total hospital bill of $129,549 compared with $294,165 for status I patients supported with pulsatile VADs before transplantation. Furthermore, commitments of time by key personnel are significant. If a separate circulatory support team cannot be made available, elective cardiac procedures may have to be curtailed, because they lead to an inappropriate allocation of personnel and resources to a small group of patients.

If more appropriate patients with a better opportunity of survival can be identified, then the survival rates should improve. This improvement should lead to an expansion of the indications for mechanical circulatory support. Presently this technology benefits a small number of patients; however, it has the potential to alter significantly the effects of acute and chronic heart failure.

REFERENCES

1. Bolooki H (ed): Clinical Application of Intra-aortic Balloon Pump, 2nd ed. Mount Kisco, NY, Futura Publishing, 1984.
2. Creswell LL, Rosenbloom M, Cox JL, et al: Intra-aortic balloon counterpulsation: Patterns of usage and outcome in cardiac surgery patients. Ann Thorac Surg 54:11, 1992.
3. Dembitsky WP, Moore CH, Holman WL, et al: Successful mechanical circulatory support for noncoronary shock. J Heart Lung Transplant 11:129, 1992.
4. Didisheim P, Olsen DB, Farrar DJ, et al: Infections and thromboembolism with implantable cardiovascular devices. ASAIO Trans 35:54, 1989.
5. DiLello F, Mullen DC, Flemma RJ, et al: Results of intra-aortic balloon pumping after cardiac surgery: Experience with the Percor balloon catheter. Ann Thorac Surg 46:442, 1988.
6. Golding LR, Jacobs G, Groves LL, et al: Clinical results of mechanical support of the failing left ventricle. J Thorac Cardiovasc Surg 83:597, 1982.
7. Joyce LD, Kiser JC, Eales F, et al: Experience with the Sarns centrifugal pump as a ventricular assist device. ASAIO Trans 36:619, 1990.
8. Kanter SR, Swartz MT, Pennington DG, et al: Renal failure in patients with ventricular assist devices. ASAIO Trans 33:426, 1987.
9. McBride LR, Swartz MT, Reedy JE, et al: Bridging to transplantation in patients with previous cardiac operations. J Heart Transplant 9:57, 1990 [abstract].
10. McBride LR, Swartz MT, Reedy JE, et al: Device related infections in patients supported with mechanical circulatory support devices greater than 30 days. ASAIO Trans 37:258, 1991.
11. Miller CA, Pae WE, Pierce WS: Combined registry for the clinical use of mechanical ventricular assist devices: Postcardiotomy cardiogenic shock. ASAIO Trans 36:43, 1990.
12. Miller CA: Combined registry for the clinical use of mechanical ventricular assist pumps and total artificial hearts. Pennsylvania State University. Personal communication.
13. Moore CH, Rubin JM, Shnitzler RN, et al: Experience and direction using cardiopulmonary support in fifty-three consecutive cases. ASAIO Trans 37:340, 1991.

14. Moroney D, Swartz MT, Reedy JE, et al: Importance of ventricular arrhythmias in recovery patients with ventricular assist devices. ASAIO Trans 37:516, 1991.
15. Naunheim KS, Swartz MT, Pennington DG, et al: Intra-aortic balloon pumping in cardiac surgical patients: Risk analysis and long-term follow-up. J Thorac Cardiovasc Surg 104:1654, 1992.
16. Naunheim KS, Fiore AC, Wadley JJ, et al: The changing mortality of myocardial revascularization: Coronary artery bypass and angioplasty. Ann Thorac Surg 46:666, 1988.
17. Norman JC, Cooley DA, Igo SR, et al: Prognostic indices for survival during postcardiotomy intra-aortic balloon pumping. J Thorac Cardiovasc Surg 74:709, 1977.
18. Parascandola SA, Pae WE, Davis PK, et al: Determinants of survival in patients with ventricular assist devices. ASAIO Trans 34:222, 1988.
19. Pennington DG, Joyce LD, Pae WE, Burkholder JA: Patient selection. Ann Thorac Surg 47:77, 1989.
20. Pennington DG, McBride LR, Kanter KR, et al: The effect of perioperative myocardial infarction on survival of postcardiotomy patients supported with ventricular assist devices. Circulation 78(Suppl III):110, 1988.
21. Pennington DG, McBride LR, Swartz MT, et al: Use of the Pierce-Donachy ventricular assist device in patients with cardiogenic shock after cardiac operations. Ann Thorac Surg 47:130, 1989.
22. Pennington DG, Merjavy JP, Codd JE, et al: Extracorporeal membrane oxygenation for patients with cardiogenic shock. Circulation 70(Suppl I):130, 1984.
23. Pennington DG, Merjavy JP, Swartz MT, et al: The importance of biventricular failure in patients with postoperative cardiogenic shock. Ann Thorac Surg 39:16, 1985.
24. Pennington DG, Reedy JE, Swartz MT, et al: Univentricular versus biventricular assist device support. J Heart Lung Transplant 10:258, 1991.
25. Pennington DG, Swartz MT, Codd JE, et al: Intra-aortic balloon pumping in cardiac surgical patients: A nine-year experience. Ann Thorac Surg 36:125, 1983.
26. Pennington DG, Swartz MT: Assisted circulation and mechanical hearts. In Braunwald E (ed): Heart Disease, 4th ed. Philadelphia, W.B. Saunders, 1991, pp 535–550.
27. Pennington DG, Swartz MT: Temporary circulatory support in patients with postcardiotomy cardiogenic shock. Card Surg: State Art Rev 5:373–392, 1991.
28. Phillips SJ, Zeff RH, Kongatahworn C, et al: Percutaneous cardiopulmonary bypass: Application and indications for use. Ann Thorac Surg 47:121, 1989.
29. Raithel SC, Swartz MT, Braun PR, et al: Experience with an emergency resuscitation system. ASAIO Trans 35:475, 1989.
30. Reedy JE, Pennington DG, Miller LW, et al: Status I heart transplant patients: Conventional vs ventricular assist device (VAD) support. J Heart Lung Transplant 11:246, 1992.
31. Reedy JE, Swartz MT, Pennington DG, et al: Bridge to cardiac transplantation: Importance of patient selection. J Heart Transplant 9:473, 1990.
32. Reichman RT, Joyo CI, Dembitsky WP, et al: Improved patient survival after cardiac arrest using a cardiopulmonary support system. Ann Thorac Surg 49:101, 1990.
33. Swartz MT, Reedy JE, Lohmann DL, et al: Cost and reimbursement rates for investigational circulatory support. ASAIO Trans 37:549, 1991.
34. Wareing TH, Kouchoukos NT: Postcardiotomy mechanical circulatory support in the elderly. Ann Thorac Surg 51:1443, 1991.

TIMOTHY B. ICENOGLE, MD[1]
DAVID J. SATO, MSBE, CCE[2]
RICHARD G. SMITH, MSEE, CCE[3]
MARILYN CLEAVINGER, MSBME[3]
DAVID LOFFING, MSBE, CCE[3]
STEPHEN A. MIKITISH[4]

TRANSPORT OF THE CRITICALLY ILL CARDIAC PATIENT

[1]Director
Inland Northwest Thoracic Organ
    Transplant Program
Spokane, Washington

[2]Circulatory Assist Program
Sacred Heart Medical Center
Spokane, Washington

[3]Department of Artificial Heart
University Medical Center
Tucson, Arizona

[4]Department of Physical
    Resources
University of Arizona
Tucson, Arizona

Reprint requests to:
Timothy B. Icenogle, MD
105 W. 8th
Suite 36
Spokane, WA 99204

Cardiac transplantation is the treatment of choice for a variety of maladies. Unfortunately, the donor supply has reached a plateau, whereas the number of referred patients continues to increase. The result is an increasing number of status I patients in the intensive care unit (ICU) waiting for transplant. Pulsatile devices extend lives but as temporary devices do not solve the shortage of donor organs.

The development of permanently implanted left ventricular assist devices (LVADs) is moving rapidly. These devices may service an estimated population of 40,000 patients with endstage heart disease each year.[5] Devices developed by Novacor (Oakland, CA) and Thermo Cardiosystems (Woburn, MA) are in the initial stages of clinical testing. The high cost of ICU care may make permanent implantation of VADs the low-cost option for many patients with endstage heart disease.

The regionalization of implant centers is nearly inevitable given the political emphasis to concentrate skills and reduce costs. Many proponents of regionalization cite the Canadian system of health care as a model.[11] Some insurance carriers preferentially refer patients to specialized centers that demonstrate superior clinical and economic results in an effort to contain costs.[3]

Regionalization of specialized cardiac systems can be accomplished only if a nearly infallible system of transport for critically ill cardiac patients can be developed. Access to specialized health care cannot be limited by a patient's proximity to the centers; candidates for permanent circulatory assist devices must be transported via a system that emulates the intensive care environment. The centers must ensure safe transport if they are the sole referral site for specialized health care in the region. This chapter explores the driving forces in the development of transport systems for the critically ill cardiac patient and describes one method of meeting this challenge.

THE CRITICALLY ILL CARDIAC PATIENT

Transport of the critically ill cardiac patient is difficult for several reasons. The "scoop-and-run" mentality common in ambulance services is not appropriate for these patients. The intra- and interhospital transport of critically ill cardiac patients is associated with severe hemodynamic changes, arrhythmias, and occasionally death.[1,18,19] Noise in the aircraft environment inhibits communication and auditory diagnostic skills.[13] Vibration introduces mechanical artifacts into monitoring waveforms and can disable equipment not hardened to this environment.[12] Altitude changes during flight result in varied atmospheric pressures that can adversely affect ventilators and intraaortic balloons.[13] Patients may require multiple infusion pumps, monitors, ventilators, and circulatory assist devices during transport. Adequate stabilization before transport, extensive monitoring and support of the patient during transport, and the attendance of ICU-trained personnel are imperative for patient safety.[1,4,14,16,18,19] Intraaortic balloon pump (IABP) transports are common, but use of other circulatory assist devices during transport is rare.[2,6,12,13] Patients have been transported on centrifugal force blood pumps for both left ventricular and biventricular support; recent reports describe transport of patients on full cardiopulmonary bypass.[7,9]

The mode of transport plays a significant role in associated difficulties. Transports within a range of 100 miles can be accomplished by ground or rotary-wing aircraft. Ground transport is less expensive, but rotary-wing aircraft have the advantage of bypassing traffic. Unfortunately, rotary-wing aircraft are associated with more untoward events than ground transport because of noise, vibrations, and accelerations.[17] Transports of over 100 miles usually dictate fixed-wing airplanes, which provide a stable, spacious environment but require ambulance transport between airport and hospital.

THE REGULATION OF AEROMEDICAL TRANSPORTS

The Federal Aviation Administration (FAA) has avoided regulation of aeromedical transport and limits its scope to the interaction of medical equipment with the operation and safety of the aircraft. The FAA rules are recorded in the Federal Air Regulations (FAR), which require that any object or mass (medical equipment) in an aircraft be secured to withstand the wind-gust and emergency crash-landing loads for a given aircraft. Emergency egress regulations stipulate that the aisle and emergency exits must be clear of medical equipment connected to the patient. Medical equipment must be tested to ensure that it does not produce electromagnetic interference (EMI) that could possibly disrupt aircraft electronics. Medical gases must be properly stored, secured, and protected to prevent rupture to containers or damage to gauges and high-pressure lines. All extraneous hardware must meet Military Specifications (Mil-Spec) that govern quality and traceability to the manufacturer. Flammable materials, such as stretcher mattresses and sheets, must meet strict fire-retardant standards.

A separate part of the FAR covers each class of aircraft: small fixed wing, large fixed wing, small rotary wing, and large rotary wing (Parts 23, 25, 27, and 29, respectively). Because the FAR evolve with aircraft technology, a given aircraft is regulated by the FAR in effect at the time of its manufacture. The FAA recommends that new installations follow the most recent regulations, regardless of the manufacture date of the aircraft. Current regulations (dated January 1, 1991) for aircraft commonly used for aeromedical transport require that items of mass be restrained to resist maximal forces of 16 G in the forward direction, 1.5 G to the rear, 8 G laterally, 20 G downward, and 4 G upward. They also require a safety factor of 1.33 for attachment points.[15] This safety factor increases a 20 G force to 26.6 G, which is equivalent to the forces exerted on a passenger in a car that accelerates from 0 to 60 mph in 0.10 seconds. The FAA does not specify the operational capabilities of medical equipment subjected to these loads but requires only that the device attachment points support these stresses.

To determine whether a system meets FAA guidelines, an FAA-designated engineering representative (DER) evaluates the system. The DER analyzes the mounting system, designs and observes pull tests, evaluates electrical requirements, determines weight and center of gravity loads, tests for EMI, and submits the appropriate documentation to the FAA.

There are two levels of FAA approval for the installation of a system in an aircraft: (1) field approval or form 337 and (2) supplemental type certificate (STC). The 337 approves installation of a system in a specific aircraft. The installation must meet FAA standards and then be inspected and approved by a local FAA officer. The STC is an FAA approval for installation of a system in a specific model of aircraft. An STC requires not only that the installation of the system meet FAA standards, but also that the manufacture, repair, maintenance, quality assurance, and testing of the system be documented.

Subcommittee F30.01 of the American Society of Testing and Materials (ASTM) established recommendations for rotary- and fixed-wing medical transport, including minimal requirements for personnel, patient care equipment, medical supplies, and vehicle configuration. Many state regulatory agencies adopt these recommendations as law. Their impact on aeromedical transport systems is significant: any surfaces that could present a hazard to patients or personnel during an aircraft crash must be recessed or padded, and medical equipment must be secured with the same structural integrity as aircraft seats. In the past medical equipment was classified as baggage and thus could be temporarily strapped to the floor or to vacant seats in the passenger compartment. Current regulations from the FAA and the ASTM require that medical equipment be installed as an integral aircraft component.

INTENSIVE CARE TRANSPORT: ONE METHOD

The management of intravenous lines, patient leads, ventilator circuits, circulatory assist devices, infusion pumps, monitors, ventilators, and circulatory support consoles creates challenging logistic problems during transport. Transfer into an aircraft of a patient connected to multiple devices is at times almost impossible. Many teams interrupt IABP and ventilator support during transfer.[2] Interruptions in support devices may not be tolerated and at best are stressful to the critically ill cardiac patient. Once in the aircraft, patient equipment must be secured in compliance with the FAR and with the configuration described in the 337 or STC. Access to the patient by the transport team leaves few options for locations of equipment that do not violate the FAR.

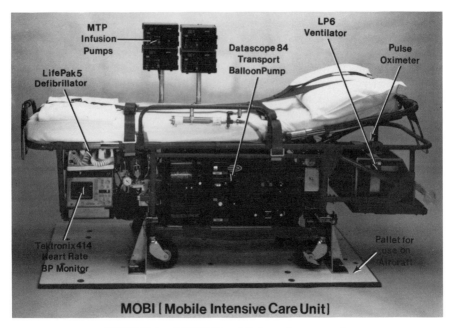

FIGURE 1.   MOBI III mobile intensive care unit.

We developed the concept of a modular mobile intensive care unit (MOBI) to transport critically ill cardiac patients without interruption of support devices and monitoring.[8] The MOBI concept uses nondedicated aircraft or aircraft not specifically modified for air ambulance missions. Purchase, maintenance, operating costs, and low utilization make a dedicated "flying ICU" aircraft impractical.[10]

The third prototype of the system, designated MOBI III, was designed for use in standard ambulances and in chartered Learjet 25 and 35 series aircraft (Fig. 1). This system had a volume ventilator, pulse oximeter, IABP, defibrillator, monitor with two pressure channels, and four infusion pumps. The platform for this equipment was a reinforced, welded, and heat-tempered stretcher frame capable of withstanding the forces stipulated by the FAA.

At the referring hospital the patient was transferred onto the stretcher frame. The self-contained design of MOBI III provided continuous support and monitoring of the patient throughout transport. The transport team consisted of a physician, two ICU registered nurses trained in IABP, and a respiratory therapist. The transport team evaluated and stabilized the patient before traveling by ambulance to the airport. MOBI III was secured to a honeycomb aluminum pallet mounted on the aircraft seat rails. Separately mounted power inverters, pneumatic support module, and liquid oxygen converter supplemented MOBI III in the aircraft and ambulance.

Thirty-five patients were transported by land and air using MOBI III (Table 1). All patients were transferred to the University Medical Center, Tucson, Arizona. No deaths occurred during transport, and deaths after transport were not attributed to the transport process. Equipment problems encountered during some transports were remedied by the transport staff. All patient equipment was

TABLE 1.   The MOBI Experience

Patient Initials	Mode of Transport	Distance One-way	Support Devices	Outcome
DB	Ground	122	IABP, V	Not listed
BC	Ground	122		TAH/Txn/TAH/Txn/died
LV	Fixed wing	515	IABP	Not listed
JM	Fixed wing	632	IABP, V	Not listed
BW	Fixed wing	400	IABP	Txn/alive
AD	Fixed wing	2431	IABP	Not listed
KT	Ground	112	IABP	Not listed
RC	Fixed wing	257	IABP, V	Not listed
JP	Fixed wing	391	IABP, V	Txn/alive
LG	Ground	122		Txn/died
KK	Ground	122	IABP	LVAD/not listed
DP	Ground	122	IABP	Txn/alive
RB	Ground	122	IABP, V	Txn/alive
SS	Fixed wing	2431	IABP	BVAD/Txn/alive
TN	Ground	122	V	Not listed
JM	Ground	122	IABP	Txn/alive
EM	Fixed wing	400	V	Donor
RS	Fixed wing	1508	IABP, V, CBVAD	BVAD/not listed
RO	Ground	122	IABP	Txn/alive
HS	Ground	122	CLVAD	BVAD/not listed
PC	Fixed wing	966		Not listed
RO	Ground	122	IABP	Txn/alive
IV	Ground	122	IABP, V	BVAD/not listed
GS	Ground	122	IABP, IABP	LVAS/not listed
PS	Ground	122	IABP, V	BVAD/Txn/alive
EL	Ground	122	IABP	BVAD/not listed
GG	Fixed wing	150	IABP, V	Meds/alive
DR	Ground	122	IABP	BVAD/alive
BN	Ground	122	IABP	CABG/alive
CC	Ground	122	IABP, V	Txn/alive
AM	Ground	122	IABP	Not listed
ML	Ground	122		Waiting
JL	Ground	122	IABP	Txn/alive
SC	Ground	122	IABP	Txn/alive
SH	Ground	122		CABG/alive

For abbreviations, see text.

expressly adapted for transport, and no disabling equipment failures occurred during transport.

Twenty-four patients transported by ground averaged one-way distances of 122 miles and durations of approximately 4 hours. Eleven fixed-wing transports averaged a one-way distance of 916 miles and an approximate duration of 6 hours. The farthest transports were 2431 miles, with a duration of approximately 17 hours.

Twenty-eight patients were transported on IABP, 12 patients on ventilator support (V), 1 patient on centrifugal force biventricular assist devices (CBVADs), and 1 patient on centrifugal force left ventricular assist device (CLVAD). All patients were transported on infusion pumps and monitors.

Once at the medical center, 15 received transplants (Txn), 1 was bridged to transplant with a total artificial heart (TAH), 7 were implanted with pulsatile biventricular assist devices (BVAD), and two were implanted with pulsatile left ventricular assist devices (LVAD). Outcomes labeled "not listed" indicate patients not listed for transplant because of the development of contraindications or patient refusal.

MOBI development has now reached the fourth prototype. The stretcher platform was reengineered to create a lighter system employing the most current technology and fulfilling new design criteria (Table 2).

The MOBI IV stretcher platform is a welded construction using 4130 Chrome Moly. Welders are certified to Mil-Spec-T-5021D for aircraft and missiles. The platform contains three bays that allow a variety of medical equipment to be mounted. The mounting and wheel hardware are manufactured from 6061-T6 aluminum. The stretcher platform measures 72″ long, 19″ wide, and 28″ high and can be loaded into most aircraft with at least a 20″ door. Tapering the leg end of the platform permits rotation of the stretcher as it passes through the aircraft door. To facilitate attachment in standard ambulances, the platform has a 22″ wide wheel base. During loading into an aircraft, a battery-powered mechanism retracts the wheels to within the 19″ width of the stretcher platform. The wheels can be retracted completely to allow the platform to be mounted directly to aircraft seat rails, thus eliminating the need for a pallet and reducing the height to 22″.

The MOBI IV stretcher platform weighs 90 pounds. The initial configuration of patient equipment, including a volume ventilator, IABP, defibrillator with external pacemaker, monitor, liquid oxygen system (LOX), and three channel infusion pumps, brings the weight to 280 lbs (Fig. 2). All equipment mounts in the stretcher platform on rails that can accommodate various configurations. Future configurations will include ventricular assist consoles, cardiopulmonary bypass equipment, or other ICU equipment. The patient rests on a mattress constructed of FAA-approved, flame-retardant material and is secured by a 4-point shoulder harness, lap belt, and lower extremities belt.

MOBI IV requires minimal modification to the aircraft. An aircraft-mounted inverter converts the 28 VDC common in aircraft electrical systems to 120 VAC. The initial MOBI IV configuration requires a 120-VAC, 800-watt power source in the aircraft or ambulance. Onboard batteries supply 2 hours of operation when AC power is not available.. The platform is secured by small mounting plates attached to the aircraft seat rails before loading MOBI IV. After MOBI IV is loaded and positioned in the aircraft, the wheels are completely retracted and the stretcher platform is locked in place. The few modifications required for MOBI transports can be accomplished on aircraft not dedicated to aeromedical transport.

CONCLUSION

The introduction of permanent left ventricular assist devices and the need to reduce health-care expenditure drive the demand for long-distance transport of prospective patients. The implementation of transport systems must follow stringent FAA and aircraft industry standards to ensure the safety of the patient and transport personnel. The MOBI concept demonstrates that a system meeting

TABLE 2.   Design Criteria

Provide continuous uninterrupted patient support
Meet and exceed current FAA load requirements
Fit most aircraft and ambulances
Allow various patient equipment configurations
Eliminate external support equipment
Use nondedicated aircraft
Minimize weight

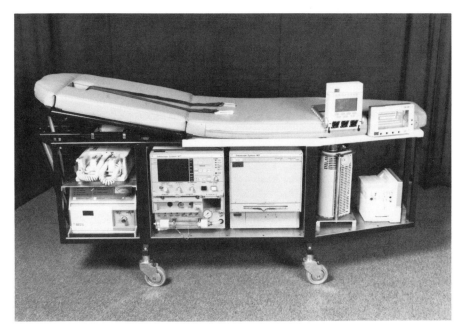

FIGURE 2. MOBI IV mobile intensive care unit.

FAA guidelines can transport critically ill cardiac patients over great distances. Transport that is both safe and cost-effective allows distant patients the chance for life.

REFERENCES

1. Braman SS, Dunn SM, Amico CA, Millman RP: Complications of intrahospital transport in critically ill patients. Ann Intern Med 107:469–473, 1987.
2. Campbell P: Air transport of the intraaortic balloon pump dependent patient. Aero Med J 1:20–21, 1986.
3. Cochran DB: One hospital's experience with the Fortune 100. Hospitals 63:17, 1989.
4. Ehrenwerth J, Sorbo S, Hackel A: Transport of critically ill adults. Crit Care Med 14:543–547, 1986.
5. Evans RW, Manninen DL, Dong FB: The National Cooperative Transplantation Study: Final Report. Publ. no. BHARC-100-90-020. Seattle, Battelle-Seattle Research Center, June 1991.
6. Gottlieb SO, Chew PH, Chandra N, et al: Portable intraaortic balloon counterpulsation: Clinical experience and guidelines for use. Cathet Cardiovasc Diagn 12:18–22, 1986.
7. Hill JG, Bennett J, Parsons J, et al: Transportation of patients on emergency cardiopulmonary bypass systems. Circulatory Support 1991, Society of Thoracic Surgeons, 1991 [abstract].
8. Icenogle TB, Machamar WF, Nelson RJ, et al: Mobile intensive care patient handling system apparatus and method of using. United States Patent: 4,957,121, September 18, 1990.
9. Icenogle TB, Smith RG, Crane S, et al: Long-distance transport of the asystolic patient. Aviat Space Environ Med 60:479, 1989.
10. Icenogle TB, Smith RG, Sato D, et al: Card Surg State Art Rev 3:499–505, 1989.
11. Iglehart JK: Canada's health care system. N Engl J Med 315:202, 1986.
12. Kramer RP: Helicopter-transported intra-aortic balloon pumping: Advance technology made airborne. Cardiac Assists 4:2, 1988.
13. Mertlich G, Quaal SJ: Air transport of the patient requiring intra-aortic balloon pumping. Crit Care Nurs Clin North Am 1:3, 1989.

14. Olson CM, Jastremski MS, Vilogi JP, et al: Stabilization of patients prior to interhospital transfer. Am J Emerg Med 6:1, 1987.
15. Petersen RD: Personal communication. Aeronautical Technologies, Inc., Boulder, CO, January 23, 1992.
16. Reeve WG, Runcie CJ, Reidy J, Wallace PGM: Current practice in transferring critically ill patients among hospitals in the west of Scotland. BMJ 300:85–87, 1990.
17. Schneider S, Borok Z, Heller M, et al: Critical cardiac transport: Air versus ground. Am J Emerg Med 6:5, 1988.
18. Waddel G: Movement of critically ill patients within hospital. BMJ 2:417–419, 1975.
19. Waddel G, Scott PD, Lees NW, Ledingham IM: Effects of ambulance transport in critically ill patients. BMJ 1:386–389, 1975.

GEORGE J. MAGOVERN, Jr, MD

USE OF BIOMEDICUS PUMP IN POSTOPERATIVE CIRCULATORY SUPPORT

From the Department of Surgery
Allegheny General Hospital
Allegheny Campus
The Medical College of
   Pennsylvania
Pittsburgh, Pennsylvania

Reprint requests to:
George J. Magovern, Jr., MD
Department of Surgery
Division of Thoracic Surgery
Allegheny General Hospital
320 E. North Avenue
Pittsburgh, PA 15212

The Biomedicus Corporation of Minnetonka, Minnesota approached Allegheny General Hospital in 1978 for laboratory testing of a new pump to replace the standard roller pump,[10] which had become associated with some of the damaging effects of cardiopulmonary bypass. The Bio-Pump (Fig. 1) has a centrifugal pump composed of valveless rotator cones made from nonthrombogenic acrylics. These cones impart a circular motion to the blood, generating centrifugal force, pressure, and flow. The hydrodynamically designed flow path of the pump eliminates turbulence, cavitation, and resulting damage to blood elements. A magnetic drive and a solid housing design prohibit induction of air or contaminants.

EARLY OBSERVATIONS

Our initial attempts at using the Bio-Pump for long-term left-heart assist were carried out by coating the Bio-Pump, tubing, and connectors with a solution of graphite, benzalkoniumchloride, and heparin. A dog was placed on left-heart assist for a planned 6-hour study. Early in the experiment we noted that the graphite material was pealing from the tubing and the Bio-Pump. After 5 hours the dog was in a state of disseminated intravascular coagulation, and the experiment was terminated.

In a follow-up experiment we used tridodecylmethyl almoniumchloride to coat the tubing, connectors, and Bio-Pump. A dog was then prepared for left-heart assist. However, when the Bio-Pump was opened to prime the circuit, we

CARDIAC SURGERY: State of the Art Reviews—Vol. 7, No. 2, 1993
Philadelphia, Hanley & Belfus, Inc.

249

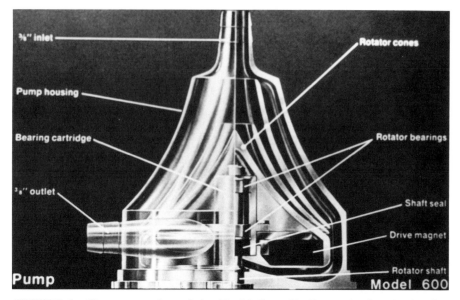

FIGURE 1. The cross-section of the Bio-Medicus Bio-Pump showing the bearing housing, which is an area of low-flow, low-shear rates, and elevated temperatures, where thrombus formation and actual binding of the mechanism occurred. Emboli also originated from the struts between rotor plates.

noted that the solvent had weakened the strut supporting the concentric cones. Because the experiment had already been started, we decided to continue, but with an untreated Bio-Pump, tubing, and connectors. The dog survived 6 hours on assist. An important outcome was normal coagulation studies.

After this observation, 5 mongrel dogs were treated with left ventricle-to-femoral artery bypass for 24 hours at a flow ranging from 1.8–3.2 L/min. No venous reservoir was used. All animals survived and recovered without sequelae. No excessive bleeding from the wounds was found. We reopened the wounds at termination of the procedure for inspection and observed no evidence of thromboembolic sequelae at autopsy. The serum hemoglobin level rose slightly during the course of the experiment, but platelet counts remained within the normal range. Fibrinogen levels were also constant, as were prothrombin time (PT) and partial thromboplastin time (PTT).

In the next experiment a 65-kg male sheep was placed on left ventricular assistance with the Biomedicus pump for 14 days. Arterial return was established through a graft sutured to the descending thoracic aorta. Flow ranged from 4.0–4.4 L/min, and cardiac output by thermodilution was 5.3–5.8 L/min during the experiment. Fibrin split products remained <40. PPT fluctuated early but stabilized to normal limits within 5 days (Fig. 2). PT was normal throughout the experiment, but serum hemoglobin levels rose gradually during the first 7 days, then stabilized. Fibrinogen levels rose quickly and then leveled after the third day. Platelet counts dropped initially but remained stable after 2 days. Levels of blood urea nitrogen (BUN) remained stable until the 14th day. Because of the sharp rise in BUN/creatinine at this point, the animal was sacrificed; postmortem study demonstrated renal infarction.

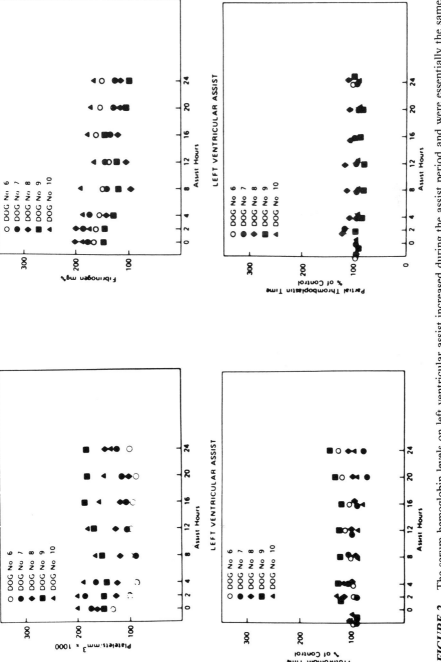

FIGURE 2. The serum hemoglobin levels on left ventricular assist increased during the assist period and were essentially the same as venoarterial membrane assist animals. Contrary to expectations, the platelet count did not fall during the left ventricular assist period despite lack of anticoagulation. Fibrinogen levels remained constant during the assist. The prothrombin time did not deviate from control levels at any time during the 24 hours of assist. Partial thromboplastin time did not fluctuate during the run.

From these animal experiments we made several interesting observations that contrasted with results from the standard roller pump: (1) no obstruction and cavitation of the inflow cannula, with resultant air embolization, occurred; (2) serum hemoglobin levels in the experimental animals remained low; and (3) no anticoagulation was needed when the Bio-Pump was run at 2,000–3,000 rpm for periods up to 2 weeks.

Early Experimental Background at Allegheny General Hospital

The vast majority of patients undergoing open-heart surgery can be effectively weaned from cardiopulmonary bypass with either pharmacologic support alone or in conjunction with intraaortic counterpulsation balloon pumping (IABP). However, a small but significant group of patients (<1%) cannot be weaned from bypass despite these conventional support mechanisms.[1]

The salutary effects of mechanical assist for the failing left ventricle after open-heart surgery have been well documented.[3] During the past three decades, various devices and modifications have been introduced to achieve assist pumping, and their merits have been detailed.[6] Dennis et al.[5] first presented mechanical left ventricular assist in 1962. They hypothesized that assist devices allowed a reduction in preload that would decrease myocardial oxygen consumption and wall tension while maintaining adequate systemic perfusion and coronary blood flow. The concept of lowering left ventricular preload to decrease wall tension and myocardial oxygen consumption is based on the law of Laplace.[11] In 1963 Liotta et al. were the first to use left ventricular assist clinically.[9] Spencer and associates reported the first survivor.[12]

The rationale for use of a ventricular assist device (VAD) after open-heart surgery is based on the premise that reversible perioperative myocardial injury has occurred. Reversibly injured postischemic heart muscle has been termed "stunned myocardium" by Braunwald and Kloner,[2] among others. In order to study the recovery of stunned myocardium, our laboratory developed a model of normothermic ischemia to produce profound global myocardial dysfunction. In the canine model, 45 minutes of global ischemia produced severe myocardial injury, which was fatal with standard resuscitative techniques.[7] Our model was developed to determine whether such an injury would be reversible when treated with biventricular support using the Biomedicus pump (Fig. 3).

In brief, the hearts of 10 dogs were exposed through a mediastinotomy and placed on biventricular support with cannulation of the femoral artery, left atrial appendage, right atrial appendage, and main pulmonary artery. The aorta was then cross-clamped for 45 minutes of normothermic ischemia, after which the cross-clamp was removed, resulting in immediate ventricular fibrillation. A beating, nonworking state was maintained for the next 24 hours. After 20 minutes of reperfusion, a brief attempt was made to wean the dogs from biventricular assist by volume-loading the heart and decreasing the flow rate of the Biomedicus pump to 500 cc/min. None of the hearts could sustain a stable rhythm or blood pressure, and biventricular support was quickly resumed. After 12 hours of biventricular assist, we again attempted to wean the dogs by volume-loading the heart. Measures of developed pressure (DP) and its first derivative dP/dt were obtained. At the end of 24 hours, a final attempt was made to wean the dogs from the assist pumps. No pressor agents were used. The final measurements of cardiac output, pulmonary capillary wedge pressure (PCWP), DP, and dP/dt were then recorded. Adenosine triphosphate (ATP) samples, obtained with a Travenol true-cut biopsy needle

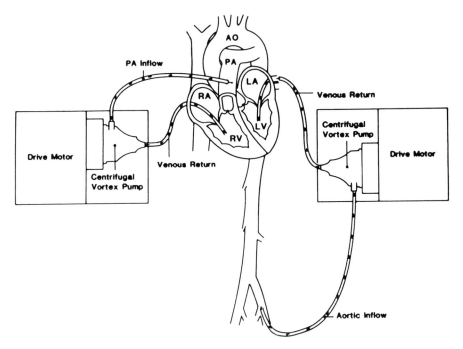

FIGURE 3. Experimental model. Heart is placed on biventricular support by cannulation of femoral artery, left atrial appendage, right atrial appendage, and main pulmonary artery. *Ao,* aorta; *PA,* pulmonary artery; *LA,* left atrium; *RA,* right atrium; *LV,* left ventricle; *RV,* right ventricle.

(Travenol Labs, Deerfield, IL), were taken at the end of ischemia, at 20 minutes of reperfusion, and after 12 and 24 hours of ventricular assist.

CONCLUSIONS OF THE STUDIES

Figures 4–7 show the results of our study. Significant ventricular recovery is possible with prompt institution of long-term biventricular assist (Figs. 4 and 5). As mentioned above, in our series of 10 dog hearts undergoing 45 minutes of normothermic ischemia, attempts to wean from biventricular assist during the first 12–24 hours were unsuccessful. Volume-loading resulted in ventricular distention and ventricular fibrillation. With complete ventricular decompression over 24 hours, however, DP and dP/dt steadily improved. At 12 hours of assist, DP had recovered to 66% of control; after 24 hours of support, 7 of the 10 animals were successfully weaned from biventricular assist. Left ventricular function parameters were essentially normal, and subsequent analysis of myocardial water content indicated no significant edema. Recovery of myocardial ATP also closely paralleled the return of ventricular function (Figs. 6 and 7). ATP concentration after 12 hours of support, while significantly less than control levels, was much improved over early reperfusion. By 24 hours of reperfusion, myocardial ATP stores had fully recovered to control levels.

Finally, an analysis of myocardial ultrastructure provided further evidence that the 45-minute ischemic insult was severe but not irreversible. After 45 minutes of normothermic ischemia, moderate ultrastructural damage occurred, with a

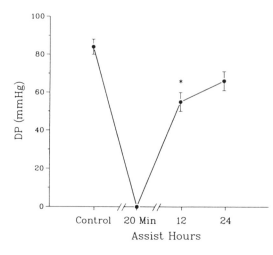

FIGURE 4. Recovery of developed pressure (DP) after 45 minutes of normothermic ischemia and 24 hours of biventricular support. After 24 hours of support, developed pressure has recovered to near control values. *, p < 0.05 vs. control.

moderate amount of nuclear chromatin clumping and margination, myocardial swelling with occasionally disrupted cristae, relaxed myofibrils, and glycogen depletion. After 20 minutes of reperfusion, further glycogen depletion was noted, along with occasional disrupted myofibrils. After 12 hours of assist, chromatin clumping and margination were significantly less and no further myocardial distortion occurred. After 24 hours of support, no major structural abnormalities were noted. Of significance, none of the tissue in any group showed severe myocardial injury with the disruption and flocculent density formation of irreversible cell injury. In conclusion, a full 24 hours of ventricular assist was required for functional, metabolic, and structural recovery. Thus, in the clinical setting of postcardiotomy pump failure, whether caused by air embolism, coronary artery spasm, myocardial infarction (MI), ventricular distention, or inadequate myocardial protection, prolonged ventricular assist pumping should be considered; in some instances it may permit recovery of reversibly injured myocardium.

In a similar model from our laboratory, Demmy et al.[4] attempted to shorten the time for hemodynamic recovery of injured myocardium by administering

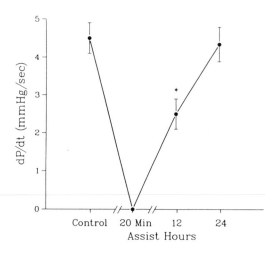

FIGURE 5. Recovery of maximal positive dP/dt at 12 and 24 hours of biventricular support. After 24 hours of assist, maximal positive dP/dt returned to near control values. *, p < 0.01 vs. control.

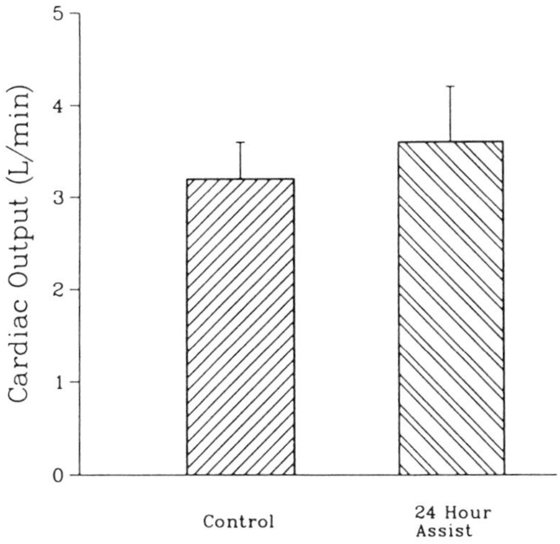

FIGURE 6. Cardiac output after 45 minutes of normothermic ischemia and 24 hours of biventricular support in the seven dogs weaned from biventricular support.

adenosine-enriched cardioplegia at the end of 45 minutes of normothermic ischemia. Animals treated with adenosine after ischemia had faster recovery of left ventricular function than control animals (Fig. 8). One hour after weaning from circulatory support, adenosine-treated animals had higher left ventricular peak systolic pressure (110 ± 21 vs. 57 ± 36 mmHg), greater dP/dt (3,407 ± 812 vs. 1,510 ± 1,376 mmHg/sec), and lower left ventricular end-diastolic pressure (23.8 ± 4.8 vs. 34.0 ± 7.2 mmHg) than the control group. Greater recovery of ATP levels in the adenosine group correlated nicely with the hemodynamic results (Fig. 9). Thus, adenosine clearly accelerated left ventricular recovery and shortened the time required for biventricular assist after uniform global ischemic

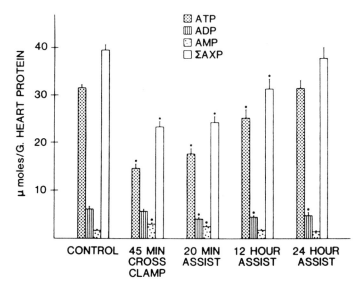

FIGURE 7. Recovery of myocardial ATP, ADP, and AMP, and total adenine nucleotide level (AXP) during 24 hours of biventricular support. *, $p < 0.01$ vs. control.

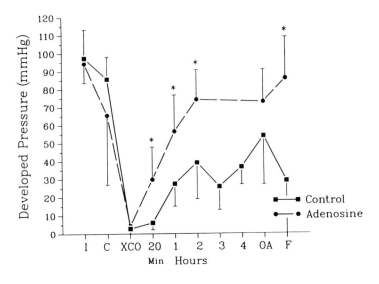

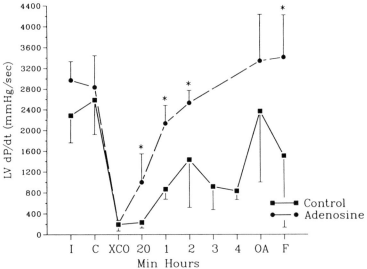

FIGURE 8. Recovery of ventricular function: relationship of left ventricular (LV) developed pressure, compliance (EDP, end-diastolic pressure), and contractility (dP/dt) versus time for adenosine and control groups. Developed pressure was calculated as systolic minus diastolic ventricular pressure. For each variable there was no significant difference between the groups before ischemia. Aggregate postischemic performance for the adenosine group was significantly better than control in each comparison ($p < 0.01$). Statistically significant differences at discrete time intervals between groups are indicated by asterisks ($p < 0.05$). Analysis for individual 3- and 4-hour time points was not performed because only 1 adenosine-treated animal was still on assist. By 2 hours the adenosine group had recovered function not statistically different from its starting values, whereas the control group remained statistically different from initial values ($p < 0.05$). (C, cannulated, assist started; F, final readings; I, initial; OA, off assist; XCO, cross-clamp off).

(Continued on facing page.)

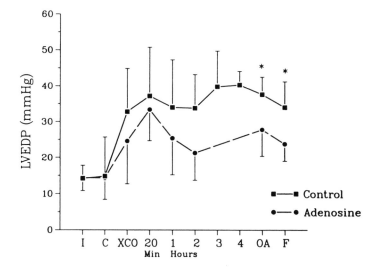

FIGURE 8. *(Continued.)*

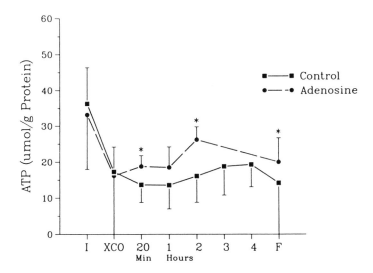

FIGURE 9. Recovery of adenosine triphosphate (ATP): relationship of myocardial ATP versus time for the adenosine and control groups. There was no significant difference between the groups at the start of the experiment or at the end of ischemia. Aggregate postischemic biopsy results in the adenosine group were significantly better than control ($p < 0.03$). Adenosine group samples at 3 and 4 hours were not compared (n = 1). Individual analysis of the 20-minute, 2-hour, and final specimens showed significant differences between the groups. Control ATP value remained less than initial values ($p < 0.05$), whereas final biopsies of adenosine-treated animals were not significantly different. (F, final biopsies; I, initial; XCO, end of 45 minute ischemic period.)

injury. The mechanism postulated for this improvement is that adenosine is extracted from the coronary circulation and used to increase intracellular adenosine nucleotides.

Based on these findings, we are considering a clinical protocol with infusion of adenosine in patients on biventricular support. Adenosine treatment may shorten the time for hemodynamic recovery of injured myocardium as well as decrease the incidence of renal, pulmonary, urologic, and infectious complications that so often intervene and cause death.

EARLY CLINICAL EXPERIENCE
AT ALLEGHENY GENERAL HOSPITAL

The first clinical use of the Bio-Pump for left ventricular assist was undertaken in July 1980 in a 59-year-old woman with triple-vessel coronary artery disease and well-preserved left ventricular function. The patient could not be weaned from cardiopulmonary bypass after double coronary artery bypass grafting (CABG), despite pressor support and IABP. Aortic cross-clamp time was 50 minutes.

Myocardial protection was achieved with moderate systemic hypothermia and 500 cc of cold crystalloid cardioplegia. The Bio-Pump was inserted with cannulas in the common femoral artery using the Gore-Tex side graft to perfuse the lower extremities. The return came from the left ventricle via the right superior pulmonary vein. The assist device was continued for 48 hours without anticoagulation. After removal of the device, postoperative progress was slow but steady, and the patient was discharged on the 46th postoperative day. Congestive heart failure was a recurrent problem at home and required several hospitalizations during the next 4 months. She died suddenly at home 4 months postoperatively.

Since that time, 15,500 adult patients have undergone open-heart surgery at Allegheny General Hospital from May 1980 to July 1991; 77 have required ventricular Bio-Pump support.

CENTRIFUGAL VENTRICULAR ASSIST PROTOCOL

Description of Device System

The ventricular assist device system used at Allegheny General Hospital consists of a commercially available centrifugal vortex pump (Bio-Pump, Biomedicus, Inc., Minnetonka, MN) and standard cannulas and tubing found in routine cardiopulmonary surgery. The system can be used for partial circulatory assist or for total replacement of right and left ventricular function.

For left-heart support, cannulation is achieved via the left atrium through either the atrial appendage or right superior pulmonary vein, with return via a cannula in the aorta. For biventricular assist, the right atrium is cannulated in standard fashion as for cardiopulmonary bypass, with return via the main pulmonary artery. The following equipment and supplies should be available:

1. Biomedicus pump console
2. Biomedicus disposable pump head
3. Biomedicus flow transducer
4. Biomedicus disposable flow probe
5. Sterile 3/8″ × 3/16″ tubing (approximately 10 ft)
6. Tubing clamps (4)
7. Priming solution (typically 3 L of Plasmalyte A)
8. Large sterile basin (5-L capacity)
9. Battery pack
10. Patient management data sheets (appendix)

Indication for Use

The Biomedicus pump is appropriate for use in several different clinical situations: patients unable to be weaned from cardiopulmonary bypass after a technically successful open-heart operation but deemed to have potentially salvageable myocardium; candidates for heart transplantation in cardiogenic shock secondary to idiopathic cardiomyopathy or to AMI; patients with postoperative development of cardiogenic shock after successful surgery with potentially salvageable myocardium; and patients in cardiogenic shock after AMI who are not surgical candidates, but who might have reversibly injured or stunned myocardium.

Contraindications

Contraindications include active systemic infection, chronic debilitating diseases, neurologic impairment, metastatic cancer, no potentially salvageable myocardium, blood dyscrasia, or any problem obviating heart transplantation.

Cannulation for Left Ventricular Assist

The left atrial cannula (usually 32- or 34-Fr Sarns venous cannula) can be placed through either the left atrial appendage, the right superior pulmonary vein, or the roof of the left atrium.

Typically the heart is retracted to expose the left atrial appendage or the right superior pulmonary vein. Pursestring sutures with Teflon pledgets are placed in the base of the appendage or in the right superior pulmonary vein and passed through rubber tourniquets. The left atrial pressure is raised by restricting the venous return, the atrium is opened, and the cannula is inserted. After the left atrial cannula is secured, it is connected to the inflow line of the Bio-Pump. All air must be excluded from the connection and tubing at this time. The aortic cannula previously placed for cardiopulmonary bypass is switched to the outflow line from the Bio-Pump at the appropriate time.

Initiation of Left Ventricular Assist

Cardiopulmonary bypass flow is reduced gradually while the left atrial pressure is monitored by either a left atrial line or pulmonary artery wedge pressure. When the left atrial pressure reaches 20 mmHg, assist flow is initiated. Cardiopulmonary bypass flow is then discontinued, and the venous line is clamped. The aortic arch cannula is clamped, and the cardiopulmonary bypass perfusion line is quickly removed. The Bio-Pump outlet line is then connected to the arch cannula. All air must be excluded from the connection and tubing at this time. Assist flow is initiated and increased incrementally. The total systemic blood flow (native ventricular output + ventricular assist pump flow) is maintained at 2.2 L/min/m². Left atrial pressure or pulmonary artery wedge pressure (PCW) is maintained in the 5–15 mmHg range by volume adjustment.

Most patients have some degree of right-heart failure when the left ventricular assist is initiated. If left ventricular assist pumping cannot maintain a cardiac index of 2.2 L/min/m² with good cannula placement and adequate volume, then right-heart failure is present, and right-heart assist may also be required.

Preparation and priming of the Bio-Pump is completed as previously described. The right atrial cannula placed for cardiopulmonary bypass is connected to the inflow line of the second Bio-Pump. A pulmonary artery catheter (typically 22-Fr Bard right-angle aortic arch cannula) is inserted into the pulmonary artery distal to the pulmonic valve and secured with pursestring sutures. Cannulas are brought out through the superior or inferior aspect of the incision. The skin is approximated while the sternum is not. The perfusion lines are securely sutured to the skin and covered with several towels and a large adhesive plastic drape.

When a patient is on biventricular assist, coordination of the left and right flow rates requires manipulation of the pumps sequentially with close monitoring of the pulmonary artery pressure. The right assist pump is gradually increased, whereas the left pump flow is incrementally raised to accommodate the right-sided output. The right assist pump must unload the right ventricle efficiently for the left assist to pump a minimum of 2.2 L/min/m². Left atrial pressure should be 5–15 mmHg.

Postinsertion Management

During ventricular assist the patient must be constantly attended by a resident in thoracic surgery, two critical care nurses, and one perfusionist. A second perfusionist should be available in the hospital in the event of an emergency.

After arrival in the surgical intensive care unit (SICU), the patient is ventilated with a positive pressure ventilator, using sufficient FiO_2 to keep the arterial PO_2 above 70 mmHg. The electrocardiogram is continually displayed to detect the presence of dysrhythmias and to permit IABP synchronization. Arterial pressure is monitored routinely via a femoral arterial catheter, and left atrial pressure is determined by either a left atrial or Swan-Ganz catheter in the pulmonary wedge position. Cardiac output determinations are performed with the Fick method and by thermodilution when appropriate.

Ideally, during ventricular assist, inotropic drugs should be discontinued for the first 24 hours. Mean arterial pressure is kept at 60–70 mmHg, and SVO_2 is maintained at > 65%.

Table 1 shows the laboratory protocol, which should be ordered as soon as possible after the patient is admitted to the unit. The dynamic nature of the patient on ventricular assist requires that the laboratory work and results be handled on an immediate (STAT) basis.

Anticoagulation Regimen and Coagulopathy

After cardiopulmonary bypass, heparin should be reversed with protamine. After returning to the ICU, the patient is not anticoagulated until clotting studies have normalized, after which he or she is started on heparin to maintain ACTs >150 sec. The perfusionist on duty is responsible for monitoring ACT and determining necessary doses of heparin. If heparin-coated cannulas and tubing are used, no heparin is to be given. Control of nonsurgical bleeding is accomplished by administration of fresh frozen plasma, cryoprecipitate, and platelets to maintain coagulation profiles within normal limits. A disseminated intravascular coagulation (DIC) profile should be obtained, and evidence of DIC, as determined by thrombocytopenia, hypofibrinogenemia, and increase in fibrin split products, should be treated with appropriate blood products.

Weaning of Ventricular Assist

Weaning is usually not attempted during the first 24 hours of assist support. When the clinical picture is stable and cardiac recovery is suspected, a weaning assessment can be completed in 3 minutes or less. Assessment parameters are documented by the perfusionist on duty, as described below. Pump flow is never decreased to <1 L/min. At 1 L/min, the ACT must be >180 seconds, and the

TABLE 1. Postinsertion Laboratory Protocol

1. White blood cell count (WBC)	11. Potassium (K)	22. Serum osmolality
2. Red blood cell count (RBC)	12. Chloride (Cl)	23. Direct bilirubin
3. Hemoglobin (Hgb)	13. Carbon dioxide (CO_2)	24. Aspartate aminotransferase (AST)
4. Hematocrit (Hct)	14. Blood urea nitrogen (BUN)	25. Alanine aminotransferase (ALT)
5. Platelets (Plts)	15. Creatinine (Cr)	26. Lactic dehydrogenase (LDH)
6. Prothrombin time (PT)	16. Glucose	27. Creatinine phosphokinase (CPK)
7. Partial thromboplastin time (PTT)	17. Calcium (Ca)	28. Creatinekinase-MB (CK-MB)
8. Fibrinogen (Fib)	18. PO_4	29. Alkylating phosphate
9. Fibrin split products (FSP)	19. Magnesium (Mg)	30. Gamma-glutamyltranspeptidase (GGTP)
10. Sodium (Na)	20. Total protein	31. Plasma Hgb
	21. Albumin	

Every 4 hr: WBC, RBC, Hgb, Hct, Plts, PT, PTT, Fib, FSP, Plasma Hgb, arterial and mixed venous blood gases. All volume in and out must be documented every 4 hr.

Every 6 hr: Na, K, Cl, BUN, Cr, glucose, Ca, Mg, total protein, albumin, serum osmolality, direct bilirubin, AST, ALT, LDH, CPK, CK-MB, alkylating phosphate, GGTP.

duration of time at this flow must not exceed 2 minutes. If the pump flow is to be kept at 1 L/min for longer than 2 minutes, the ACT must be extended to 200 seconds. BVADs may be weaned concomitantly in the same manner as single assist devices or separately in a stepwise manner.

ASSESSMENT PROCEDURE

Left Ventricular Assist Device.   Assist pump flow should be decreased to a rate that induces a rise in left atrial or PCW pressure to 20–25 mmHg. At the same time, arterial pressure waveform should be recorded and the patient monitored for signs of left ventricular ejection.

Right Ventricular Assist Device.   Assist pump flow should be decreased to a rate that induces a rise in right atrial pressure to 20–25 mmHg. At the same time, the pulmonary artery pressure should be recorded in waveform and the patient monitored for signs of right ventricular ejection.

If, after 1 minute of reduced flow, no native ventricular ejection is evident, the assist pump flow is returned to previous levels. *The combined flow of the native ventricle and the assist pump should always deliver a minimal cardiac index of 2.2 L/min/m².*

If ventricular ejection is noted during weaning, cardiac output should be calculated by both thermodilution and Fick methods. If significant recovery is noted, a transesophageal echocardiography (TEE) should be ordered as a STAT procedure and the patient returned to full VAD support. The TEE should be performed at bedside with the assist pump at a flow of 1 L/min.

Staged weaning is guided by the degree of cardiac recovery as documented by cardiac output and TEE results. If native ventricular output minus assist pump flow is >2.2 L/min and all other patient parameters are stable, a gradual stepdown weaning procedure is instituted. Over 4–8 hours, pump flow is reduced by 1 L every 2 hours until a minimal pump flow of 1 L/min is reached.

At each decrement in flow, cardiac output should be determined and hemodynamic stability assessed. Inotropes are used throughout weaning to maximize ventricular function. When the surgeon determines that the native ventricle can support the required cardiac output, the assist cannulas are removed in the SICU or operating room under strict aseptic technique.

CLINICAL RESULTS

From June 1980 to July 1991, 15,500 patients underwent cardiopulmonary bypass support for cardiac surgery at Allegheny General Hospital. Seventy-seven (0.5%) developed refractory cardiac failure that required extended support with a centrifugal VAD. Of the 77 patients, 37 received a left VAD, 4 a right VAD, and 36 a BVAD. The 52 men and 25 women ranged in age from 34–74 years with an average of 56.5 years.

The primary surgical procedures consisted of 52 coronary revascularizations, 8 valve replacements, 9 combined valve–coronary procedures, 3 combined coronary–left ventricular aneurysmectomy procedures, 2 left ventricular aneurysm resections alone, and 3 miscellaneous cases. Nine patients had undergone previous cardiac surgery. All patients were protected with cold cardioplegic solution, topical Ringer's flush, and systemic hypothermia. Concomitant IABP and pharmacologic support were implemented in all cases. The median sternotomy incision was either left open and packed or sealed with an Esmarck patch. Pump flow rate, which is critically dependent on preload, was manipulated to maintain a cardiac index ≥ 2.2. High flows were maintained not only to unload and rest the ventricle but also to minimize or eliminate the need for heparin. Flows <2 L/min were allowed only intermittently for assessment of ventricular recovery. ACTs were managed between 150–200 seconds. The assist device was implanted in 65 patients immediately after initial surgery and in 12 patients who suffered subsequent hemodynamic deterioration 2–48 hours after surgery.

Overall duration of assist ranged from 6.5–184 hours, with a mean of 52 hours. Average length of assist for LVAD, RVAD, and BVAD were 45, 49, and 60 hours, respectively.

Of the 77 patients, 34 (44%) died on the device (NS = nonsurvivors), 16 (21%) were weaned but died before discharge (STS = short-term survivors), and 27 (35%) were discharged (LTS = long-term survivors). Length of assist was not significantly different among the 3 groups. LTSs were equally distributed among LVADs and BVADs (34% vs. 37%).

Cardiac failure with associated organ failure was the cause of death for all unweanable patients (NS). Four STS patients died of sepsis, 1 patient died from a ruptured infected femoral artery secondary to prior IABP insertion, and the remaining deaths were due to progressive cardiac failure.

Postoperative bleeding, which required frequent reexploration and multiple transfusions, was the primary complication of VAD support (83% of cases). Sepsis was the second most frequent complication, resulting in 3 deaths. Renal dysfunction (creatinine >2.0) occurred in approximately 35% of all patients, but only 7 patients required dialysis while on support (1 LTS, 5 STS, 1 NS). Permanent neurologic deficits were documented in 6 cases (4 LTS, 2 STS). Etiology (embolic or ischemic) could be determined only in 1 early case; it was thought to be embolic because the event occurred shortly after weaning.

Survival was not significantly influenced by age, sex, primary procedure, aortic cross-clamp time, type of assist, length of assist, or complications of VAD support. Survival increased significantly ($p < 0.05$) when analyzed by operative era. From 1980–1984 the survival rate was 25% compared with 45% for 1985 through April 1991. This improvement is attributed to increased physician and perfusionist expertise with the system, more aggressive institution of assist support, and better patient selection.

Of the 27 LTSs, 17 are alive and 10 are dead. The length of hospital stay for LTSs ranged from 15–199 days after weaning. The follow-up period after hospital discharge ranged from 0.14–10.8 years with a mean of 4.0 years. Observation time for the 17 alive patients in follow-up ranges from 0.4–10.8 years with a mean of 5.4 years. The cumulative 5-year survival rate for all discharged survivors is 59%.

Six LTSs died within 1 year after weaning. Before death all 6 patients were New York Heart Association (NYHA) class III. Four NYHA class III patients died late at 3.1, 3.3, 3.4, and 4.5 years. Cardiac failure was responsible for 9 deaths; respiratory failure and pneumonia accounted for the remaining deaths.

Before operation 13 of the 17 alive patients were NYHA class IV, 2 were NYHA class III, and 2 were NYHA class II. Three NYHA class IV patients were in cardiogenic shock, 1 from AMI and 2 from acute failed percutaneous transluminal coronary angioplasties. The latter 3 patients included 2 who were NYHA class II and 1 who was NYHA class I. At follow-up, 14 patients are NYHA class I, 2 are NYHA class II, and 1 is NYHA class III. Ten patients have returned to full working and recreational activities. Four NYHA class I patients are disabled by noncardiac postsurgical sequelae. One LTS patient returned 2 years after VAD support, underwent uneventful reoperative CABG, and is now classified as NYHA class I with no limitations.

A significant number of patients with postcardiotomy ventricular failure have reversible injuries, as demonstrated by our overall salvage rate of 35% (27/77), our long-term survival rate (>3 years) of 67% (18/27), and our 59% cumulative survival rate at 5 years for discharged LTSs. After 10 years of clinical experience with a centrifugal VAD, we have not yet discovered specific variables that predict recovery in a majority of VAD patients. Our experience also supports the long-term efficacy of VAD support for postcardiotomy patients.

Survivors can reasonably expect to have an excellent quality of life. We therefore advocate a continued effort in the development of more effective VADs for application after open-heart surgery.

FUTURE DIRECTIONS

The Allegheny General Hospital ventricular assist program continues to evolve. Most recently, we have used the Medtronic/Carmeda (Minneapolis, MN/ Stockholm, Sweden) extracorporeal membrane oxygenator (ECMO) system in 4 postcardiotomy patients. This system essentially consists of a heparin-coated fiber oxygenator, a disposable biopump, sterile tubing, and various heparin-coated cannulas for the femoral artery or aortic arch and for the femoral vein or right atrium.

In one of the more promising recent breakthroughs in the field of biocompatible materials, Olle Larm, chief chemist at Carmeda, developed a technique to bond heparin covalently to foreign surfaces.[8] Larm noted that the heparin molecule has an active component that must be freely exposed to the blood if the chemical chain reactions that prevent coagulation are to take place. Heparin must stand up from the surface as a result of a covalent binding process known as endpoint attachment.

Heparin is a naturally occurring polysaccharide with an anticoagulant effect due primarily to activation of the enzyme antithrombin. Antithrombin then inactivates thrombin, the enzyme needed in the final pathway for clot formation. The covalent bond developed by Carmeda is situated at the terminal aldehyde group of heparin, allowing the antithrombin binding sites to remain free. Of importance, the process is nonleaching while in contact with blood, saline, or albumin. The resulting surface is stable and thrombin-resistant.

The Allegheny General Hospital group has used the system in treating 4 patients with no device failures. The system effectively decompresses both the left and right sides of the circulation. Cannulas have been inserted via the femoral artery-femoral vein approach as well as through the aortic arch and right atrium. Insertion is not technically difficult. If the device is implanted through the chest, the midsternotomy incision is left open. The femoral approach allows for chest closure. Bleeding has not been a problem, and the oxygenator has been both reliable and effective for nearly 60 hours. The assist device has not required additional heparin, the flow rate has been at least 4 L/min, and the average assist time has been 41 hours. Coagulation profiles, including ACT, platelet count, PTs, PPTs, levels of fibrinogen, and levels of fibrin split products have not demonstrated any damage to blood elements. Of importance, no problem with disseminated intravascular coagulation has occurred.

All 4 patients placed on the device after cardiotomy were successfully weaned. Two of the 4 are considered to be LTSs. Both underwent CABG for cardiogenic shock complicated by AMI. A third patient was placed on the Carmeda system after mitral valve repair and concomitant CABG for severe ischemic mitral regurgitation. Although weaned from the device, the patient ultimately died of cardiac failure. A fourth patient developed acute right-heart failure after heart transplantation. The device was used as a bridge for 48 hours, at which time a second donor heart was procured. The patient ultimately died of right-heart failure.

At this point the clinical indications for use of ECMO are not defined; however, the system appears to have promise in treating patients with postcardiotomy cardiogenic shock. In addition, it may have a role in treating patients suffering from cardiogenic shock after AMI or cardiac or multisystem trauma.

REFERENCES

1. Bernhard WF, Berger RL, Steiz JP, et al: Temporary left ventricular bypass: Factors affecting patient survival. Circulation 60:131, 1979.
2. Braunwald E, Kloner RA: The stunned myocardium: Prolonged, postischemic ventricular dysfunction. Circulation 66:1146–1149, 1982.
3. Cooley DA, Akutsu T, Norman JC, et al: Total artificial heart in two-staged cardiac transplantation. Cardiovasc Dis Bull Texas Heart Inst 8:305, 1981.
4. Demmy TL, Magovern JA, Kao RL, et al: Resuscitation of injured myocardium with adenosine and biventricular assist. Ann Thorac Surg 52:1044–1051, 1991.
5. Dennis C, Hall DP, Moreno JP, et al: Reduction of the oxygen utilization in the heart by left heart bypass. Circ Res 10:298–305, 1962.
6. Dixon CM, Sakert T, Magovern GJ: Improved myocardial preservation with nifedipine cardioplegia. J Extracorpor Technol (in press).
7. Ebert PA, Greenfield LJ, Austen WG, et al: Experimental comparison of methods for protecting the heart during aortic occlusion. Ann Surg 155:25–32, 1962.
8. Arnander C, Olsson P, Larm O: Influence of blood flow and the effect of protamine on the thromboresistant properties of a covalently bonded heparin surface. J Biomed Mater Res 22:859–868, 1988.
9. Liotta D, Hall CW, Walter SH, et al: Prolonged assisted circulation during and after cardiac or aortic surgery: Prolonged partial left ventricular bypass by means of extracorporeal circulation. Am J Cardiol 12:399–405, 1963.
10. Osborn JJ, Cohn K, Hait M et al: Hemolysis during perfusion: Sources and means of reduction. J Thorac Cardiovasc Surg 43:499, 1962.
11. Park SB, Liebler GA, Burkholder JA, et al: Mechanical support of the failing heart. Ann Thorac Surg 42:627–631, 1986.
12. Spencer FC, Eiseman B, Trinkle JK, et al: Assisted circulation for cardiac failure following intracardiac surgery with cardiopulmonary bypass. J Thorac Cardiovasc Surg 49:56–73, 1965.

LI-CHIEN HSU, PhD

DURAFLO II HEPARIN-IMMOBILIZED CARDIOPULMONARY BYPASS CIRCUITS

Li-Chien Hsu, PhD
Senior Baxter Scientist
Bentley Division
Baxter Healthcare Corporation
Irvine, California

Reprint requests to:
Li-Chien Hsu, PhD
Senior Baxter Scientist
Bentley Division
Baxter Healthcare Corporation
17511 Armstrong Avenue
Irvine, CA 92714

For the past decades, extracorporeal blood circulation has been used with increasing frequency for cardiac surgery, hemodialysis, extracorporeal life support, organ transplants, and other procedures. Technical improvements in extracorporeal devices and surgical procedures have significantly reduced the mortality of patients undergoing cardiopulmonary bypass to less than 3%.[26] Despite these improvements, patients undergoing bypass procedures still have associated coagulopathies, increased pulmonary capillary permeability, neurologic disorders, anaphylactic reactions, and to various degrees, renal and other organ dysfunction.[2,6,18,61,62] These profound physiologic effects of bypass procedures have been attributed in large part to the exposure of blood to large areas of synthetic surfaces.

The cardiopulmonary bypass circuit represents the most complex extracorporeal circuit used clinically (Fig. 1). It consists of an oxygenator, blood filters, venous/cardiotomy reservoir, heat exchangers, suction wands, hemoconcentrator, pumps, tubing, connectors, cannulas, and various monitoring devices. The design of some devices has been improved significantly over the years, e.g., from bubble oxygenator, to internal blood-flow hollow-fiber membrane oxygenator, to external blood-flow hollow-fiber oxygenator. However, the materials used in the construction of these devices have essentially remained unchanged. The materials are chosen primarily for their physical properties rather than for biocompatibility. Extracorporeal blood

CARDIAC SURGERY: State of the Art Reviews—Vol. 7, No. 2, 1993
Philadelphia, Hanley & Belfus, Inc.

265

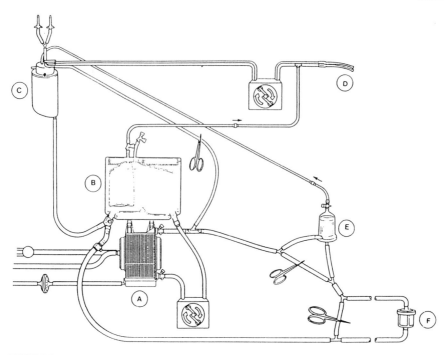

FIGURE 1. Extracorporeal circuit for cardiopulmonary bypass. A: oxygenator; B: venous reservoir; C: cardiotomy reservoir; D: suction wands; E: arterial filter; F: recirculation filter.

circulation cannot be regarded as a physiologic process, as damaging effects always occur.

Numerous efforts have been made in the past to enhance the blood compatibility of synthetic surfaces. These efforts range from "passive" surfaces to surfaces incorporating biologically active substances. Passive properties such as surface morphology, surface texture, electrocharge, and wetability have been found to affect blood compatibility. However, none of these properties or combination thereof has consistently produced thromboresistance. The most thromboresistant surface continues to be the endothelial lining, which is known to provide diverse antithrombotic mechanisms. Active substances involved in the endothelial cell layer include heparan sulfate, thrombomodulin, and prostacyclin (PGI_2), all of which actively interact with circulating blood in response to changes in hemostatic status.[40] A reproduction of endothelial lining on synthetic surfaces continues to be the ultimate goal of biomaterial scientists. It seems that the closer the normal interface between blood and endothelium is reproduced, the more compatible the surface with blood.

Heparin, urokinase, prostacyclin (PGI_2), hirudin, and other biologically active substances have been incorporated onto various synthetic surfaces.[4,10,44] Of the various biologically active substances, heparin is the most popular substance immobilized onto synthetic surfaces. Heparin is a catalytic cofactor that markedly accelerates the action of antithrombin III (AT III) to inactivate several serine proteases of the blood coagulation system. These proteases include thrombin, factor IXa, factor Xa, factor XIa, factor XIIa, factor XIIf, and plasma kallikrein.[8] The catalytic action of heparin allows the heparin molecule to repeat its action on

AT III. In theory, immobilized heparin should have a prolonged activity on the surface compared with other substances that may become inactivated upon blood contact.[41]

Heparin can be immobilized onto synthetic surfaces by physical entrapment or by adsorption, ionic bonding, and covalent bonding. The techniques of heparin coating have been reviewed extensively in the literature.[22,43]

DEVELOPMENT OF HEPARIN-COATED DEVICES

Catheters and Shunts

The original work of heparin coating was that of Gott[13] in preparing a graphite benzalkonium heparin (GBH) surface. Gott's discovery of GBH was a major breakthrough in the development of thromboresistant materials. GBH was initially applied to the polycarbonate housing of a hinged leaflet prosthetic valve[12] and to aneurysm shunts.[50] These coated devices were used in a number of patients with improved clinical results. Grode et al.[15] subsequently eliminated the use of graphite and developed a TDMAC-heparin (tridodecylmethyl ammonium heparin). Various investigational devices coated with TDMAC-heparin were evaluated.[30] In one study, Piepgras[38] showed the absence of thrombus formation on TDMAC-heparin coated silicone shunts for carotid endarterectomy, compared with noncoated shunts, in which they routinely found thrombus deposition during clinical procedures.

Heparin-coated catheters and shunts became commercially available in the early 1980s. Benzalkonium heparin, TDMAC-heparin, and Toray's Anthron[33] heparin coating have been applied to catheters and shunts. Hoar et al.[20] evaluated the thrombogenicity of heparin-coated and noncoated pulmonary-artery catheters in patients undergoing coronary artery bypass surgery. When the catheters were examined during bypass (through an atriotomy), no thrombi were observed on any of the heparin-coated catheters; however, thrombi were found on the surface of all non-heparin-coated catheters. Nichols et al.[35] reported the prevention of fibrin formation and catheter-induced platelet alpha-granule release on heparin-coated catheter surfaces in patients undergoing percutaneous cardiac catheterization. Many catheters and shunts used clinically now are heparin coated. Uncoated catheters continue to have thrombus formation on catheter surfaces in clinical uses.[9,34]

Blood Filters

Filtration of arterial blood is used during cardiopulmonary bypass to prevent the infusion of fibrin clots or microemboli into the patient's circulation. Use of an arterial blood filter has been shown to reduce micro- and macroembolization and to improve neurologic outcomes. On the other hand, platelet depletion, fibrin formation on the filter, and other thromboembolic complications that lead to the occlusion of the filter during CPB have been observed.

Heimbecker et al.[19] demonstrated that an arterial blood filter could be a grave source of platelet and fibrin destruction when the filter was subjected to 3 to 5 LPM of blood flow in the arterial line during clinical cardiopulmonary bypass (CPB). In patients investigated, there was an improvement in platelet counts and a reduction in chest drainage when an arterial filter was not used. It was suggested that this was due to the elimination of a degree of consumptive coagulopathy. Longmore et al.[32] used heparin for anticoagulation during experimental CPB and reported platelet depletion, platelet deposits on the arterial filter, and pressure fluctuations across the filter. The findings suggested that material was periodically being released from the filter. The phenomenon did not occur when both heparin and prostacyclin were used. The observations led Longmore[31] to conclude the following: whereas it is probably malpractice to use arterial line filtration with heparin alone, it may be similarly negligent not to use arterial line filtration when prostacyclin comes into general use. The excessive platelet depletion due to arterial filter led Gervin et al.[11] to suggest the use of an arterial filter to produce acute thrombocytopenia in animals.

The clinical reports led us to evaluate the thrombogenicity of arterial filter materials and to devise methods for improving the thromboresistance of the filter. In an in-vitro blood recirculation loop test and ex-vivo bovine studies, platelet depletion, thrombus formation, and pressure fluctuations across the standard polyester screen filter were observed.[22,23,46] Using a laser light scattering technique, Reynolds et al.[42] demonstrated that thrombi were formed on the filter screen during a period of increasing inlet filter pressure until a sudden decrease in pressure was preceded by a release of thrombi. The pressure fluctuation across a filter observed experimentally and clinically was related to the release of thrombi from the downstream side of the filter.

Arterial filters coated with benzalkonium heparin and TDMAC-heparin were found to have limited thromboresistant properties when they were evaluated in a simulated in-vitro recirculation loop test.[22] The relatively weak ionic bonding between benzalkonium and heparin results in dissolution of the coating material in saline during prime.[36] Because of the instability of benzalkonium-heparin-coated arterial filters, their perceived clinical advantages have been limited to the ease of priming and debubbling. The same in-vitro and ex-vivo tests conducted with filters coated with Duraflo II heparin, after vigorous priming and recirculation, showed a significant improvement in blood compatibility as indicated by improved platelet counts and the absence of thrombus formation or shedding.[21]

Cardiopulmonary Bypass Circuits

The thrombogenicity of cardiopulmonary bypass circuit requires the use of systemic heparin during surgery. Even with heparinized blood, plasma proteins and cells are activated as blood leaves its normal endothelialized vascular channels and enters the bypass circuit. The activated cells and plasma proteins have the capacity to cross-activate one another, act in concert, resulting in a complex array of postoperative sequelae such as coagulopathies, a systemic inflammation-like reaction, and organ dysfunction. These damaging effects of CPB have been collectively termed postpump syndrome or whole body inflammatory response.[5,27,49]

Heparin coating of cardiopulmonary bypass devices and circuits presents specific challenges. Devices such as oxygenator, cardiotomy reservoir, and hemoconcentrator are of complex configuration and have substantial surface areas. The devices are made from a variety of synthetic materials. Heparin coating for CPB circuits must:

- have high affinity for all plastics and metallic materials
- retain biologic activities of heparin on the surfaces
- be stable in crystalloid solution and other physiological solutions
- have low toxicity
- not de-laminate or generate particular matters in high flow conditions
- not effect the performance characteristics of the devices
- be applicable to complex devices such as cardiotomy reservoir.

Based on these considerations, a heparin-coating system applicable to CPB circuits was developed. The coating system, tradenamed Duraflo II, consists of unfractionated USP heparin and a hydrophobic binding agent. The binding agents are incorporated into the structure of heparin in such a way that the modification affects the physicochemical but not biologic properties of heparin. A sub-micro-thin layer of coating material can be applied to virtually all surfaces. Duraflo II heparin has been applied to the entire CBP circuit, including oxygenators, cardiotomy reservoirs, blood filters, hemoconcentrators, tubing, connectors, and cannulas.

EXPERIMENTAL EVALUATION OF DURAFLO II HEPARIN-COATED EXTRACORPOREAL CIRCUITS

The thromboresistance of Duraflo II coated surfaces has been evaluated extensively. In-vitro tests using freshly-drawn heparinized blood have shown reduced platelet depletion and platelet adhesion, reduced thrombus formation and thromboemboli shedding, and lower fibrinogen adsorption on Duraflo II-coated surfaces compared with noncoated control surfaces.[23,24,42]

The Duraflo II heparin-coated CPB circuit was compared with an noncoated control circuit using a calf model under simulated clinical conditions.[47] The activated clotting times (ACT) were maintained above 480 seconds for both groups. Better preserved platelet counts and platelet function, and lower fibrino-peptide A generation were observed in the heparin-coated group relative to the control group. Heparin-coated arterial filters were free of thrombus formation, whereas two of the five noncoated filters developed extensive clotting shortly after the initiation of bypass. Palatianos et al.[37] evaluated the heparin-coated CPB circuit in conjunction with Iloprost using a pig model and found better preserved platelets and reduced platelet adhesion in the oxygenator of the heparin-coated group. Taylor,[45] in a canine study, found substantially reduced white cell activation and sequestration in lung with the Duraflo II-coated circuit.

With the use of Duraflo II heparin-coated circuits, investigations have been made into the reduction and elimination of systemic heparin during CPB, extracorporeal membrane oxygenation (ECMO), and continuous arteriovenous hemofiltration (CAVH). von Segesser et al.[55] evaluated the performance characteristics of heparin-coated oxygenators in an open-chest dog model without systemic anticoagulation. The results were compared with those from noncoated membrane and bubble oxygenators with standard systemic heparinization (300 units/kg). Lower hemolysis and higher platelet counts were noted in the heparin-coated group. The heparin-coated oxygenators performed well throughout the 6 hours of bypass. When heparin-coated oxygenators were replaced with noncoated control oxygenators, major clotting occurred. von Segesser et al.[53,54] also evaluated the heparin-coated cardiotomy reservoir and heparin-coated hemofilter using a calf model without the use of systemic anticoagulant. In both cases, heparin-coated devices performed significantly better than the corresponding noncoated devices.

Toomasian et al.[48] evaluated Duraflo II-coated ECMO circuits with heparinless sheep for 96 hours without complications. The oxygenators performed well throughout the test period. Small amounts of clots were, however, noted in areas of blood stagnation. von Segesser et al.[56] performed prolonged CPB (24 hours) without systemic heparinization in an open-chest dog model with the heparin-coated circuits and observed a reduced level of plasma free hemoglobin and improved platelet preservation in the heparin-coated group.

A bifurcation circuit, in which a heparin-coated device and a noncoated device were connected in parallel, was used to evaluate the effectiveness of the heparin treatment ex vivo. The experimental design minimizes the animal-to-animal variation and allows direct comparison between the two devices under identical testing conditions. In one set of experiments, venous blood from a fully heparinized calf (ACT >600 sec) was bifurcated into two membrane oxygenators with integrated cardiotomy reservoirs: one control and one heparin coated. Both control and coated oxygenators were stressed by purging large quantities of air into the open-shell reservoirs throughout the 6-hours of venoarterial bypass. Postbypass examination of the oxygenators indicated that, despite the extensive blood-air interactions, few thrombi were noted in the reservoir of the coated device, whereas extensive red thrombi were observed on the heat exchanger, defoamers, and reservoir housing of the noncoated oxygenator. In a similar set of bifurcation ex-vivo bovine experiments with ACT reduced to 240 sec, extensive clots were noted on the hollow-fiber membrane of the noncoated oxygenator; whereas the heparin-coated oxygenator was free of thrombus formation.[22]

Using a bifurcated circuit of similar design, we have evaluated the relative efficacy of Duraflo II-coated and noncoated Avercor/SciMed solid silicone membrane oxygenators (model 0600) at a low-dose heparin (ACT = 180 sec) and without systemic anticoagulant in a bovine model.[26] Pressure differentials across the oxygenators and oxygen transfer properties were monitored. In all cases, the noncoated silicone oxygenators developed high inlet pressure shortly after the

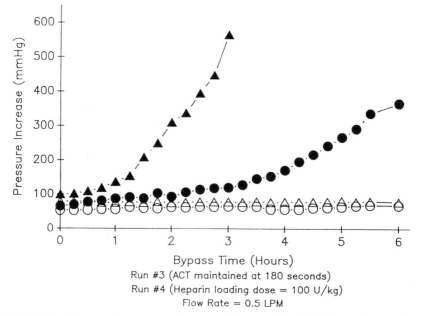

FIGURE 2. Comparative pressure increases between Duraflo II heparin-coated and noncoated Avercor/SciMed silicone membrane oxygenators in bovine bifurcation studies (ACT = 180 sec); blood flow rate = 0.5 L/min each.

Run 3: Noncoated ●——●   Duraflo II ○——○
Run 4: Noncoated ▲——▲   Duraflo II △——△

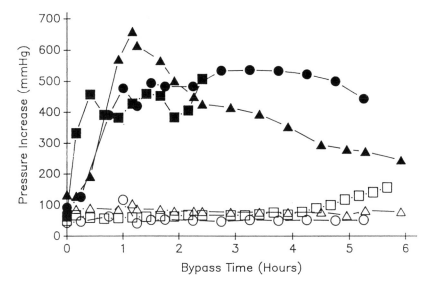

FIGURE 3. Comparative pressure increases between Duraflo II heparin-coated and noncoated Avecor/SciMed silicone membrane oxygenators in bovine heparinless bifurcation studies; blood flow rate = 0.96 L/min each.

Run 1: Noncoated ●━━━●   Duraflo II ○━━━○
Run 2: Noncoated ■━━━■   Duraflo II □━━━□
Run 3: Noncoated ▲━━━▲   Duraflo II △━━━△

initiation of bypass. The pressure increase was accompanied by a rapid loss of gas transfer. On the other hand, the heparin-coated silicone oxygenators exhibited little increase in pressure and maintained the gas transfer properties throughout the bypass period. Figures 2 and 3 show the relative increases in inlet pressure of the oxygenators under low and no systemic anticoagulation, respectively, in the bifurcation studies. Extensive clots were observed in the noncoated oxygenators after six hours of bypass.

The effectiveness of Duraflo II heparin-coated and noncoated hemofilters was evaluated using bilateral circuits in a heparinless sheep model.[46] The heparin treatment did not change the mass transfer properties of the hemofilter. The improved blood compatibility due to the heparin treatment was demonstrated by the significant reduction in thrombus formation, prolonged work life in a continuous arteriovenous hemofiltration mode, and superior performance in heparinless sheep. The stability of Duraflo II heparin on the hemofilter in plasma was further assessed by using radioactively-labeled Duraflo II heparin. The total amounts of heparin detected in circulating plasma at 1 hour, 20 hours, and 68 hours were 60 units (7% of total), 140 units (17%), and 220 units (27%), respectively. The relative thrombus formation on a coated hemofilter and a noncoated hemofilter after 24 hours of heparinless arteriovenous hemofiltration is shown in Figure 4.

The overall experimental results support the thromboresistant properties of the Duraflo II heparin-coated devices and circuits. Reduced coagulation activation or thrombus formation, improved platelet function and preservation, and reduced hemolysis are frequently observed. The performance characteristics of various

Arterial End

Control   D - II

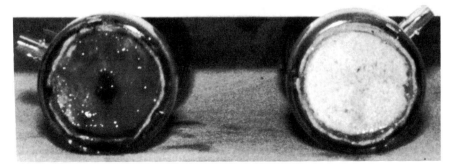

FIGURE 4. Duraflo II coated and noncoated control hemofilters after heparinless CAVH in a sheep model using bilateral circuits. (From: Tong SD, et al: ASAIO Trans 38:702–706, 1992, with permission.)

devices, including gas transfer properties of oxygenators,[3] defoaming capability of cardiotomy reservoir, filtration efficiency of blood filters, and clearance rates or ultrafiltration rates of hemofilter are not affected by the heparin treatment. The experimental results further suggest that, with the use of heparin-coated circuits, it is possible to reduce or eliminate the use of systemic anticoagulant and, thus, reduce surgical bleeding. Clotting may, however, occur in areas of blood stagnation during prolonged heparinless bypass. This finding is not unexpected, as stagnant blood clots even on undamaged endothelial-lined surfaces.

CLINICAL APPLICATIONS OF DURAFLO II
HEPARIN-COATED CPB CIRCUITS
Duraflo II heparin-coated bypass circuits have been used clinically for patients undergoing CPB with varying levels of systemic heparin. Heparinless bypass has also been performed on patients with high bleeding potentials.

Gu et al.[17] compared the heparin-coated and noncoated circuits in a group of 30 patients undergoing elective coronary artery bypass grafting. All patients received a standard dose of heparin (300 units/kg). Significantly lower thrombin-antithrombin (TAT) level was observed throughout the bypass period in the Duraflo II group. Reduced complement activation (C3a level), elastase release, and lower tumor necrosis factor after administration of protamine were also observed in the Duraflo II group.[16] The results thus suggest the inhibition of coagulation activation and reduction in complement and leukocyte activation. The postoperative bleeding was lower in the Duraflo II group, but the difference was not statistically significant. Cohen[7] compared the heparin coated and noncoated control circuits in a group of 56 patients undergoing CPB. The total postoperative chest drainage volume was less in the Duraflo II group (1020 ± 395 ml) compared with the control (1402 ± 877 ml). Pradhan et al.[39] in a similar study also found a reduction in TAT complex in the Duraflo II patient group. No differences in retinal microembolization between control and heparin-coated groups were observed. Gravlee et al.[14] found no differences in bleeding, fibrinopeptide A, and beta-thromboglobulin. All these studies involve the use of a traditional level of systemic heparin with ACT maintained at greater than 480 sec. Because of the unavailability of heparin-coated cardiotomy reservoir at the time of these studies, either a noncoated cardiotomy reservoir or an autotransfusion device was used in the studies.

von Segesser et al.[51,57] used the heparin-coated circuits with substantially reduced systemic anticoagulation levels in over 100 patients and found significantly reduced blood loss and blood transfusion requirements. In one study,[59] patients undergoing coronary artery revascularization were randomly divided into a low systemic heparinization group (total heparin loading 8041 ± 1247 units; ACT >180 sec) and a full systemic heparinization group (total heparin loading 52,500 ± 17,100 units; ACT >480 sec). The low-dose systemic heparin resulted in reduced protamine requirements, reduced blood loss, and reduced blood transfusion requirements (Fig. 5). The D-dimer levels were found to be significantly lower in the low-dose heparin group. No macroscopic clots were noted in any of the devices. To avoid blood stagnation in the low-dose group, a shunt was used to recirculate blood between arterial and venous lines immediately after weaning from bypass.

Based on this experience, von Segesser et al.[58] successfully performed coronary artery revascularization in patients who refused any transfusion of blood products (Jehovah's witnesses) using heparin-coated bypass circuits and low systemic heparin. Partial cardiopulmonary bypass with heparin-coated circuits and low systemic heparinization has also been used on patients with aneurysms of the descending thoracic aorta and thoraco-abdominal aorta.[60] These procedures with low systemic heparin were performed without the use of a cardiotomy reservoir, and an autotransfusion device was used to handle the shed blood.

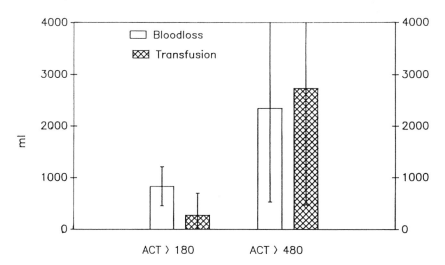

FIGURE 5. A comparison between low level (ACT >180 seconds) and normal level (ACT >480 seconds) systemic anticoagulation in patients undergoing coronary revascularization with Duraflo II heparin coated circuits. (From von Segesser LK, et al: J Thorac Cardiovasc Surg 103:790–799, 1992, with permission.)

Similar improvements in blood loss and transfusion requirements were found in recent clinical procedures with the heparin-coated circuit including coated cardiotomy reservoir.[51] Ahlvin et al.[1] found that the heparin-coated cardiotomy reservoirs performed satisfactorily at reduced systemic heparinization (ACT = 200–250 sec) on 33 patients undergoing coronary artery grafting, resection of aneurysms, valve replacements, and other procedures. No problems related to the techniques of cardiopulmonary bypass with low systemic heparinization were experienced. The postoperative blood loss was reported to be low.

Laub et al.[29] reported a heparinless ECMO case using a Duraflo II-coated circuit on a patient with intractable postoperative cardiopulmonary failure. A heparinless cardiopulmonary bypass was also performed on a patient with accidental deep hypothermia and cardiorespiratory arrest.[52] Both patients survived. No macroscopic clots were found in the bypass circuits.

Clinical extracorporeal CO_2 removal ($ECCO_2R$) procedures have been performed with low or no systemic heparin on patients with acute respiratory failure (ARF) using heparin-coated circuits. Because patients with ARF often have multiple trauma with bleeding complications, the use of heparin-coated extracorporeal circuits appears to have significant advantages. Clinical experience with the use of heparin-coated circuits for prolonged bypass does seem to confirm the advantages of reduced blood loss and blood transfusion requirements.[28] However, since only microporous membrane oxygenators are heparin-coated at this time, plasma leakage may occur during prolonged extracorporeal blood circulation. The need for replacing the oxygenator presents considerable clinical problems, particularly in infants and children. The development of heparin-coated nonporous membrane oxygenators would be highly desirable.

Experimental and clinical results suggest that heparin coating improves the blood compatibility of extracorporeal circuits by minimizing blood trauma caused by blood-material interactions. The use of heparin-coated circuits also allows the modification of systemic anticoagulation, which may result in reduced blood loss and blood transfusion requirements. It is believed that the transition to blood-compatible extracorporeal circuits will continue and that the circuits will contribute to the overall safety of extracorporeal procedures.

REFERENCES

1. Ahlvin E, Thorno E, Hagman L, Thelin S: Experimental and clinical experience with a heparin-coated cardiotomy reservoir and reduced systemic heparinization. Pathophysiology and Techniques of Cardiopulmonary Bypass. San Diego, CA, Cardiothoracic Research and Education Foundation, 1993, p 172.
2. Blauth CI, Arnold JV, Schulenberg WE, et al: Cerebral microembolism during cardiopulmonary bypass. J Thorac Cardiovasc Surg 95:668–676, 1988.
3. Boonstra PW, Akkerman C, Tigchelaar I, et al: Heparin surface treatment does not impair gas and heat transfer of an extracorporeal circuit. Perfusion 7:109–114, 1992.
4. Breillat J, Johnson RJ, Ku C, et al: Recombinant hirudin analog designed for attachment to polymers. FASEB J 6:A1320, 1992.
5. Butler J, Rocker GM, Westaby S: Inflammatory response to cardiopulmonary bypass. Ann Thorac Surg 55:552–559, 1993.
6. Chenoweth DE, Cooper SW, Hugli TE, et al: Complement activation during cardiopulmonary bypass: Evidence for generation of C3a and C5a anaphylatoxins. N Engl J Med 304:497–503, 1981.
7. Cohen S: Reduction in post-operative bleeding: Use of Duraflo II-treated circuit. Clinical studies. Lake Tahoe, CA, AmSECT Region X Meeting, October 1990.
8. Colman RW, Scott CF, Pixley RA, Cadena RA: Effect of heparin on the inhibition of contact enzymes. Ann NY Acad Sci 556:95–103, 1989.

9. Donefan JH, Rupp S: Should multiorifaced central venous catheters be heparin bonded? Anesthesiology 68:178–179, 1988.
10. Ebert CD, Lee LS, Kim SW: The antiplatelet activity of immobilized prostacyclin. J Biomed Mater Res 16:629–638, 1982.
11. Gervin AS, Manson K, Limbird T, Silver D: Ultrapore filter-induced thrombocytopenia. Surgery 75:566–572, 1974.
12. Gott VL, Daggett RL, Whiffen JD, et al: A hinged-leaflet valve for total replacement of the human aortic valve. J Thorac Cardiovasc Surg 48:713–725, 1964.
13. Gott VL, Whiffen JD, Dutton RC: Heparin coating on colloidal graphite surfaces. Science 142:1297–1298, 1963.
14. Gravlee GP, Phipps J, Mills SA, et al: Hematologic evaluation of a heparin-coated circuit for cardiopulmonary bypass [abstract]. Anesthesiology 77:A99, 1992.
15. Grode GA, Anderson SG, Grotta HM, Falb RD: Nonthrombogenic material via a simple coating process. ASAIO Trans 15:1–5, 1969.
16. Gu YJ, van Oeveren W, Akkerman C, et al: Reduction of inflammatory response during cardiopulmonary bypass by the use of heparin-coated extracorporeal circuit. Ann Thorac Surg (in press).
17. Gu YJ, van Oeveren W, van der Kamp KWHJ, et al: Heparin-coating of extracorporeal circuits reduced thrombin formation in patients undergoing cardiopulmonary bypass. Perfusion 6:221–225, 1991.
18. Hashimoto K, Miyamoto H, Suzuki K, et al: Evidence of organ damage after cardiopulmonary bypass. J Thorac Cardiovasc Surg 104:666–673, 1992.
19. Heimbecker R, Rober A, McKenzie FN: The extracorporeal pump filter—saint or sinner? Ann Thorac Surg 21:55–58, 1976.
20. Hoar PF, Wilson RM, Mangano DT, et al: Heparin bonding reduces thrombogenicity of pulmonary-artery catheters. N Engl J Med 305:993–995, 1981.
21. Hsu LC: Duraflo II heparin-treated extracorporeal devices. Proc Am Acad Cardiovasc Perfusion 13:135–139, 1992.
22. Hsu LC: Heparin-coating of bypass circuits: Principles of heparin-coating techniques. Perfusion 6:209–219, 1991.
23. Hsu LC, Loar ME, Tong SD: Thromboresistant properties of surface modified arterial filter materials. Trans Soc Biomater 14:112, 1991.
24. Hsu LC, Tong SD: Evaluation of thromboresistant properties of Duraflo II heparin coated membrane oxygenator materials. Trans Soc Biomater 13:99, 1990.
25. Hsu LC, Tong SD, Patterson WR: A direct method for evaluation of ECMO circuit. Chicago, IL, ASAIO Abstracts, 1991, p 61.
26. Kirklin JK: Prospect for understanding and eliminating the deleterious effects of cardiopulmonary bypass. Ann Thorac Surg 51:529–531, 1991.
27. Kirklin JK, Westaby S, Blackstone EH, et al: Complement and the damaging effects of cardiopulmonary bypass. J Thorac Cardiovasc Surg 86:845–857, 1983.
28. Knoch M, Kollen B, Dietrich G, et al: Progress in veno-venous long-term bypass techniques for the treatment of ARDS. Int J Artif Organs 15:103–108, 1992.
29. Laub GW, Muralidharan S, Clancy R, et al: Use of ECMO for intractable cardiopulmonary failure [abstract]. San Francisco, CA, Circulatory Support, 1991.
30. Leininger RI, Crowley JP, Falb RD, Grode GA: Three years' experience in-vivo and in-vitro with surfaces and devices treated by the heparin complex method. ASAIO Trans 18:312–315, 1972.
31. Longmore DB: The value of prostacyclin in cardiopulmonary bypass. In Longmore DB (ed): Towards Safer Cardiac Surgery. Boston, G.K. Hall, 1981, pp 355–377.
32. Longmore DB, Bennet G, Gueirrara D, et al: Prostacyclin: A solution to some problems of extracorporeal circulation. Lancet 1:1002–1005, 1979.
33. Miyama H, Harymiya N, Mori Y, Tanzawa H: A new antithrombogenic heparinized polymer. J Biomed Mat Res 11:251–265, 1977.
34. Mollitt DL, Golladay ES: Complications of TPN catheter-induced vena caval thrombosis in children less than one year of age. J Pediatr Surg 18:462, 1983.
35. Nichols AB, Owen J, Grossman A, et al: Effect of heparin bonding on catheter-induced fibrin formation and platelet activation. Circulation 70:843–849, 1984.
36. Palanzo DA, Kurusz M, Butler B: Surface tension effects of heparin coating on arterial line filters. Perfusion 5:277–284, 1990.
37. Palatianos GM, Dewanjee MK, Smith W, et al: Platelet preservation during cardiopulmonary bypass with Iloprost and Duraflo II heparin-coated surfaces. ASAIO Trans 37:620–622, 1991.

38. Piepgras DG, Sundt TM: Clinical and laboratory experience with heparin-impregnated silicone shunts for carotid endarterectomy. Ann Surg 184:637–641, 1976.
39. Pradhan MJ, Fleming JS, Nkere UU, et al: Clinical experience with heparin-coated cardiopulmonary bypass circuits. Perfusion 6:235–242, 1991.
40. Preissner KT: Physiological role of vessel wall related antithrombotic mechanisms: Contribution of endogenous and exogenous heparin-like components to the anticoagulant potential of the endothelium. Hemostasis 20(Suppl 1):30–49, 1990.
41. Remy MH, Poznansy MJ: Immunogenicity and antigenicity of soluble crosslinked enzyme/albumin polymers. Lancet 2:68, 1978.
42. Reynolds L, Clark R, Drumm G: In-vitro efficacy test for arterial filter materials. Trans Soc Biomater 11:115, 1985.
43. Sefton MV, Cholakis CH, Llanos G: Preparation of nonthrombogenic materials by chemical modification. In Williams DF (ed): Blood Compatibility. Boca Raton, FL, CRC Press, 1987, pp 151–198.
44. Senatore FF, Bernath FR, Meisner K: Clinical study of urokinase-bound fibrinocollagenous tubes. J Biomed Mater Res 20:177, 1986.
45. Taylor KM: Personal communication.
46. Tong SD, Hsu LC: Nonthrombogenic hemofiltration system for acute renal failure treatment. ASAIO Trans 38:M702–M706, 1992.
47. Tong SD, Rolfs MR, Hsu LC: Evaluation of Duraflo II heparin immobilized cardiopulmonary bypass circuits. ASAIO Trans 36:654–656, 1990.
48. Toomasian JM, Hsu LC, Hirschl RB, et al: Evaluation of Duraflo II heparin coating in prolonged extracorporeal membrane oxygenation. ASAIO Trans 34:410–414, 1988.
49. Utley JR: Pathophysiology of cardiopulmonary bypass: Current issues. J Cardiac Surg 5:177–188, 1990.
50. Valiathan MS, Weldon CS, Bender CS, et al: Resection of aneurysms of the descending thoracic aorta using a GBH-coated shunt bypass. J Surg Res 8:197–205, 1968.
51. von Segesser LK: Cardiopulmonary bypass with low or no systemic heparin. The 23rd Annual Meeting of the Japanese Society for Cardiovascular Surgery, March 3–5, 1993, Fukuoka, Japan.
52. von Segesser LK, Garcia E, Turina M: Perfusion without systemic heparinization in accidental hypothermia. Ann Thorac Surg 52:560–561, 1991.
53. von Segesser LK, Pasic M, Leskosek B, et al: Heparin coated cardiotomy reservoirs with improved thromboresistance: Experimental evaluation ex-vivo. Les Cahiers du CECEC 36:9–16, 1991.
54. von Segesser LK, Pasic M, Olah A, et al: Performance characteristics of hemofilters with heparin surface coating: An experimental study. J Extracorp Technol 24:81–85, 1992.
55. von Segesser LK, Turina M: Cardiopulmonary bypass without systemic heparinization. J Thorac Cardiovasc Surg 98:386–396, 1989.
56. von Segesser L, Turina M: Long-term cardiopulmonary bypass without systemic heparinization. Int J Artif Organs 13:687–691, 1990.
57. von Segesser LK, Weiss BM, Garcia E, et al: Reduced blood loss and transfusion requirements with low systemic heparinization: Preliminary clinical results in coronary artery revascularization. Eur J Cardiothorac Surg 4:639–643, 1990.
58. von Segesser LK, Weiss BM, Garcia E, Turina M: Clinical application of heparin-coated perfusion equipment with special emphasis on patients refusing homologous transfusions. Perfusion 6:227–233, 1991.
59. von Segesser LK, Weiss BM, Garcia E, Turina M: Perfusion with low systemic heparinization during resection of descending thoracic aortic aneurysms. Eur J Cardiothorac Surg 6:246–250, 1992.
60. von Segesser LK, Weiss BM, Garcia E, et al: Reduction and elimination of systemic heparinization during cardiopulmonary bypass. J Thorac Cardiovasc Surg 103:790–799, 1992.
61. Wenger RK, Lukasiewicz H, Mikuta BS, et al: Loss of fibrinogen receptors during cardiopulmonary bypass. J Thorac Cardiovasc Surg 97:235–239, 1989.
62. Woodman RC, Harker LA: Bleeding complications associated with cardiopulmonary bypass. Blood 76:1680–1697, 1990.

THOMAS X. AUFIERO, MD
WALTER E. PAE, JR, MD

EXTRACORPOREAL PNEUMATIC VENTRICULAR ASSISTANCE FOR POSTCARDIOTOMY CARDIOGENIC SHOCK

From the Department of Surgery
Division of Cardiothoracic Surgery
The Pennsylvania State University
The Milton S. Hershey Medical Center
Hershey, Pennsylvania

Reprint requests to:
Walter E. Pae, Jr., MD
Department of Surgery
Division of Cardiothoracic Surgery
The Pennsylvania State University
The Milton S. Hershey Medical Center
Hershey, PA 17033

Significant advances continue to be made in techniques for myocardial preservation and perioperative management of the cardiac surgical patient. Nonetheless, postcardiotomy cardiogenic shock (PCCS) continues to occur in 2–6% of all patients undergoing myocardial revascularization or valvular heart surgery.[10] Prompt institution of intraaortic balloon pumping (IABP) and appropriate inotropic and vasodilatory support allow 80% of these patients to be weaned from cardiopulmonary bypass (CPB), with a hospital survival of 50%.[3,12] Therefore, approximately 1% of patients undergoing open-heart surgery are refractory to such therapy; for this group, more aggressive forms of circulatory support have been employed.[11] For example, temporary mechanical ventricular assistance has provided support of systemic and/or pulmonary circulation while unloading the depressed myocardium. By decreasing myocardial oxygen consumption, circulatory support may allow time for the metabolic recovery of so-called stunned myocardium. At the same time, systemic perfusion and end-organ function are maintained. Various devices have been proposed to this end. Reasonable clinical experience has been obtained with three types of assist pumps: (1) roller; (2) centrifugal (Vortex); and (3) pulsatile pneumatic. Recently, limited experience has been obtained with transvascular, Archemede's screw-type devices. The comparative features of these devices are outlined in Table 1.

TABLE 1.   Comparison of Pulsatile, Centrifugal, and Roller Pump Systems

System Type	Advantages	Disadvantages
Pulsatile device	Decreased risk of thromboembolic event Little or no anticoagulation required Little or no hemolysis occurs Good long-term support performance	IDE required Expensive system
Centrifugal pump (Vortex)	Relatively inexpensive User familiarity Readily available	Questionable long-term performance Risk of hemolysis Heparin requirement uncertain Continuous pump control required
Roller pump	Relatively inexpensive User familiarity Readily available	Poor long-term performance Risk of hemolysis Heparin required Continuous pump control required

IDE = investigational device exemption, required from the FDA before clinical application.

Currently, two types of external pneumatic pulsatile pumps are available: The Pierce-Donachy pulsatile ventricular assist pump and the Abiomed Pump (Abiomed Cardiovascular, Inc., Danvers, MA). The Abiomed BVS System 5000 has been used clinically in a small group of patients. Recently, Jett reported its use in 7 patients, 3 of whom had PCCS.[4] Most of our experience has been with the Pierce-Donachy pump; we await further reports from investigators using the Abiomed pump. The Pierce-Donachy pump, developed at the Pennsylvania State University, has been used clinically for more than 15 years. Its use is still limited because an investigational device exemption from the Food and Drug Administration (FDA) is required. However, its advantages are significant: decreased need for systemic anticoagulation, less trauma to formed blood elements, and longer-term support capabilities. Effective support of both systemic and pulmonary circulations has been demonstrated clinically.[8,9]

POSTCARDIOTOMY CARDIOGENIC SHOCK

Profound refractory heart failure is a cause of death after 1% of technically successful open-heart operations, despite conventional medical therapy and attempts at support with IABP. When a patient is unable to be weaned from CPB, accurate hemodynamic monitoring is instituted, including right atrial pressure (RAP), pulmonary artery pressure (PAP), left atrial pressure (LAP), and aortic pressure (AoP). A means for accurately determining cardiac output is also necessary to make accurate decisions about each subsequent intervention (Table 2). Patients with a cardiac index (CI) $<1.8–2.0$ L/min/m^2, an LAP >18 mmHg, an RAP <15 mmHg, and a systolic AoP <90 mmHg, despite conventional therapy, are candidates for left ventricular assistance.

TABLE 2.   Guidelines for Assist Device Insertion

Device	RAP (mmHg)	LAP (mmHg)	AoP Sys (mmHg)	CI (L/min/m^2
LVAD	<15	>25	<90	$<1.8–2.0$
RVAD	>25	<15	<90	$<1.8–2.0$

LVAD = left ventricular assist device; RVAD = right ventricular assist device; RAP = right atrial pressure; LAP = left atrial pressure; AoP Sys = systolic aortic pressure; CI = cardiac index.

Similarly, right ventricular failure is evidenced by a CI <1.8–2.0 $L/min/m^2$ and an LAP <15 mmHg despite an RAP ≥25 mmHg. Right ventricular failure is manifest as pulmonary blood flow that is insufficient to provide adequate preload to the left ventricle. Right ventricular failure may occur as an isolated event and may not be evident until left ventricular assistance unmasks right ventricular failure. Less significant right ventricular failure may be managed initially by correcting acidosis, hypoxia, and hypercarbia, in an attempt to lower pulmonary vascular resistance. Additionally, pharmacologic support of the right ventricle and lowering of pulmonary vascular resistance can be modulated with amrinone[2] or prostaglandin E1.[1] Pulmonary artery balloon counterpulsation has generally not been successful. If these methods fail, mechanical circulatory support is certainly indicated. Once ventricular failure has been determined to be refractory, further delays in the institution of ventricular support are only detrimental, prolonging CPB at the risk of well-known sequelae such as multiple organ failure and bleeding complications.

VENTRICULAR ASSIST SYSTEM AND INSERTION TECHNIQUES

The Pierce-Donachy pulsatile ventricular assist pump, developed and employed by the Pennsylvania State University, is an extracorporeally placed, pneumatically driven device (Fig. 1). A flexible, seam-free blood sac of segmented polyurethane is enclosed within a rigid polysulfone outer case. The inner chamber of the case has the shape of an oblate sphenoid. A flexible diaphragm separates the driveline inlet port from the thin-walled blood sac. Pumping is activated by pulses of compressed carbon dioxide introduced between the pump housing and the flexible diaphragm from an external power source through a 2-meter polyvinyl chloride tube.

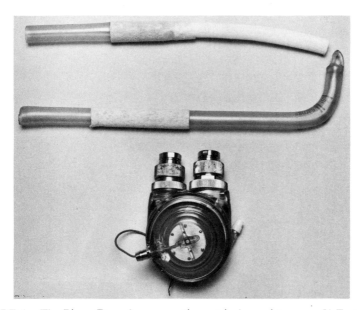

FIGURE 1.   The Pierce-Donachy pneumatic ventricular assist pump, 51-Fr angled left atrial cannula, and composite aortic cannula.

Unidirectional flow of blood through the blood sac is ensured by inlet and outlet tilting disk valves constructed of Derlin. The stroke volume is approximately 70 cc.

For left ventricular assistance, a 51-Fr, angled, lighthouse-tipped, polyurethane-coated cannula (Sarns 3M) is used to remove blood from the left atrium. Blood is returned to the ascending aorta through a composite segmented polyurethane, 14-mm, woven Dacron graft sutured directly to the ascending aorta. Right ventricular assistance is accomplished by cannulating the right atrium and pulmonary artery in a similar fashion. These cannulas exit through stab wounds created below the costal margins. The pump housing itself lies outside the body on the anterior abdominal wall and is connected to the power console by means of a vinyl driveline and a wire from a Hall effect switch. This switch, located between the rigid housing and diaphragm, detects complete pump filling. The control panel of the drive unit (Fig. 2) has adjustments to control both systolic driveline pressure and diastolic vacuum. In addition to manual rate control, the duration of the systolic pulse can be adjusted also. A monitoring port spliced into the driveline allows the airwave to be observed and thus confirms both complete filling and complete emptying of the pump. The flexible control unit allows the device to be run in a fixed-rate manual mode, full-to-empty automatic mode, and R-wave synchronous mode for counterpulsation.

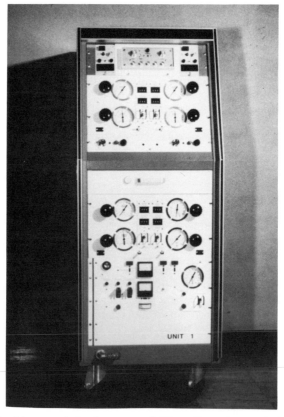

FIGURE 2.   The drive console for the pneumatic Pierce-Donachy ventricular assist device.

Because a diastolic vacuum is employed almost routinely to balance pump filling, the presence of a patent foramen ovale (PFO) is associated with a marked right-to-left shunt.[5] Therefore, before instituting support in our early experiences, we placed two venous cannulas to allow for atriotomy and visualization of the foramen. We now determine patency of the foramen by palpation through a pursestring suture in the right atrium or via transesophageal Doppler echocardiography, both of which allow more rapid employment of the assist device. Obviously, if a PFO exists, it must be closed.

Pump insertion is begun by creating the tunnels from the mediastinum to the upper abdomen. Two concentric felt-backed pursestring sutures are then placed in the left atrium, either at the base of the left atrial appendage, between the right superior and right inferior pulmonary veins, or in the roof of the left atrium (Fig. 3). A stab wound is made in the atrium and dilated with a finger or a Hegar dilator. The 51-Fr lighthouse cannula is then inserted to a depth of 3 cm, with the tip directed toward the mitral valve. Position can be optimized and confirmed by transesophageal echocardiography. The pursestrings are tightened with long rummel keepers and then tied over polypropylene buttons, thus negating the need for new pursestrings when the device is removed. The composite graft is anastomosed to the ascending aorta. The cannulas are brought through the skin and connected to the pump (Fig. 4). Small amounts of air remaining in the pump are removed by clamping the Dacron portion of the outflow graft and inserting an 18-gauge needle. Pumping at a slow rate with the inflow cannula unclamped deairs the system. Except in patients undergoing assistance as a bridge to transplantation, we no longer use the left ventricular apex as a cannulation site.[7] This avoids additional myocardial damage and the need to obturate and leave in place the apical cannula if myocardial recovery occurs.

If hemodynamic parameters indicate the need for right ventricular support, the right pump is united with inflow from the right atrium and outflow to the pulmonary artery (Fig. 5). CPB is slowly discontinued, and the surgeon should

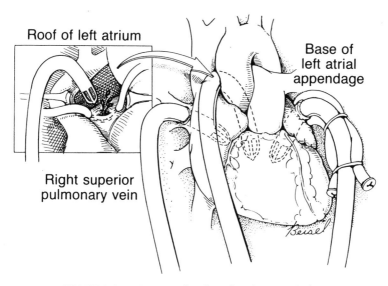

FIGURE 3.   Alternate sites for left atrial cannulation.

Roof of left atrium

Base of
left atrial
appendage

Right superior
pulmonary vein

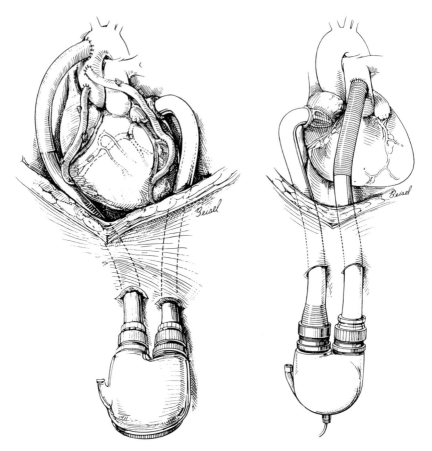

FIGURE 4 *(left).*   Placement of the Pierce-Donachy VAD for left ventricular assistance. The left atrial appendage is used for atrial cannulation.

FIGURE 5 *(right).*   Configuration for right ventricular assistance. The inflow cannula is placed in the right atrial appendage; the outflow graft is anchored with the main pulmonary artery.

achieve meticulous hemostasis at this point. Diastolic vacuum is avoided until the chest is closed. Placement of biventricular assist devices is shown in Figure 6.

MANAGEMENT OF THE VENTRICULAR ASSIST PATIENT

The initial postoperative management is similar to that for any critically ill open-heart patient. Invasive monitoring includes a thermodilution pulmonary artery catheter and left atrial line. Once the chest is closed, a small amount of diastolic vacuum is applied so that the pump inflow cannula removes the entire atrial blood volume and pump output is maintained in the range of 2.2–3.0 L/min/m². The pump is run in a full-to-empty mode to ensure complete washout of the blood sac. This, along with a smooth polyurethane surface and high interfacial shear rates, helps to prevent thrombus. Protamine sulfate is routinely administered after cessation of bypass, and when chest-tube drainage has decreased to <50 ml/hr,

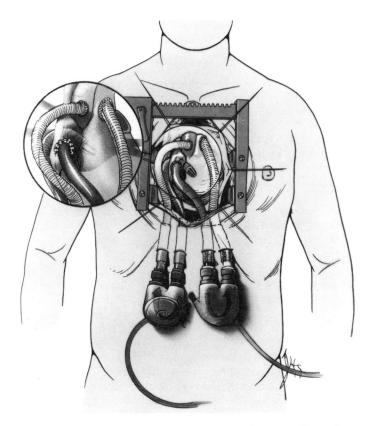

FIGURE 6.   Configuration of assist devices for both right and left ventricular assistance.

low-molecular-weight dextran is infused to decrease platelet adhesion. We currently recommend heparin to maintain the activated clotting time in the range of 150–250 seconds after the first 24–48 hours and during weaning.

In patients with a severely depressed left ventricle, the left VAD usually pumps the entire output delivered to the left atrium from the pulmonary circulation. In this situation, right ventricular function is the usual factor that limits cardiac output, and some right ventricular dysfunction is invariably present. The right ventricle can be supported initially with dobutamine, dopamine, or amrinone. A left atrial pressure between 10–15 mmHg is usually required for satisfactory pumping, if the cannula is properly positioned. *Prompt* support of the right ventricle with a device is mandatory if drug therapy fails in the operating room.

Assist pumping is briefly discontinued each day to evaluate the patient's native ventricular function. Pumping is discontinued initially for only 15 seconds; the right and left atrial pressures are not allowed to rise above 30 mmHg. When pumping can be discontinued for 60-second periods with atrial pressure <20 mmHg, AoP >100 mmHg, and cardiac output index >2.0 L/min/m^2, weaning is considered. Additional data can be obtained by performing transesophageal echocardiography while pump flow is decreased. Adequate systemic anticoagulation is mandatory for weaning.[9] The pump is now run in the manual

TABLE 3. Ventricular Assistance for Postcardiotomy Cardiogenic Shock, 1975–1991

System Type	Total No. of Patients	Age (Range in Years)	Length of Support (Range in Days)
Pneumatic	243	54 (3–83)	5.4 (0–69)
Centrifugal	582	56 (0–85)	2.9 (0–33)

mode, and VAD output is gradually decreased to a minimum of 30 beats per minute. When adequate ventricular function has been maintained at these levels for 24 hours with a minimum of inotropic agents, the patient is returned to the operating room for device removal through a reentry sternotomy. CPB is unnecessary for removal.

CONCLUSIONS

In 1985 a Combined Registry for the Clinical Use of Mechanical Ventricular Assist Devices and Total Artificial Hearts was established under the auspices of the International Society for Heart Transplantation and the American Society of Artificial Internal Organs. Data have been collated from information voluntarily provided by the implanting surgeons up to December 31, 1991. Table 3 shows the total number of patients, their average age, and the average length of support for both pneumatic and centrifugal pump use for PCCS. Of the 743 patients registered, 162 were men, 80 were women, and no gender was identified in the remainder. The number of patients weaned and discharged after pneumatic VADs is listed in Table 4. Although 44% of patients were weaned from circulatory support, only 23% survived to be discharged from the hospital. Although this rate may seem disappointing, all patients would have died in the operating room without an assist device. Survival and hospital discharge are independent of the original operation, suggesting that myocardial recovery is possible in a variety of situations.[6] Patients requiring the least amount of support, right or left univentricular, generally had a better outcome than patients requiring biventricular support. This can be explained by the relative extent of ventricular dysfunction. The frequency of reported complications and reported causes of death is listed in Table 5. These results are similar to those that we reported previously.[6] Our report showed little demonstrable difference between a pneumatic or a centrifugal system. Duration of circulatory support is relatively short; most patients who survive to discharge are weaned in <1 week. Patients with centrifugal devices are generally supported for a shorter period of time, although the survival rates are similar.[6] The reasons are not clear. Multiple complications are seen in both groups. In both groups, however, the long-term survival of discharged patients is

TABLE 4. Number of Patients Not Weanable, Weanable, and Discharged after Pneumatic Ventricular Assistance

	RVAD	LVAD	BVAD
Not weaned	14	72	54
Weaned	9	75	19
Discharged	7	37	13
Total	23	147	73

RVAD = right ventricular assist device; LVAD = left ventricular assist device; BVAD = biventricular assist device.

TABLE 5. Complications and Causes of Death in Pneumatic Ventricular Assist Patients

Event	Complications (%)	Cause of Death (%)
Bleeding	75 (34)	37 (21)
Renal failure	70 (32)	51 (29)
Respiratory failure	42 (19)	39 (23)
Mechanical failure	4 (2)	1 (0.6)
Embolic	15 (7)	7 (4)
Ventricular failure	62 (28)	104 (60)
Infection	38 (17)	26 (15)
Hemolysis	15 (7)	
Thrombosis	14 (6)	
Cannula obstruction	16 (10)	
Neurologic (nonembolic)	21 (10)	

excellent, with most patients classified as New York Heart Association functional class I or II.[6]

These data indicate that in a select group of patients ventricular assist pumping can provide satisfactory support for the circulation while decreasing myocardial work and allowing satisfactory recovery of the stunned myocardium. Although the overall survival approximates only 1 of 4 patients, these patients were certain to die without use of a device. Long-term survival of discharged patients is excellent; most have only minimal or no cardiac disability. In spite of major engineering differences between centrifugal and pneumatic assist systems, the overall results for both groups are similar. Further analysis of data in the ASAIO/ISHLT Combined Registry may suggest that centrifugal systems are adequate for support of PCCS and that pneumatic support systems are best reserved for longer support times, as in bridging to transplantation.[6] The relatively short times of circulatory support, coupled with the expense of pneumatic systems and the need to obtain an investigational device exemption for their use, may favor use of the centrifugal device. Most importantly, considerable future work is needed to improve accuracy and timing in patient selection, prospective determination of the reversibility of myocardial injury, and control of bleeding associated with device implantation.

REFERENCES

1. D'Ambroa MN, LaRara PJ, Rhilbin DM, et al: Prostaglandin E1: A new therapy for refractory right heart failure and pulmonary hypertension after mitral valve replacement. J Thorac Cardiovasc Surg 89:567–572, 1985.
2. Deeb GM, Boling SF, Guynn TP, Wicklas JM: Amrinone versus conventional therapy in pulmonary hypertensive patients awaiting cardiac transplantation. Ann Thorac Surg 48:665–669, 1989.
3. Downing TP, Miller DC, Stoffer R, Shumway NE: Use of the intra-aortic balloon pump after valve replacement. J Thorac Cardiovasc Surg 92:210–217, 1986.
4. Jett GK: Circulatory support utilizing the Abiomed BVS System 5000. Cardiovascular Science and Technology: Basic and Applied: II. 1990, p 305 [abstract].
5. Magovern JA, Pae WE, Rickenbacher WE, Pierce WS: The importance of a patent foramen ovale in left ventricular assist pumping. ASAIO Trans 32:449–453, 1986.
6. Miller CA, Pae WE, Pierce WS: Combined Registry for the Clinical Use of Mechanical Ventricular Assist Devices. Post-cardiotomy cardiogenic shock. ASAIO Trans 36:43–46, 1990.
7. Oaks TE, Pae WE, Rosenberg G, et al: The use of a paracorporeal ventricular assist device as a bridge-to-cardiac transplantation. ASAIO Trans 33:408–411, 1987.
8. Pae WE, Pierce WS, Pennock JL, et al: Long-term results of ventricular assist pumping in postcardiotomy cardiogenic shock. J Thorac Cardiovasc Surg 93:434–441, 1986.

9. Pennington DG, Samuels LD, Williams G, et al: Experience with the Pierce-Donachy ventricular assist device in post-cardiotomy patients with cardiogenic shock. World J Surg 9:37–46, 1985.

10. Pennington DG, Swartz M, Codd JE, et al: Intra-aortic balloon pumping in cardiac surgical patients: A nine-year experience. Ann Thorac Surg 36:125–131, 1983.

11. Rose DM, Colvin SB, Sulliford AT, et al: Long-term survival with partial left heart bypass following perioperative myocardial infarction and shock. J Thorac Cardiovasc Surg 83:483–492, 1982.

12. Sanfelippo PM, Baker NH, Ewy HG, et al: Experience with intra-aortic balloon counterpulsation. Ann Thorac Surg 41:36–41, 1986.

R.A. OTT, MD
D.E. GUTFINGER, PhD
T.C. MILLS, PhD*
J. EUGENE, MD,
E.TOVAR, MD
M. VANA, Jr, MD,
P. FOPIANO, BS, RN
A.B. GAZZANIGA, MD

THE ROLE OF PNEUMATIC VADs IN REVERSIBLE MYOCARDIAL INJURY

From the Department of
  Cardiothoracic Surgery
University of California–Irvine
  Medical Center
Orange, California

*Baxter L.I.S. Division
Advanced Development
Irvine, California

Reprint requests to:
Richard A. Ott, MD
Division of Cardiothoracic
  Surgery
University of California–Irvine
  Medical Center
Orange, CA 92668

Mechanical support of the failing heart continues to capture the imagination and to challenge the skill of surgeons worldwide. Since the early reports of clinical success with ventricular assistance,[10,53] a confusing array of overlapping technology has evolved, featuring systems based on roller pumps,[51] centrifugal pumps,[4] pneumatic heterotopic pumps,[13,17,46] and electrically powered implantable devices.[9,30,49,50]

Initially, ventricular assist devices (VADs) were developed to treat refractory postcardiotomy cardiogenic shock (PCCS). More recently, the success of cardiac transplantation has dramatically increased the recipient pool, creating a subset of patients who require mechanical cardiac assistance as a bridge to transplantation (BTT). Use of pneumatic VADs as a BTT has yielded gratifying results.[33] However, application of pneumatic VADs for patients with potentially reversible myocardial injury has been disappointing.[40] The overall survival equals the results obtained with simpler, less expensive centrifugal extracorporeal systems. As a result, enthusiasm was lost for pneumatic VADs as an effective technology for bridge to recovery (BTR).

Historically, VADs have successfully reversed cardiogenic shock with recovery of the native heart in four clinical conditions: (1) the syndrome of a stunned myocardium,[2,5] (2) cardiogenic shock associated with perioperative myocardial infarction,[54] (3) allograft failure after cardiac transplantation,[20,21,35] and (4) myocarditis with acute cardiopulmonary failure.[18] Of these, PCCS related to perioperative infarction is associated with the poorest survival.[41]

Numerous studies[1-3,5,11,22,24,39,41-44,48,52,54] have shown that infarct size is reduced by early institution of ventricular assistance. Direct left ventricular (LV) cannulation results in complete LV decompression and maximal reduction in infarct size.[22,24,27,52] However, it also results in additional injury to the myocardium and clinically has been supplanted by techniques using left atrial (LA) cannulation and partial preload reduction. Our interest has been to reexamine the use of pneumatic VADs in recoverable myocardial injury and to define the optimal method of support to protect end-organ function and to promote myocardial recovery. For this goal we have developed a two-phased approach. The initial phase consists of optimizing device output to reverse the effects of cardiogenic shock. This is accomplished through asynchronous pneumatic VAD pumping, which also maximally reduces myocardial consumption of O_2. After hemodynamic stabilization and evidence of end-organ recovery, synchronous VAD counterpulsation is emphasized to focus specifically on recovery of the heart. Through augmentation of diastolic coronary blood flow, improved subendocardial perfusion aids recovery. To explore this concept, a series of theoretical formulations were derived and in-vitro experiments performed, the results of which are described below.

DEVICE IMPEDANCE AND OPTIMIZING OUTPUT

In-vitro Experiments and Device Impedance

To explore the impact of various parameters on device output, a series of in-vitro experiments were carried out on a mock circulation.[14] Two devices were evaluated: the Jarvik-7-70 (J-7-70) (Symbion, Inc., Salt Lake City, UT) total artificial heart (TAH) and the Symbion acute ventricular assist device (AVAD) (Symbion, Inc., Salt Lake City, UT).

Function curves were produced for average device output (ADO) as related to rate, vacuum, and systolic duration. Figures 1 and 2 illustrate the curves produced for the J-7-70 and AVAD, respectively. All curves show characteristics similar to typical Frank-Starling curves. Although the J-7-70 and Symbion AVAD have the same stroke volume (70 cc), these data show substantially larger device outputs for the J-7-70. This difference results from the higher device inflow and outflow impedance associated with the cannulas used to attach the AVAD to the native heart.

Using the data gathered from the in-vitro experiments, estimates were obtained for the inflow and outflow impedances of J-7-70 and AVAD.[15] Inflow impedance, Z_{in}, and outflow impedance, Z_{out}, are computed as follows:

$$Z_{in} = \frac{\text{Fill pressure}}{\text{Fill rate}} = \frac{(AP + VAC) \cdot \text{Fill duration}}{\text{Fill volume}}$$

$$Z_{out} = \frac{\text{Drive pressure}}{\text{Ejection rate}} = \frac{DP \cdot \text{Ejection duration}}{\text{Stroke volume}} \qquad (1)$$

AP, VAC, and DP are the atrial pressure, applied vacuum, and driveline pressure, respectively. The impedance estimates obtained are summarized in Table 1; as an example, Figure 3 shows the data points used in obtaining the inflow impedance of the AVAD.

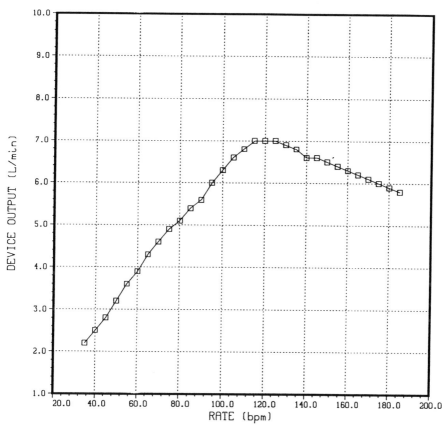

FIGURE 1. In-vitro J-7-70 output curves. Artificial heart: Jarvik-7-70. Right drive pressure = 50 mmHg; left drive pressure = 140 mmHg; Vacuum = 0 mmHg; right atrial pressure = 15 mmHg; % systole = 50.

Drive Pressure, Vacuum, $\frac{dP}{dt}$, and Hemolysis

To compensate for the increased inflow impedance in the AVAD, vacuum is often applied to aid in device filling, and the percent of device systole is typically reduced.[12] In the J-7-70, by contrast, adequate device filling is generally obtained passively.[45] The increased outflow impedance in the AVAD, along with the tendency to use a reduced percent of device systole, forces the use of higher drive pressures (i.e., >160 mmHg). Thus, in comparison with the J-7-70, the AVAD requires the higher vacuum and drive pressures.

The use of higher vacuum and drive pressures in the AVAD causes the pressurization and depressurization rates, $\frac{dP}{dt}$, to be larger. Clinical trials have shown that an increase in $\frac{dP}{dt}$ is correlated with an increase in hemolysis.[16,25] Current guidelines maintain average $\frac{dP}{dt}$ below 3500 mmHg/sec.[25]

The in-vitro mock circulation system was used to estimate $\frac{dP}{dt}$ as a function of drive pressure and vacuum for the J-7-70 and AVAD. Both devices were driven with the same driver. The estimates obtained are shown in Figure 4. The Cardiac Output and Monitoring Diagnostic Unit (COMDU) (Symbion, Inc., Salt Lake City, UT) estimated $\frac{dP}{dt}$ from the driveline pressure waveforms.

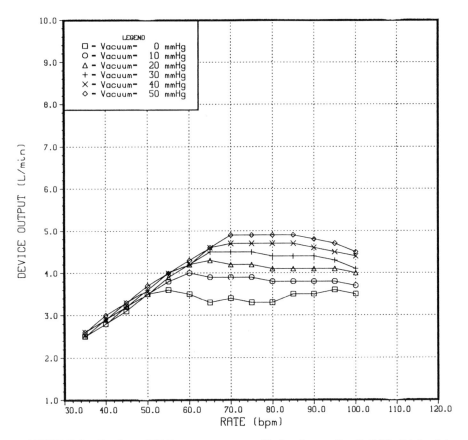

FIGURE 2. In-vitro AVAD output curves. Native heart: Jarvik-7-70. Right drive pressure = 35 mmHg; left drive pressure = 0 mmHg; vacuum = 0 mmHg; right atrial pressure = 16 mmHg; rate = 120 bpm; % systole = 50. Left assist device: Symbion AVAD. Drive pressure = 200 mmHg; % systole = 50.

Analysis of the data has shown similar $\frac{dP}{dt}$ characteristics for the J-7-70 and AVAD, suggesting dependency on the drive system rather than the device driven. In particular, for both devices a linear correlation between $\frac{dP}{dt}$ and the pressurization gradient was determined. The following model was formulated:

$$\frac{dP}{dt} = \frac{DP + VAC}{\Delta t} \tag{2}$$

DP and VAC denote the applied drive pressure and vacuum, respectively; Δt denotes a constant estimated to be 0.057 ± 0.003 seconds and represents the lost time associated with isovolumetric pressurization and depressurization. According to the in-vitro experiments the variation in Δt as a function of the applied vacuum and drive pressure is negligible.

An upper limit on the permissible clinical drive pressure and vacuum can be determined from equation (2) by setting $\frac{dP}{dt}$ to 3500 mmHg/sec and solving for the quantity (DP + VAC). The limit determined for (DP + VAC) is 200 mmHg.

TABLE 1. Inflow and Outflow Device Impedances

Device	Z_{in} mmHg*min/L	Z_{out} mmHg*min/L
Symbion AVAD	3.2 ± 0.4	12.5 ± 1.5
Jarvik-7-70	0.83 ± 0.04	7.8 ± 1

Thus, in optimizing hemodynamics clinically, the maximal allowable vacuum is derived as follows:

$$\text{Maximum VAC} = 200 - \text{DP} \qquad (3)$$

Prediction of Optimal Device Output

A model for predicting optimal device output was formulated[15] by using the estimates obtained for the inflow and outflow impedances as well as the lost time associated with isovolumetric pressurization and depressurization. Valve

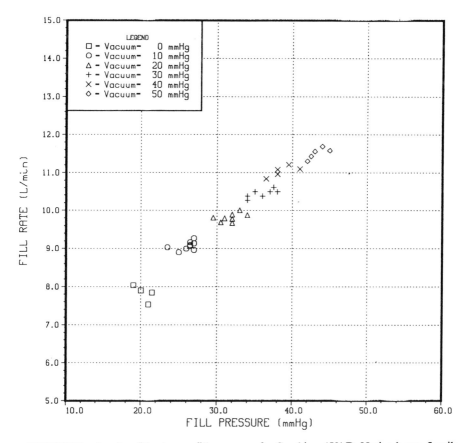

FIGURE 3. In-vitro fill rates vs. fill pressures for Symbion AVAD. Native heart: Jarvik-7-70. Right drive pressure = 35 mmHg; left drive pressure = 0 mmHg; vacuum = 0 mmHg; right atrial pressure = 16 mmHg; rate = 120 bpm; % systole = 50. Left assist device: Symbion AVAD. Drive pressure = 200 mmHg; % systole = 50.

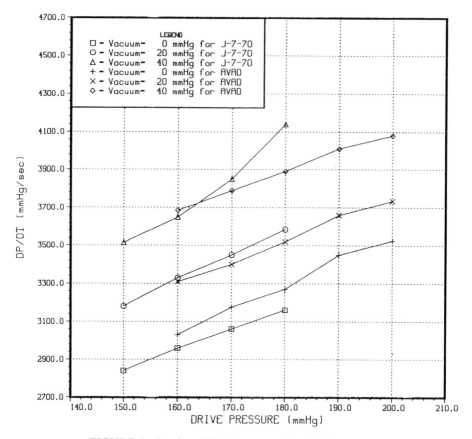

FIGURE 4. In-vitro dP/dt data curves for AVAD and J-7-70.

regurgitation of the prosthetic valves was not included in the model and was assumed to be negligible.

Using equation (1), the fill volume, stroke volume, and ADO can be predicted for various values of AP, VAC, DP, fill duration, and ejection duration. Maximal ADO can be determined from these predictions, and an analytical solution can be derived by rewriting equation (1) as follows and solving for the fill and ejection durations:

$$\text{Optimal ADO} = \frac{(AP + VAC) \cdot \text{Fill duration}}{Z_{in}} = \frac{DP \cdot \text{Ejection duration}}{Z_{out}} \quad (4)$$

Let d denote the ratio of the time spent in device diastole to the time of a complete device cycle. Let RATE denote the device rate in beats per minute (bpm). Then the fill duration and ejection duration can be expressed as:

$$\text{Fill duration} = d - \Delta t \cdot RATE \quad\quad \text{Ejection duration} = 1 - d - \Delta t \cdot RATE \quad (5)$$

Substituting equation (5) into equation (4) and solving for d yields:

$$d = \frac{DP \cdot Z_{in} \cdot (1 - 2 \cdot \Delta t \cdot RATE)}{(AP + VAC) \cdot Z_{out} + DP \cdot Z_{in}} + \Delta t \cdot RATE \quad (6)$$

Substituting equation (6) into equation (4) yields:

$$\text{Optimal ADO} = \frac{(AP + VAC) \cdot DP \cdot (1 - 2 \cdot \Delta t \cdot RATE)}{(AP + VAC) \cdot Z_{out} + DP \cdot Z_{in}} \qquad (7)$$

A solution for the optimal RATE can be obtained by setting

$$\text{Optimal ADO} = RATE \cdot SV_{max} \qquad (8)$$

(where SV_{max} denotes the maximal stroke volume of the device) and solving equations (7) and (8), which yields:

$$\frac{1}{\text{Optimal RATE}} = \frac{SV_{max} \cdot [(AP + VAC) \cdot Z_{out} + DP \cdot Z_{in}]}{(AP + VAC) \cdot DP} + 2 \cdot \Delta t \qquad (9)$$

A computer used the solution provided in equations (4) through (9) to produce function curves of ADO as related to rate and vacuum (Figs. 5 and 6). In addition, the computer produced function curves of optimal ADO as related to drive pressure and fill pressure (Figs. 7 and 8) and a quick reference table for determining

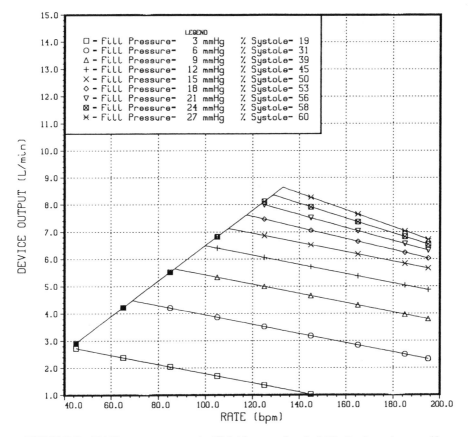

FIGURE 5. TAH output curves. Artificial heart = Jarvik-7-70. Stroke volume = 65 cc; drive pressure = 140 mmHg; inflow impedance = 0.83 mmHg*min/L; outflow impedance = 7.8 mmHg*min/L.

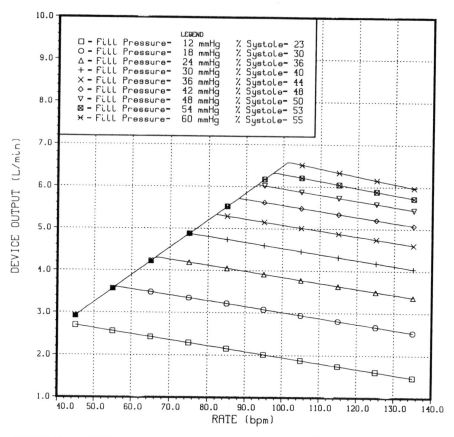

FIGURE 6. AVAD output curves. Assist device: Symbion AVAD. Stroke volume = 65 cc; drive pressure = 180 mmHg; inflow impedance = 3.2 mmHg*min/L; outflow impedance = 12.5 mmHg*min/L.

parameter settings for maximizing device output. Table 2 provides an example for the AVAD (with DP = 180 mmHg) and J-7-70 (with DP = 140 mmHg). Fill pressure refers to the quantity (AP + VAC). Similar reference tables with different DPs can also be easily produced.

For example, if the atrial pressure is 12 mmHg with a maximal vacuum of 20 mmHg, the fill pressure will be 32 mmHg, and the maximal achievable AVAD output is about 5 L/min, with a device rate of 77 bpm and 42% systole. On the other hand, with the same atrial pressure, but using the J-7-70 with no vacuum, the maximal achievable TAH output is 6.5 L/min, with a device rate of 100 bpm and 46% systole. With DP = 180 mmHg and VAC = 20 mmHg, the AVAD $\frac{dP}{dt}$ is 3500 mmHg/sec, whereas for the J-7-70 (with DP = 140 mmHg and no vacuum) the $\frac{dP}{dt}$ is 2460 mmHg/sec.

This approach for predicting optimal device parameters has been useful in clinical applications. A quick reference parameter table is used perioperatively as a guide to establish initial settings. Minor adjustments are made to the parameter settings as necessary to ensure proper device filling and emptying (i.e., partial device fill and full device ejection). Postoperative estimates are obtained for the

TABLE 2. Optimal Device Parameters

Fill Pressure (AP + VAC) mmHg	Symbion AVAD DP = 180 mmHg			Jarvik-7-70 DP = 140 mmHg		
	ADO L/min	HR bpm	SYS %	ADO L/min	HR bpm	SYS %
2	0.59	9	5	2.00	31	14
4	1.11	17	9	3.42	53	24
6	1.58	24	13	4.48	69	31
8	2.01	31	17	5.30	82	37
10	2.39	37	20	5.95	92	42
12	2.74	42	23	6.49	100	46
14	3.06	47	26	6.93	107	49
16	3.35	52	28	7.31	112	51
18	3.62	56	30	7.63	117	54
20	3.87	59	32	7.91	122	56
22	4.10	63	34	8.15	125	57
24	4.31	66	36	8.37	129	59
26	4.51	69	38	8.56	132	60
28	4.70	72	39	8.73	134	61
30	4.87	75	41	8.88	137	62
32	5.03	77	42	9.02	139	63
34	5.19	80	44	9.14	141	64
36	5.33	82	45	9.26	142	65
38	5.47	84	46	9.36	144	66
40	5.60	86	47	9.46	146	67
42	5.72	88	48	9.55	147	67
44	5.83	90	49	9.63	148	68
46	5.94	91	50	9.71	149	68
48	6.05	93	51	9.78	150	69
50	6.15	95	52	9.85	152	69

DP = drive pressure; AP = atrial pressure; VAC = vacuum; ADO = average device output; HR = heart rate; SYS = systole.

device inflow and outflow impedances, and a patient-specific quick reference table is produced.

Although the quick reference parameter table is not essential for success, it has been helpful in predicting the effects of altering vacuum and estimating atrial pressure. In addition, it has been particularly useful for staff inservicing and bedside training.

The automatic fill-to-empty (i.e., variable rate) pumping mode commonly employed in the Thoratec VAD (Thoratec, Inc., Berkeley, CA) results in the same selection of device rate and % systole. However, a decision regarding the selection of the drive pressure and vacuum is still required; this decision is facilitated with use of the quick reference parameter table.

EKG SYNCHRONOUS COUNTERPULSATION

In-vitro Experiments

To determine the impact of EKG synchronous counterpulsation and asynchronous pumping on myocardial workload and endomyocardial perfusion, a series of in-vitro experiments were performed.[36]

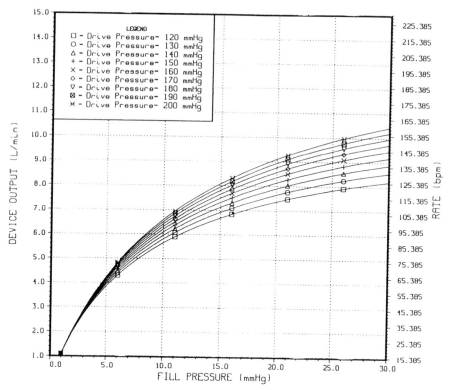

FIGURE 7. Optimal TAH output curves. Artificial heart: Jarvik-7-70. Stroke volume = 65 cc; inflow impedance = 0.83 mmHg*min/L; outflow impedance = 7.8 mmHg*min/L.

In the experimental setup the J-7-70 and the AVAD are configured in parallel (Figs. 9 and 10). The J-7-70 simulates the failing heart and the AVAD the left ventricular assist device (LVAD). Separate circulatory support system consoles with COMDUs drive each device. The LVAD can be operated in both the asynchronous and the EKG synchronous pumping modes. In the synchronous mode an EKG simulator signal is fed to each controller through a Cardiosync module, and a programmable input-delay parameter permits offsetting the trigger times of the J-7-70 and LVAD.

Atrial and arterial pressures are monitored through pressure transducers attached to a pressure monitor. A computer with an analog-to-digital converter permits digitization and processing of the pressure waveforms. ADO is estimated with a flowmeter, along with the COMDUs. Figures 11 and 12 show a series of pressure waveforms recorded for the asynchronous and synchronous pumping modes, respectively.

Endomyocardial Viability Ratio

During systole, endomyocardial perfusion is reduced as coronary vascular resistance increases with contraction. The subendocardium is the most vulnerable and the first injured in any ischemic event. Therefore, delivery of O_2 is maximized

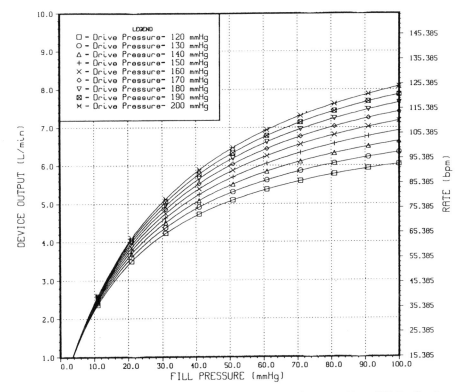

FIGURE 8. Optimal AVAD output curves. Assist device: Symbion AVAD. Stroke volume = 65 cc; inflow impedance = 3.2 mmHg*min/L; outflow impedance = 12.5 mmHg*min/L.

with EKG synchronous counterpulsation so that, during pneumatic VAD support, device output is coordinated with diastolic relaxation. EKG synchronous counterpulsation may also affect native heart consumption of O_2 by reducing afterload similar to intraaortic balloon counterpulsation.

Endomyocardial viability ratio (EVR) is defined as:

$$\frac{DPTI}{TTI} = \frac{\text{Diastolic pressure time index}}{\text{Tension time index}} \qquad (10)$$

EVR provides a measure of subendocardial perfusion as well as ventricular unloading and afterload reduction. In the unassisted heart EVR is <1. However, with EKG synchronous counterpulsation the EVR of the assisted heart can be made >1. The greater the EVR, the more O_2 is delivered in the presence of reduced myocardial work.

EVR and ADO were computed as a function of vacuum and trigger delay.[36] The data show that EVR is maximized for a trigger delay between 0.05–0.2 seconds. A comparison between synchronous and asynchronous pumping appears in Table 3. These data clearly show that EKG synchronous counterpulsation is superior to asynchronous pumping for increasing EVR. Our clinical experience in PCCS[31,32,35] also supports this conclusion (Table 4).

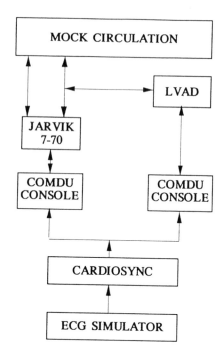

FIGURE 9.   Block diagram of in-vitro experimental setup.

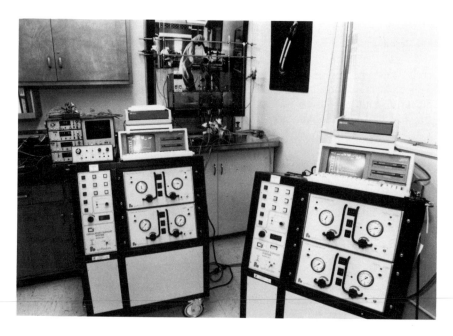

FIGURE 10.   In-vitro experimental setup.

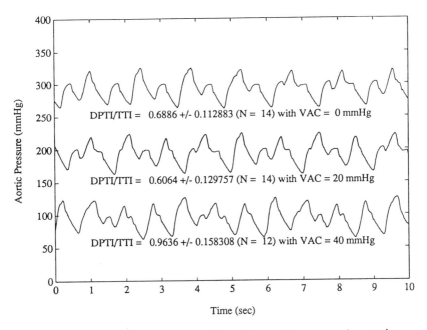

FIGURE 11.   In-vitro pressure waveforms for asynchronous mode pumping.

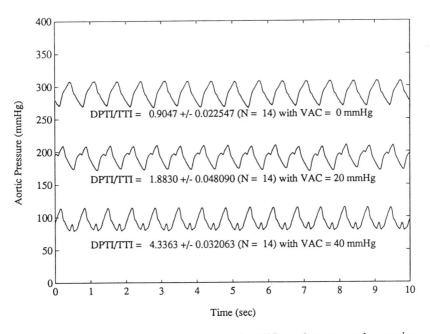

FIGURE 12.   In-vitro pressure waveforms for EKG synchronous mode pumping.

TABLE 3. Synchronous and Asynchronous Pumping Data

| VAC mmHg | Synchronous: Delay = 0.15 sec | | | | Asynchronous | | | | |
	DPTI/TTI Rate = 90	ADO L/min	LAP mmHg	MAP mmHg	DPTI/TTI	ADO L/min	Rate bpm	LAP mmHg	MAP mmHg
0	$0.90 \pm 0.02^{\dagger}$	2.0	15	89	0.69 ± 0.11	2.9	42	20	92
20	$1.88 \pm 0.05^{\dagger}$	3.1	3	91	0.61 ± 0.13	4.0	56	8	94
40	$4.34 \pm 0.03^{\dagger}$	5.0	-2	93	0.96 ± 0.16	4.9	70	-4	95

$\dagger$ $p < 0.005$ (n = 14).

Rate = device rate in bpm; native heart rate = 90 bpm in all experiments; AVAD drive pressure = 180 mmHg; AVAD % systole = 50; J-7-70 left drive pressure = 120 mmHg; J-7-70 right drive pressure = 50 mmHg; J-7-70 % systole = 50; VAC = vacuum; DPTI = diastolic pressure time index; TTI = tension time index; ADO = average device output; LAP = left atrial pressure; MAP = mean arterial pressure.

Device Output

Although EKG synchronous counterpulsation maximizes the EVR, ADO is reduced when compared with asynchronous pumping.[6] This relates to the rate for maximizing ADO, which is generally lower than the native heart rate. The data show that the reduction in ADO increases with an increase in the difference between the native rate and the desired asynchronous rate. Our clinical data show a reduction of 1 L/min with 1:1 EKG synchronous pumping. The reduction in ADO is due to lost time associated with isovolumetric pressurization and depressurization of the VAD as well as regurgitation of the prosthetic valves. The reduction in ADO can be minimized by using higher vacuum, as illustrated in the in-vitro experiments. However, for native rates above 100 bpm, this becomes increasingly difficult.

PROTOCOL

The use of mechanical cardiac assist devices as a BTR and as a BTT requires careful evaluation and analysis. Patient selection is most important for successful outcome.[17,46] Device selection is also important,[34] but often the number of available devices is limited, and the best results are probably obtained with the device with which the center has the most experience. Once a decision is made to institute a cardiac assist device, implantation should proceed quickly. Delays in intervention have typically been associated with unfavorable outcomes.[1,41] The following protocol is based on our experience with the Symbion AVAD; however, many of the concepts also apply to pneumatic VADs in general.

Device Implantation

Implantation of pneumatic VADs is indicated as a BTR or a BTT (Table 5). In the BTT, implantation may occur without use of cardiopulmonary bypass

TABLE 4. Clinical Comparison of AVAD Pumping Modes

Pumping Mode	DPTI/TTI	ADO (L/min)	MAP (mmHg)	VAD Rate (bpm)	Native Rate (bpm)
Async	0.7	5.5	108	85	130
Sync 1:1	2.5	4.5	109	90	90
Sync 1:2	2.7	4.2	114	65	130
Sync 1:3	1.8	2.3	91	35	105

DPTI = diastolic pressure time index; TTI = tension time index; ADO = average device output; MAP = mean arterial pressure; Async = asynchronous; Sync = synchronous.

TABLE 5. Device Implantation Categories

Category	Typical Support	Therapeutic Goal
Bridge to recovery	<3 weeks	Minimize myocardial O_2 consumption and maximize myocardial O_2 delivery
Bridge to transplant	>3 weeks	Maintain stable hemodynamics and adequate end-organ perfusion

(CPB), whereas in BTR (i.e., PCCS) CPB is in place and discontinuation results in hemodynamic collapse. Avoiding CPB reduces blood trauma and may impact on perioperative bleeding.[7] However, with a severely depressed left ventricle, partial CPB for a short period provides hemodynamic control with little threat of subsequent coagulopathy.[34]

In BTR inotropic agents and vasodilators are used first in an attempt to wean the patient from CPB. If unsuccessful, an intraaortic balloon pump (IABP) is inserted. If no improvement occurs, a VAD is considered. As soon as a decision to implant a VAD is made, implantation proceeds immediately.

In BTT inotropic agents and occasionally an IABP are in place. If the patient cannot be successfully maintained, a VAD is considered. This decision should be made early, because patients under prolonged support with inotropes and an IABP may be subjected to complications from marginal perfusion and immobility.[33,41]

In both BTR and BTT, a decision is made whether BVAD, LVAD, or RVAD will be implanted. BVADs are favored in cases with global injury, because better hemodynamic control results, whereas univentricular assist may suffice in patients with a substantial difference in function between the native ventricles. An LVAD should be implanted selectively because univentricular support can often result in right ventricular failure.[13] On the other hand, implantation of BVADs in patients with a properly functioning right ventricle may be unnecessary. In any event, a decision should be made intraoperatively after placement of an LVAD and observation.

Operative Technique

For implantation of biventricular heterotopic prosthetic ventricles, a partially occluding clamp is placed on the ascending aorta and the main pulmonary artery, and a longitudinal arteriotomy is performed. The previously measured and beveled pulmonary artery and aortic cannula grafts are anastomosed end-to-side to the ascending aorta and the proximal main pulmonary artery in conventional fashion by means of continuous 4.0 polypropylene suture. The outflow grafts are prepared by either preclotting or soaking in 25% albumin and autoclaving for 3 minutes to reduce bleeding from the Dacron graft.[34]

For BTT patients the aortic outflow graft is placed on the greater curve of the ascending aorta at the lowest possible site near the aortic valve. Similarly, the pulmonary artery outflow is placed just beyond the pulmonic valve. These sites allow excision of all foreign material at the time of explantation and leave sufficient length of great vessel for transplantation. In BTR patients, the site of the aortic anastomosis is largely dictated by the presence of proximal vein grafts; at the time of explantation, removal of all prosthetic material is not mandatory.

Two pledgeted 2.0 pursestring sutures are placed in the patient's left atrium beyond the intraatrial groove, and a 51-Fr right-angle venous cannula is inserted into the left atrium to lie transversely. The pursestring sutures are then tied (not snared) and secured around the cannula. This protects against aspiration of air when applying high levels of vacuum intraoperatively. The right atrial cannula is similarly placed through a suitable site in the right atrium and again secured by means of 2.0 pursestring sutures tied to the cannula. The cannulas are then attached to the prosthetic ventricles.

Deairing is accomplished with a commercial Jejunostomy catheter inserted through the pulmonary artery and aortic grafts. The conventional method for deairing the Symbion AVAD through its dorsal port is not used because this procedure may result in thrombus formation within the VAD.[37]

AVAD pumping is initiated, and device flows ranging from 4–4.5 L/min are obtained with the use of a vacuum of 15 mmHg. If the combined cardiac index remains below 2.5 L/min/m², vacuum is serially increased up to 35 mmHg to improve device filling and output. To counter even further the potential for air aspiration, the mediastinum is filled with warm saline solution, as the vacuum is increased. The goal is to drive the device at high flow rates during the initial recovery period to allow for maximal organ perfusion. In this initial period, asynchronous pumping is used, and when satisfactory hemodynamics are achieved, the patient is weaned from CPB.

It is important to obtain hemostasis rapidly with early and vigorous infusion of coagulation factors before prolonged bleeding results in uncontrollable coagulopathy.[7] Only after hemostasis is achieved and all surgical bleeding has been eliminated is the sternum closed, whenever possible, to promote hemostasis and to allow possible early extubation.

Postoperative Management

Anticoagulation is generally started only after several hours following chest closure or when the outflow from the chest tubes is <100 ml/hr for 2–3 hours. At this time 5% dextran is begun at 40 ml/hr for the first 24 hours. Intravenous heparin is then used with the goal of maintaining the activated clotting time between 160–200 seconds. In addition, dipyridamole at 100 mg is given 4 times daily as antiplatelet therapy. For prolonged implantation Coumadin and dipyridamole have become the preferred therapy.

To counter the potential for infectious complications, all patients are placed in strict reverse isolation. Short-term, broad-spectrum antibiotic coverage (vancomycin and/or cefotaxime) is given with the goal of early extubation and mobilization. Infections related to driveline and cannulation sites, although uncommon, are treated aggressively with local debridement and appropriate antibiotic therapy. Prophylactic care of the exit sites with dressing changes, using Betadine preparations, is given daily.

During the perioperative period and the initial postoperative phase an engineer is responsible for technical matters related to the device. The nursing staff and/or perfusionists who have been formally inserviced then make adjustments and monitor the AVAD control system around the clock, with clinical and technical advice provided by the surgeon and engineer.

Bridge to Recovery and Weaning

VADs are generally left in place for at least 24 hours. Although quite often the heart appears to recover during the early postoperative period, most attempts to wean and remove devices within 24 hours have been unsuccessful.[29] With pneumatic VADs the first 24 hours are dedicated to asynchronous pumping with high vacuum to achieve maximal flow rates. The goal during this initial postoperative phase is to obtain rapid hemodynamic stability and to provide a favorable setting for end-organ recovery.

Once the patient is stable with improvement in organ function, EKG synchronous counterpulsation is instituted using 1:1 pumping to provide diastolic augmentation and enhanced subendocardial perfusion with modest afterload reduction. This pumping mode requires the presence of sinus or paced rhythm at a rate of preferably <100 bpm and hence may be delayed beyond the first 24 hours. During EKG synchronous counterpulsation, drive pressures and vacuum are reduced to minimize hemolysis. In the presence of a high heart rate (>80 bpm) some reduction in ADO is expected. This pumping mode is maintained until weaning is considered. During EKG synchronous pumping, whenever the rhythm and/or EKG signal become unstable, the control system is immediately switched to asynchronous pumping.

Determining when to wean from AVAD assistance is based almost exclusively on hemodynamic evidence that recovery is present and sustained. Reduced pump flows and the ability of the native heart to assume increased workload, without significant elevation of left atrial or pulmonary pressures, are critical to successful weaning. When reducing pump flows, heparin is increased to minimize the increased potential for thromboembolism. When the native heart is capable of generating a cardiac index of at least 2.2 L/min/m^2 in the absence of AVAD pumping, it is likely that successful explantation is possible. In addition, echocardiographic data are used to assess ventricular function and to aid in deciding when to wean.

Weaning is accomplished by gradually reducing (over 24 hours) the device output to achieve approximately 50% of the maximal support previously required. Pump flow is not allowed to fall below 2 L/min at any time because of the increased likelihood of thrombus formation. Hemodynamics are closely monitored to determine that cardiac output is maintained. AVAD outputs are decreased by serially reducing the applied vacuum and device rate and/or using the 1:2 EKG synchronous pumping mode. The 1:3 EKG synchronous pumping mode is used when echocardiographic studies are carried out.

When clinical, hemodynamic, and echocardiographic evidence of recovery is present, the AVAD is explanted. Explantation may be facilitated by using femorofemoral partial bypass.[34]

CLINICAL EXPERIENCE

Our clinical experience at the University of California Irvine Medical Center consists of 5 patients (Table 6). Two patients required BVAD support for PCCS related to perioperative infarction; 2 patients required BVAD support secondary to allograft failure after orthotopic heart transplantation; and 1 patient required BVAD support as a bridge to transplantation. Our overall survival rate for patients supported by the Symbion AVAD is 20% (2 patients were weaned with 1 long-term survivor). Our only long-term survivor (3 years to date) was a 61-year-old man, weighing 85 kg, who required BVAD support after orthotopic heart transplantation.[35]

Table 7 shows some of the hemodynamic parameters used in this patient. High drive pressures and vacuum maximized device output during the first 5 days of support. During the last 3 days of support, vacuum was reduced and EKG

TABLE 6.   Clinical Summary of Patient Support by Symbion AVAD

Patient (Age/sex)	Event	Device Implanted	Days of Assistance	Outcome
JG (51/M)	PCCS	BAVADs	13	Weaned, but died shortly after
AC (47/M)	AF	BAVADs	<1 (45 min)	Died shortly after implantation
MB (61/M)	AF	BAVADs	8	Long-term survivor
LL (32/F)	PCCS	LAVAD and RCVAD	2	Open sternum, CVA, died
GM (61/M)	MI, CHF	BAVADs	16	MOF, S, died

PCCS = postcardiotomy cardiogenic shock; AF = allograft failure; CVA = cerebrovascular accident; MOF = multiorgan failure; S = sepsis; CHF = congestive heart failure; MI = myocardial infarction; AVAD = Symbion acute ventricular assist device; RCVAD = right Biomedicus centrifugal pump.

synchronous counterpulsation was employed to aid in weaning by maximally reducing afterload and increasing myocardial delivery of O_2. During the first 5 days a native heart rate >100 bpm precluded use of EKG synchronous counterpulsation. Table 7 also illustrates that during the first 6 days plasma free hemoglobin levels were elevated. This is most likely due to CPB and the use of high drive pressures and vacuum. However, the elevated plasma free hemoglobin levels normalized during the last 2 days after reducing vacuum.

CONCLUSIONS

Clinical and experimental studies continue to demonstrate the importance of early institution of ventricular assistance with the goal of minimizing myocardial O_2 demand and maximizing myocardial O_2 supply.[2,11,22,41] Nonetheless, the clinical results in treating PCCS continue to be disappointing. Pierce et al.[48] showed that

TABLE 7.   Hemodynamic Parameters

	Postop	Day 1	Day 2	Day 3	Day 4	Day 5	Day 6	Day 7	Day 8
VAD rate (bpm)	85	85	85	85	85	85	100	65	55
Heart rate (bpm)	160	120	120	133	120	114	100	88	104
BP (mmHg)	120/75	125/75	125/70	120/70	130/75	150/80	145/70	130/80	135/70
RAP (mmHg)	25	21	18	16	15	19	18	10	12
ADO (L/min)	5.5	5.3	5.3	5.2	5.2	4.8	4.0	4.0	3.5
VAC (mmHg)	30	25	25	25	25	25	15	10	0
SYS (%)	42	41	41	43	46	44	45	39	36
LDP (mmHg)	200	200	195	195	195	195	195	195	195
PFHG (mg/dl)	100	45	35	30	91	36	18	6	5

BP = blood pressure; RAP = right atrial pressure; ADO = average device output; VAC = vacuum; SYS = systole; LDP = left drive pressure; PFHG = plasma free hemoglobin.

for recovery to occur, at least 4–12 days (with an average of 7 days) of pulsatile ventricular assistance were required. This time frame is consistent with experimental studies examining the condition of the stunned myocardium[5] and is believed to be associated with the time required to restore myocardial ATP as well as to reverse the ultrastructural abnormalities that occurred with injury. The clinical data for recovery from allograft failure[20,35] also show a minimal support interval of at least 7 days. In one instance of recovery from myocarditis with acute cardiopulmonary failure, 70 days of pulsatile ventricular assistance was required.[18] Thus, a prerequisite for improving survivability in PCCS is a VAD that can safely provide circulatory support for a period of at least 7 days.

The pneumatic VADs, in comparison with the market-approved roller and centrifugal pumps, are superior in providing the required support for BTR.[8,38] The data show that the roller and centrifugal pumps have significantly higher hemolysis and bleeding complications as well as thromboembolic accidents. The limited capability of centrifugal pumps to provide long-term support is exemplified in the mean durations of LVAD support for bridging to transplantation.[33] The mean centrifugal LVAD support duration is 6.1 days, compared with 31.9 days for pneumatic LVADs and 48.1 days for electric LVADs.

One explanation for the greater complications associated with roller and centrifugal pumps is that the use of long tubing and cannulas causes a significant increase in impedance to flow, which must be overcome with higher pump rates. This results in greater hemolysis and requires more power, which is associated with greater heating and thermal deformation of proteins. The impedance estimate for the common tubing used with centrifugal pumps can easily be 10 times greater than the impedance of the atrial cannula of the Symbion AVAD.

If centrifugal pump rates are lowered to reduce hemolysis, inadequate flow rates affect organ function and increase the risk of thrombus formation. The potential for thromboembolic events can be counteracted with increased anticoagulation; however, this may not be feasible if active bleeding persists.[7,28] The introduction of the heparin-coated tubing with the centrifugal pump systems[23] may be a welcome advance; however, a broader experience is necessary before its usefulness can be determined.

Regardless of the anticoagulation issue, no evidence suggests that centrifugal pumps can be employed for longer than a few days without complications; hence clinicians consider them effective for support periods of <1 week.[45] This clearly indicates that for BTR the choice for circulatory assistance should be pneumatic heterotopic VADs. Although the evidence is substantiated, pneumatic VADs continue to be challenged and to undergo strict experimental and clinical investigations to meet the approval of the FDA for widespread market release. Another important advantage of pneumatic VADs is that in the event of inadequate myocardial recovery, the appropriate long-term support system is in place for BTT.

Our approach for BTR with pneumatic VADs consists of two phases. Initially (first 24 hours) asynchronous pumping with high vacuum is used to achieve maximal flow rates to ensure hemodynamic stability and end-organ perfusion. Once this is accomplished and the native rate is <100 bpm, 1:1 EKG synchronous counterpulsation is used to increase subendocardial blood flow. We successfully applied this approach to a patient requiring BVAD support secondary to allograft failure after orthotopic heart transplantation.[35] However, Icenogle et al.[20] show the same results for a similar case by using the asynchronous pumping mode alone. At first glance this might indicate that the added trouble of device optimization and EKG synchronous counterpulsation is unnecessary. However, studies[2,5,11,22,24,43,52,54] continue to show that maximal ventricular unloading and EKG synchronous counterpulsation are important in minimizing infarct size; therefore, improved survival would be expected when optimal device output and EKG synchronous pumping are used for recoverable injury, particularly after infarction.

Our experimental and clinical data show that EKG synchronous pumping leads to a reduction in ADO, which can be as large as 1 L/min. However, this is with the added benefit of providing diastolic augmentation and reduction in afterload. Our approach for dealing with this limitation has been to employ EKG synchronous counterpulsation only when the native heart rate is <100 bpm, which might occur during the later stages of the initial recovery period. In addition, we use vacuum to compensate for the reduction in ADO. This may tend to increase the hemolysis; however, alterations in drive pressure can counteract this effect.

The experimental data clearly demonstrate that pneumatic VADs with EKG synchronous counterpulsation provide the ideal setting for recovery from an ischemic injury. The superiority of pneumatic VADs over centrifugal VADs is clear. The reasoning for continued strict regulation of pneumatic VADs is obscure. Certainly this technology is safer than centrifugal pumps for long-term patient care, and continued restrictions exacerbate the considerable economic burden associated with treatment. Certainly, with our present experience, every effort should be made to deregulate superior technology and to let expanding markets reduce cost and improve availability. Only with widespread access will the true value of pneumatic VADs as a BTR be known.

REFERENCES

1. Al-Mondhiry H, Pierce WS, Richenbacher W, Bull A: Hemostatic abnormalities associated with prolonged ventricular assist pumping: Analysis of 24 patients. Am J Cardiol 53:1344–1348, 1984.
2. Bavaria JE, Furukawa S, Kreiner G, et al: Effect of circulatory assist devices on stunned myocardium. Ann Thorac Surg 49:123–128, 1990.
3. Bellotoo F, Johnson RG, Watanabe J, et al: Mechanical assistance of the left ventricle: Acute effect on cardiac performance and coronary flow of different perfusion patterns. J Thorac Cardiovasc Surg 104:561–568, 1992.
4. Bolman RM, Cox JL, Marshall W, et al: Circulatory support with a centrifugal pump as a bridge to cardiac transplantation. Ann Thorac Surg 47:108–112, 1989.
5. Braunwald E, Kloner RA: The stunned myocardium: Prolonged, postischemic ventricular dysfunction. Circulation 66:1146–1149, 1982.
6. Cohen DJ, Genecov DG, Clen MF, et al: Effect of synchronous and asynchronous pulsatile flow during left, right and biventricular bypass. ASAIO Trans 37:363–364, 1991.
7. Copeland JG, Harker LA, Joist JH, DeVries WC: Bleeding and anticoagulation. Ann Thorac Surg 47:88–95, 1989.
8. Cribbs RK, Campbell DB, Pierce WS: Vacuum effects on cellular integrity in a pulsatile ventricular assist system. ASAIO Abstr 19:63, 1990.
9. Dasse KA, Chipman SD, Sherman CN, et al: Clinical experience with textured blood contacting surfaces in ventricular assist devices. ASAIO Trans 33:418–425, 1987.
10. Debakey ME: Left ventricular bypass for cardiac assistance: Clinical experience. Am J Cardiol 27:3, 1971.
11. Eugene J, Ott RA, Moore-Jeffries EW, et al: Left atrial-to-aortic assistance: Effect of in-line venting on myocardial oxygen consumption. Heart Transplant 3:329–335, 1984.
12. Farrar DJ, Compton PG, Lawson JH, et al: Control modes of a clinical ventricular assist device. IEEE Eng Med Biol 5:19–25, 1986.
13. Farrar DJ, Hill JD, Gray LA, et al: Heterotopic prosthetic ventricles as a bridge to cardiac transplantation: A multicenter study in 29 patients. N Engl J Med 318:333–340, 1988.

14. Gutfinger DE, Ott RA, Gazzaniga AB: Design for in-vitro testing of pneumatic VAD assistance. ASAIO Abstr 21:41, 1992.
15. Gutfinger DE, Ott RA, Eugene J, et al: Prediction of optimal pneumatic TAH/VAD function using device impedance. ASAIO Abstr 21:40, 1992.
16. Henker R, Murdaugh C: Effects of pneumatic artificial heart driver on the rate of isovolumic pressure rise. Artif Organs 12:519–525, 1988.
17. Hill JD: Bridging to cardiac transplantation. Ann Thorac Surg 47:113–120, 1989.
18. Holman WL, Bourge RC, Kirklin JK: Circulatory support for seventy days with resolution of acute heart failure. J Thorac Cardiovasc Surg 102:932–934, 1991.
19. Icenogle TB, Smith RG, Cleavinger M, et al: Thromboembolic complications of the Symbion AVAD System. Artif Organs 13:532–538, 1989.
20. Icenogle TB, Williams RJ, Smith RG, et al: Extracorporeal pulsatile biventricular support after cardiac transplantation. Ann Thorac Surg 47:614–616, 1989.
21. Jurmann MJ, Wahlers T, Coppola R, et al: Early graft failure after heart transplantation: Management by extracorporeal circulatory assist and retransplantation. J Heart Transplant 8:474–478, 1989.
22. Laks H, Ott RA, Standever J, et al: Servo-controlled cardiac assistance: Effect of left ventricular-to-aortic and left atrial-to-aortic assistance on infarct size. Am J Cardiol 42:244–250, 1978.
23. Larm O, Arrader L, Olsson P: Influence of blood flow and the effect of protamine on the thrombo resistant properties of a covalently bonded heparin surface. J Biomed Mater Res 22:859–868, 1988.
24. Laschinger JC, Grossi EA, Cunningham JN, et al: Adjunctive left ventricular unloading during myocardial reperfusion plays a major role in minimizing myocardial infarct size. J Thorac Cardiovasc Surg 90:80–85, 1985.
25. Levinson MM, Copeland JG, Smith RG, et al: Indexes of hemolysis in human recipients of the Jarvik-7 total artificial heart: A cooperative report of fifteen patients. J Heart Transplant 5:236–248, 1986.
26. Levinson MM, Smith RG, Cork RC, et al: Thromboembolic complications of the Jarvik-7 total artificial heart: Case report. Artif Organs 10:236–244, 1986.
27. Lohmann DP, Swartz MT, Pennington DG, et al: Left ventricular versus left atrial cannulation for the Thoratec ventricular assist device. ASAIO Trans 36:545–548, 1990.
28. Magovern GJ, Sang BP, Maher TD: Use of the centrifugal pumps without anticoagulants for postoperative left ventricular assist. World J Surg 9:25–36, 1985.
29. Magovern GJ, Golding LAR, Oyer PE, Cabrol C: Weaning and bridging: Circulatory support, 1988. Ann Thorac Surg 47:102–107, 1989.
30. McGee M, Parnis S, Nakatani T, et al: Extended clinical support with an implantable left ventricular assist device. ASAIO Trans 35:614–616, 1989.
31. Mills TC, Ott RA: Effectiveness of synchronous mode pneumatic ventricular assistance in reversible myocardial injury. ASAIO Abstr 19:59, 1990.
32. Mills TC, Ott RA: Techniques for optimization of pulsatile ventricular assist device support. Artif Organs 16:218–221, 1992.
33. Oaks TE, Pae WE Jr, Miller CA, Pierce WS: Combined Registry for the Clinical Use of Mechanical Ventricular Assist Pumps and the Total Artificial Heart in Conjunction with Heart Transplantation: Fifth official report—1990. J Heart Lung Transplant 10:621–625, 1991.
34. Ott RA, Mills TC, Eugene J, Gazzaniga AB: Clinical choices for circulatory assist devices. ASAIO Trans 36:792–798, 1990.
35. Ott RA, Mills T, Allen B, et al: Successful treatment of acute allograft failure using pneumatic biventricular assistance. J Heart Lung Transplant 10:264–268, 1991.
36. Ott RA, Gutfinger DE, Eugene J, et al: Superior endomyocardial perfusion with synchronous VAD pumping. ASAIO Abstr 21:40, 1992.
37. Ott RA, Mills T: A simple method to avoid thrombus formation at the de-airing port of the acute ventricular assist device. J Heart Lung Transplant 11:136–138, 1992.
38. Pae WE Jr: Temporary ventricular support: Current indications and results. ASAIO Abstr 33:4–7, 1987.
39. Pae WE Jr, Pierce WS, Pennock JL, et al: Long-term results of ventricular assist pumping in postcardiotomy cardiogenic shock. J Thorac Cardiovasc Surg 93:434–441, 1987.
40. Pae WE, Miller CA, Matthews Y, Pierce WS: Ventricular assist devices for postcardiotomy cardiogenic shock: A combined registry experience. J Thorac Cardiovasc Surg 104:541–553, 1992.
41. Parascandola SA, Pae WE, Davis PK, et al: Determinants of survival in patients with ventricular assist devices. ASAIO Trans 34:222–228, 1988.

42. Park SB, Liebler GA, Burkholder JA, et al: Mechanical support of the failing heart. Ann Thorac Surg 42:627–631, 1986.
43. Pennock JL, Pierce WS, Prophet A, et al: Myocardial oxgen utilization during left heart bypass: Effect of various percentage of bypass flow rates. Arch Surg 109:635–641, 1974.
44. Pennock JL, Pierce WS, Wisman CB, et al: Survival and complications following ventricular assist pumping for cardiogenic shock. Ann Surg 198:469–478, 1983.
45. Pennington DG, Swartz MT: Management: By circulatory assist devices. Cardiol Clin 7:195–204, 1989.
46. Pennington DG, McBridge LR, Swartz MT: Use of the Pierce-Donachy ventricular assist device in patients with cardiogenic shock after cardiac operations. Ann Thorac Surg 47:130–135, 1989.
47. Pierce WS: Clinical left ventricular bypass: Problems of pump inflow obstruction and right ventricular failure. ASAIO Trans 2:1–9, 1979.
48. Pierce WS, Rosenberg GG, Donachy JH, et al: Postoperative cardiac support with a pulsatile assist pump: Techniques and results. Artif Organs 11:247–251, 1987.
49. Portner PM, Jassawalla JS, Oyer PE, et al: A totally implantable ventricular assist system for terminal heart failure. ASAIO Trans 34:57–76, 1988.
50. Portner PM, Oyer PE, Pennington DG, et al: Implantable electric left ventricular assist system: Bridge to transplantation and the future. Ann Thorac Surg 47:142–150, 1989.
51. Rose DM, Connolly M, Cunningham JN, et al: Technique and results with roller pump left and right assist device. Ann Thorac Surg 47:124–129, 1989.
52. Ruf W, Smith GT, Geary G, et al: Effects of left ventricular-to-aortic bypass on infarct size in infarct microcirculation in baboons. J Thorac Cardiovasc Surg 81:408–418, 1981.
53. Spencer FC, Eiseman UG, Trinkle JK, et al: Assisted circulation for cardiac failure following intracardiac surgery with cardiopulmonary bypass. J Thorac Cardiovasc Surg 45:56, 1965.
54. Zumbro GL, Kitchens WR, Shearer G, et al: Mechanical assistance for cardiogenic shock following cardiac surgery, myocardial infarction, and cardiac transplantation. Ann Thorac Surg 44:11–13, 1987.

BRUCE J. SHOOK, MS Eng

THE ABIOMED BVS 5000 BIVENTRICULAR SUPPORT SYSTEM
System Description and Clinical Summary

Vice President of Clinical and
Regulatory Affairs
ABIOMED, Inc.
Danvers, Massachusetts

Reprint requests to:
Bruce J. Shook, MS Eng
Vice President of Clinical and
Regulatory Affairs
ABIOMED, Inc.
33 Cherry Hill Drive
Danvers, MA 01923

The treatment of cardiogenic shock with mechanical circulatory assist devices has taken many different directions since early attempts at prolonged assist with the roller pump.[7] Numerous devices have evolved to support the circulation, each of which is targeted to meet a unique subset of both patient and physician needs.

This chapter reviews the ABIOMED BVS 5000 Biventricular Support System. The BVS 5000 has been specifically designed to provide biventricular, pulsatile assist at a reasonable cost and with a minimum of operational complexity. Meeting this challenge requires satisfying the primary needs of the patient with cardiogenic shock and the clinical staff providing care.

Achievement of these design goals has made the BVS 5000 the most widely used biventricular assist device since its clinical introduction in 1987. The dedicated efforts of 16 clinical investigators also made the BVS 5000 the first circulatory assist device to receive premarket approval from the Food and Drug Administration (FDA) (November, 1992).

SYSTEM DESCRIPTION

The BVS 5000 is a pulsatile ventricular assist device capable of providing either left, right, or biventricular support. The system consists of single-use blood pumps that are actuated by a pneumatic drive console (Fig. 1). The pump is placed at the bedside; blood drains from the patient's left or right atrium into the top of the pump and returns to the patient's aorta or pulmonary artery from the bottom of the pump.

CARDIAC SURGERY: State of the Art Reviews—Vol. 7, No. 2, 1993
Philadelphia, Hanley & Belfus, Inc.

309

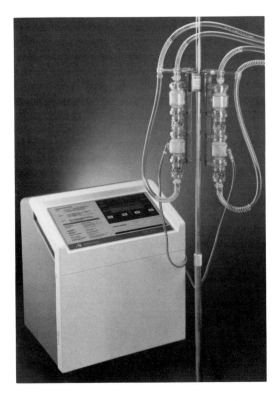

FIGURE 1. ABIOMED BVS 5000 drive console and single-use blood pumps.

The blood pumps are unlike any other ventricular assist device in three primary respects:

1. The blood pump is a dual-chamber device that incorporates an atrial (filling) chamber and a ventricular (pumping) chamber;

2. Unidirectional flow is ensured by two trileaflet polyurethane valves (Fig. 2) fabricated from Angioflex, an ultrapure biomaterial; and

3. System controls are essentially limited to "on" and "off." A highly automated control system constantly optimizes pump performance to adapt to changing patient conditions.

Dual-chamber Design

Both the atrial and ventricular chambers contain a smooth surfaced polyurethane bladder (volume = 100 ml). The atrial chamber fills passively from the patient throughout pump systole and diastole. This dual-chamber design produces continuous flow from the patient to the pump and pulsatile flow from the pump back to the patient. The patient's heart is continuously drained, even when the pump is ejecting. The ventricular chamber alternately collapses and fills in response to delivery of compressed air from the console. Figure 3 illustrates the operation of the blood pump.

The continuous drainage produced by the action of the atrial chamber also simplifies system operation and enhances safety. Vacuum is not needed to assist filling with the dual-chamber BVS blood pump. This eliminates the operational complexity associated with controlling vacuum and minimizes the risk of atrial collapse and aspiration of air into the system.

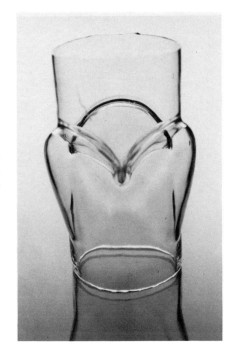

FIGURE 2. Angioflex polyurethane tri-leaflet valve. Two valves are used in each BVS 5000 blood pump to provide unidi-rectional flow.

Polyurethane Trileaflet Valves

The polyurethane trileaflet valve (Fig. 2) used in the BVS 5000 blood pump was originally developed by Lederman and coworkers[6] for use in implantable devices. The valve is fabricated from Angioflex, with no seam between the valve leaflets and conduit walls. Behind each leaflet is a contoured sinus, which is designed to minimize regurgitation on closure, cusp flapping during midsystole, and the generation of thrombi in regions where shear might otherwise be low.[6]

The unique combination of mechanical durability, hemodynamic performance, and low cost made these trileaflet valves ideal for the BVS 5000. The valve made possible a significant reduction in the cost of the blood pump relative to competitive technologies using prosthetic heart valves without compromise of excellent performance.

Control System

Advanced computer technology and a closed-loop control algorithm, developed by Bolt and coworkers,[1] allow full automation of the control system with no direct electrical connection to the patient. The control system monitors the flow of air to and from the blood pumps through the driveline tubing. Data regarding driveline air flow provide important information about blood pump performance: stroke volume (during pump systole) and ventricular bladder filling (during pump diastole). By continuously monitoring air flow, the computer can accurately adjust the duration of pump systole and diastole, pump beat rate, and pump flow. These parameters are controlled to accommodate the flow of blood coming from the patient and to maintain the pump stroke volume near its target value of 80 ml.

The net result of this automation is a system that needs only to be turned on. Once the system is running, the clinical staff do not need to adjust timing, rate, or flow. Clinicians need be concerned only with maintaining appropriate patient hydration

ABIOMED BVS 5000 BLOOD PUMP

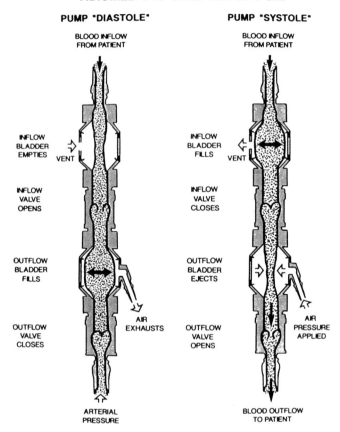

FIGURE 3. Cross-section of the BVS 5000 blood pump during the diastolic and systolic phases of pump operation.

and proper pump height relative to the patient. The pumps are typically positioned so that the top of the pump is 0–25 cm below the level of the patient's atria (Fig. 4).

The clinician may easily adjust pump flow downward through use of the weaning controls. Flow through each pump can be independently decreased in increments of 0.1 L/min from the prevailing flow down to a minimal value of 0.5 L/min. If the patient fails to tolerate the reduced blood flow, the weaning mode is simply turned off, and the pump automatically returns to the full-flow operating mode.

Cannulation

Vascular access is achieved with 46-French, wire-reinforced cannulas. The atrial cannula has a lighthouse tip and is placed through double pursestring sutures directly into the left or right atrium. Left atrial cannulation can be performed behind the interatrial groove, through the left atrial dome, or through the left atrial appendage. Right atrial cannulation can be performed through the mid-free wall or right atrial appendage. The arterial cannula incorporates a 14-mm, woven Dacron graft in place of the lighthouse tip. The graft's exterior is coated with

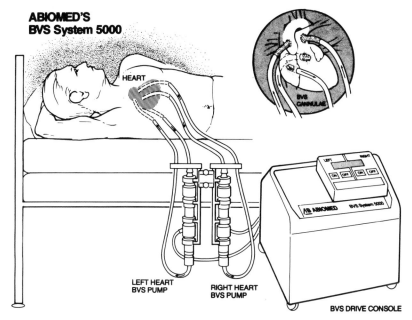

FIGURE 4. Placement of the BVS 5000 blood pump at the bedside.

an elastomer, which greatly reduces interstitial bleeding and eliminates the need for preclotting before implantation. The graft is attached to the ascending aorta or pulmonary artery via an end-to-side anastomosis. Figures 5 and 6 illustrate typical cannulation arrangements for left- and right-heart support, respectively.

The cannulas are externalized subcostally through tunnels from the pericardial space through the skin. This subcostal externalization is designed to permit sternal closure. A Dacron velour sleeve on the exterior of each cannula promotes hemostasis at the skin interface.

CLINICAL EXPERIENCE

Clinical use of the BVS 5000 began in 1987 after the successful completion of extensive animal studies.[4] Since that time, the BVS 5000 has been used in 15 countries and more than 50 centers and has resulted in the salvage of more than 100 patients who otherwise would have died. Worldwide usage of the BVS 5000 currently includes at least 352 patients and spans a variety of indications for use (Fig. 7). The dominant indication is postcardiotomy shock, which accounts for almost half of all supported patients. Most of the remaining patients received BVS 5000 support as a bridge to transplant after cardiomyopathy, massive acute myocardial infarction (AMI), or failed heart transplant (voluntary worldwide registry maintained by ABIOMED, Inc.). The BVS 5000 has also been used successfully to treat patients who suffer acute cardiac failure secondary to myocarditis.[3]

The majority (65%) of patients required biventricular support (Fig. 8). Thirty percent received left univentricular support only, and 4% received right ventricular support only.

The outcome of BVS 5000 support for any of these indications is inextricably linked to patient selection. The best survival statistics are associated with bridge

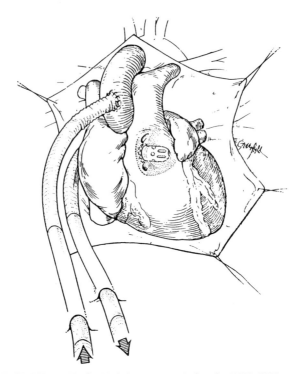

FIGURE 5.   Typical left-heart cannulation for BVS 5000 support.

to transplant. Fifty-seven patients (69%) with cardiomyopathy underwent successful transplantation, and 35 patients (42%) survived to hospital discharge. In one institution that has acquired significant experience with the BVS 5000, 100% of supported patients underwent successful transplantation, and 70% survived to hospital discharge.[2]

The worldwide statistics for postcardiotomy support demonstrate that 62 patients (37%) were successfully weaned from BVS 5000 support, 24 (14%) underwent transplantation, and 45 (27%) survived to hospital discharge. These data compare favorably with the voluntary international registry compiled by Penn State University,[5] which reports that among 965 patients treated for postcardiotomy shock with various assist devices, 24.6% survived to discharge. These survival statistics represent what centers with all levels of experience can expect, on average, from the application of mechanical assist after cardiac surgery. However, the BVS 5000 clinical trial conducted for FDA approval has demonstrated that careful patient selection can make a dramatic difference (data pending publication). Patients enrolled in this study were retrospectively segregated into two groups: those who had experienced at least one cardiac arrest before BVS 5000 support (group I) and those who had experienced no cardiac arrest (group II). The discharged survival rate within group II was 47%—significantly higher than any other group within the study population.

Quality of life for survivors of BVS 5000 support is excellent. The majority of patients in the clinical study who were discharged home were alive and well at 1-year follow-up. These patients were in New York Heart Association functional class I or II and had resumed their normal activities.

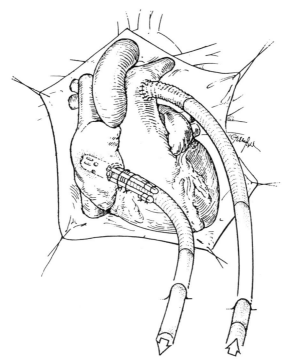

FIGURE 6.   Typical right-heart cannulation for BVS 5000 support.

WORLDWIDE POPULATION (N=352)

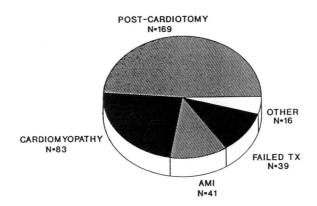

FIGURE 7.   Distribution of patients supported with the BVS 5000 by indication for use. Included are all patients in the voluntary registry maintained by ABIOMED, Inc. as of November, 1992.

MODE OF SUPPORT
(N = 352)

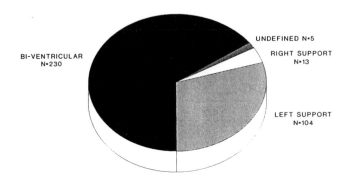

FIGURE 8. Distribution of patients supported with the BVS 5000 by mode of support. Included are all patients in the voluntary registry maintained by ABIOMED, Inc. as of November, 1992.

CONCLUSION

The BVS 5000 was developed to address the needs of both the patient and the clinical support team. This design approach has led the BVS 5000 to become one of the most widely used pulsatile cardiac assist devices in the world. Clinical experience spans numerous indications for use and involves many investigators. Included in the experience is a highly controlled, prospective clinical trial, which has provided much insight into the performance of the BVS 5000 and the factors that ultimately influence success.

Because of this experience, the BVS 5000 has become the first cardiac assist device to receive premarket approval in the U.S. The FDA's action will make this life-saving technology available to all cardiac surgeons and their patients.

Widespread use of the BVS 5000 not only will save lives, but also represents a meaningful step toward the ultimate goal of total heart replacement. The lessons we learn today with the BVS 5000 are invaluable as we move forward with the development of completely implantable systems.

REFERENCES

1. Bolt WJ, Singh PI, Cumming RD: Closed loop control of a new pulsatile biventricular support system. Presentation at CECEC, Paris, June 27, 1987.
2. Champsaur G, Ninet J, Vigneron M, et al: Use of the ABIOMED BVS System 5000 as a bridge to cardiac transplantation. J Thorac Cardiovasc Surg 100:122–128, 1990.
3. Jett GK, Miller A, Savino D, Gonwa T: Reversal of acute fulminant lymphocytic myocarditis with combined technology of OKT3 monoclonal antibody and mechanical circulatory support. J Heart Lung Transplant 11:733–738, 1992.
4. Lederman DM: Technical considerations in the development of clinical systems for temporary and permanent cardiac support. In Akutsu T (ed): Artificial Heart 2. Tokyo, Springer Verlag, 1988, pp 115–127.
5. Pae WE, Miller CA, Matthews Y, Pierce WS: Ventricular assist devices for postcardiotomy shock. J Thorac Surg 104:541–553, 1992.
6. Russell FD, Lederman DM, Singh PI, et al: Development of seamless trileaflet valves. ASAIO Trans 26:66–70, 1980.
7. Spencer FC, Eiseman B, Trinkle JK, Rossi NP: Assisted circulation for cardiac failure following intracardiac surgery with cardiopulmonary bypass. J Thorac Cardiovasc Surg 49:56–73, 1965.

J. DONALD HILL, MD
DAVID J. FARRAR, PhD
NINA TOPIC, RN,MS

THE THORATEC EXPERIENCE IN BRIDGE TO CARDIAC TRANSPLANTATION

From the Department of
Cardiac Surgery
California Pacific Medical Center
San Francisco, California

Reprint requests to:
J. Donald Hill, MD
Department of Cardiac Surgery
California Pacific Medical Center
2100 Webster, Suite 512
San Francisco, CA 94115

The use of artificial devices to support patients until the procurement of a suitable donor heart was first reported in 1969.[3] Just as cardiac transplantation has moved from an experimental procedure to an accepted therapy for the treatment of endstage cardiac disease, the use of prosthetic ventricles and artificial hearts in patients at imminent risk of dying before a donor heart becomes available has become a standard method of supporting the circulation until heart transplantation.[16] Bridge to transplantation is a two-step process: implantation of the support device and subsequent orthotopic cardiac transplantation.

The Thoratec ventricular assist device (VAD) system was first used successfully as a bridge to transplant in September 1984.[11] We have previously reported the results with this device in the first 29 patients[7] and in the first 72 patients.[8] This chapter summarizes our experience to date in 154 patients who had left-sided or biventricular support with Thoratec VADs as a bridge to heart transplantation and compares trends in its use with the previous reports.

The Thoratec VAD system consists of prosthetic ventricles with a 65-ml stroke volume, appropriate cannulas for atrial and/or ventricular inflow and arterial outflow connections, and a pneumatic drive console (Figs. 1 and 2). The blood pumping chamber and cannulas are fabricated from Thoratec's BPS-215M polyurethane

CARDIAC SURGERY: State of the Art Reviews—Vol. 7, No. 2, 1993
Philadelphia, Hanley & Belfus, Inc.

317

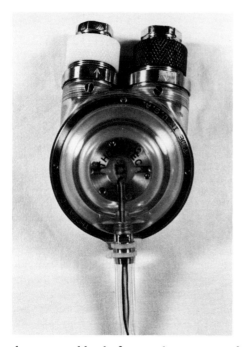

FIGURE 1. The Thoratec VAD consists of a 65-ml flexible polyurethane blood-pumping chamber in a rigid plastic housing.

elastomer, a blend of two polymers, one of which provides extensive flex life and strength, whereas the other provides thromboresistance.[5] The pneumatic drive console (Fig. 2) provides alternating positive and negative air pressure to empty and fill the blood pump and has three control modes depending on the needs of the patient: asynchronous (fixed rate), volume (full-to-empty variable rate), and synchronous.[6] The full-to-empty mode is used in most bridge cases, because it automatically adjusts beat rate and thus flow output in accordance with venous return and the needs of the body.

These heterotopic prosthetic ventricles are placed in a paracorporeal position on the anterior abdominal wall and are connected to the heart and great vessels with cannulas that cross the chest wall. For support of the left side of the heart, inflow cannulation can be achieved from the left atrial appendage, from the left atrium via the interatrial groove,[2] or from the left ventricular apex, depending on the patient's anatomy or the surgeon's preference. VAD outflow is through a polyurethane cannula attached to a preclotted 14-mm polyester graft anastomosed to the ascending aorta. For support of the right side, cannulation is from the right atrium with return blood flow to the pulmonary artery.[9]

STUDY DESIGN

The studies in the United States were carried out under the regulations for investigational device exemption (IDE) of the Food and Drug Administration (FDA). The protocol and patient consent forms were approved by institutional review boards and by the FDA. Informed consent was obtained from either the patient or the next of kin.

Excluded from the study were patients with known contraindications to cardiac transplantation other than those considered to be reversible after restoration of adequate cardiac output. At the time of device implant patients

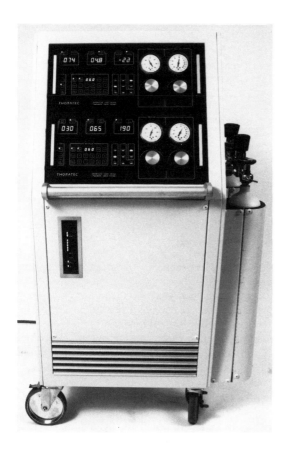

FIGURE 2. The drive console of the Thoratec VAD, containing two independent pneumatic drive modules, may be used for univentricular or biventricular support.

must be judged at imminent risk of death before obtaining a suitable donor heart on the basis of the following hemodynamic guidelines: (1) a cardiac index <1.8 L/min/m², (2) a systolic arterial pressure <90 mmHg, and (3) a left atrial pressure >20 mmHg despite appropriate use of conventional therapies such as inotropic agents, vasodilators, and intraaortic balloon pumps (IABPs).

Patients in whom contraindications developed during the bridging period and whose condition could not be stabilized by circulatory support with VADs did not receive a heart transplant and ultimately died.

As of October 1991, 154 patients awaiting heart transplantation and at imminent risk of dying before donor heart procurement have received Thoratec VADs for left or biventricular support at 39 medical centers in 10 countries (Fig. 3). Coronary artery disease was diagnosed in 65 patients (endstage ischemic heart disease in 43 patients and acute myocardial infarction [AMI] in 22) and cardiomyopathy in 73 patients (2 hypertrophic, 7 viral, 9 postpartum, and 55 idiopathic) (Fig. 4). An additional 16 patients received devices because of graft failure after prior orthotopic cardiac transplantation (8), valvular disease (3), myocarditis (3), adriamycin toxicity (1), or transposition of the great vessels (1). The 121 men and 33 women had an average age of 42 years (range: 11–64 years), an average body surface of 1.84 m² (range: 1.06–2.41 m²), and an average weight of 73 kg

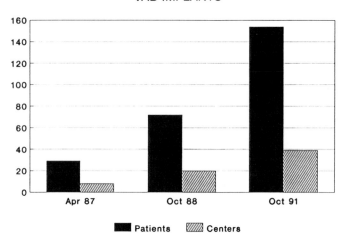

FIGURE 3. As of October 1991, the Thoratec experience with bridge to transplant includes 154 patients from 39 centers.

(range: 30–123 kg). Despite increased use of the device over time, the basic makeup of the patient population has remained relatively constant.

All patients undergoing implantation were receiving maximal inotropic support. In addition, 64 (42%) had experienced 1 or more cardiac arrests, 99 (64%) received cardiac assistance with IABPs, and 89 (58%) were receiving mechanical ventilation. Despite this therapy, the average cardiac index in the current patient population was 1.4 ± 0.9 L/min/m² with a pulmonary capillary wedge pressure of 30 ± 8 mmHg. The decision to implant VADs was made when the clinical and hemodynamic status indicated that the patient would probably die or sustain

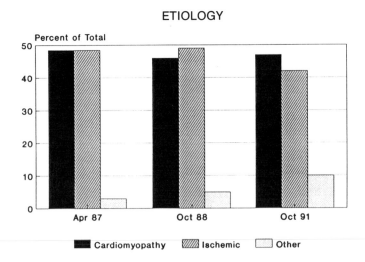

FIGURE 4. The etiology of heart failure in bridge-to-transplant patients has remained constant over time.

permanent end-organ damage before a donor heart could be located. As with the criteria defining patient population, the baseline hemodynamics have remained constant over time.

RESULTS

Of the 154 patients implanted with Thoratec VADs, 3 remain on support as of this analysis, awaiting a suitable donor heart. Results are reported for 151 patients, in whom the Thoratec VAD supported circulation for up to 226 days until a donor heart could be located and transplantation performed. Blood flow from the left VADs (LVADs) averaged 5.0 ± 0.9 L/min (flow index: 2.7 ± 0.5 L/min/m²), whereas flow from the right VADs (RVADs) averaged 4.3 ± 0.8 L/min (flow index: 2.3 ± 0.4 L/min/m²).

Of the 151 patients who received VADs for bridging to transplantation, 98 (65%) recovered sufficiently to receive transplants. Of the patients undergoing transplantation, 82 were eventually discharged from the hospital. The early posttransplant survival rate was 84% (Fig. 5), and the overall survival rate from implant to patient discharge was 54%. As the device is used in more centers, pretransplant survival appears to decrease slightly, but the difference is not statistically significant. The 1-year actuarial survival for patients bridged to transplantation with the Thoratec VAD was 82%, compared with 81% for conventional transplantation, as reported by the Registry of the International Society for Heart Transplantation.[13]

In 34 patients (22%) univentricular LVADs were sufficient to support circulation. The survival rates for the LVAD patients (87% posttransplant, 63% overall) were not statistically different from those for the 119 patients with biventricular support (83% posttransplant, 52% overall). The fraction of patients receiving biventricular support devices has increased over the past 4 years to 78% (Fig. 6).

Overall survival from VAD implant to patient discharge showed a slight decrease with age (63% in patients below 40 years, 53% in patients 40–49 years,

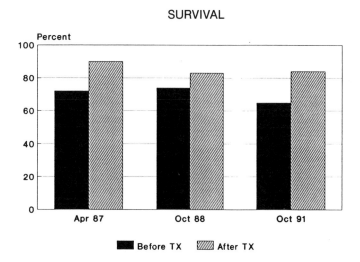

SURVIVAL

FIGURE 5.   Since our first report, there have been no statistically significant differences in survival in the bridge procedure.

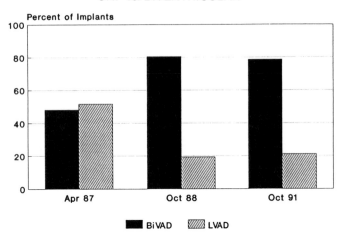

FIGURE 6. The percentage of patients receiving biventricular support has increased from 48% to 79%.

and 49% in patients 50 years and over), and posttransplant survival for patients 50 and over (83%) was actually better than for patients 40–49 (76%) but not as good as for patients under 40 (91%).

The median duration of all bridge cases was 7 days (mean: 17 days). Since our first report the maximal duration of support has increased from 31 days to 226 days (Fig. 7). Sixty-nine patients had VADs for <7 days, 43 patients for 7–30 days, and 25 patients for 30–226 days. The percentage of patients who underwent transplantation was not statistically different (65–68%) among these groups. Posttransplant

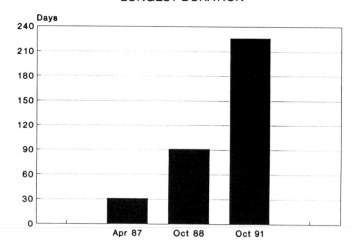

FIGURE 7. The maximal duration of VAD support has increased since 1987, reflecting the widening gap between donor-organ availability and patients awaiting transplantation.

survival for patients supported < 7 days was 89%. Survival in this group appeared to be higher compared with that of patients supported for 7–30 days (79%) or for >30 days (76%), but the differences did not reach statistical significance. The overall survival rate was similar for the 3 groups (58–52%).

COMPLICATIONS

Complete data on complications are available for 137 patients who received Thoratec VADs for bridge to transplantation. The percentage of patients undergoing reoperation for bleeding after device insertion has decreased since our initial report (from 38% to 23%), as has the percentage of patients who died from this complication (from 14% to 7%) (Fig. 8). Surgical bleeding and coagulopathies resulting in excessive chest-tube drainage, tamponade, hemothorax, or reoperation remain the most common complications during the bridge period and were reported in 42% of patients. Infection was another major complication, occurring in 49 patients (36%) and causing death in 11 (8%). Renal failure was reported in 50 patients (36%), 24 of whom required dialysis during the bridge period. Fifteen patients succumbed to multiorgan failure, which was the most common cause of death in patients who did not survive to transplantation. Hepatic failure was reported in 24% of patients. Hemolysis (defined as a plasma free hemoglobin measurement >40 mg/dl) was seen in 26 patients (19%), usually only transiently in the first week or two of support. Only 3 patients required transfusion. Respiratory failure occurred in 24 patients. Nonthromboembolic neurologic events were reported in 19 patients, including 4 who died before transplantation from brain death, believed in retrospect to be present prior to VAD insertion. Embolic events occurred in 11 patients (8%), 8 of whom had simultaneous infections. Two patients died from cerebrovascular accidents (CVAs) before transplantation. One patient with an LVAD died before transplantation with right ventricular failure, and 1 patient died when adequate inflow through the LVAD cannula could not be achieved.

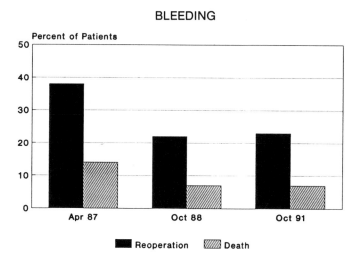

FIGURE 8.   Bleeding is the most frequently reported complication. Since 1987, however, the percentage of patients requiring reoperation for bleeding and the number of deaths from bleeding have decreased.

Seven patients who underwent transplantation died from graft failure before discharge from hospital. Additional deaths reported after transplantation but before discharge were due to infection in 4 patients, bleeding in 3 patients, and rejection in 1 patient.

DISCUSSION

From the outset important questions arose from both the medical community and ethicists over the role of bridging in cardiac transplantation. Some questioned whether the intervention should be allowed[1] because it was an untested therapy involving mechanical devices that were able to pump blood effectively when used for myocardial recovery but only sporadically had shown a positive effect on patient outcome. Then, as now, donor hearts were in short supply, and some feared that hearts would be "wasted" if the success rate in bridged patients was less than that in nonbridged recipients. By 1988 this was clearly not the case, at least with the Thoratec system.[7] Patients who have undergone heart transplantation after VAD support have survival rates equivalent to those of patients not requiring VADs.

Infection

Infection is still a concern in bridge to transplantation. Four general categories of infection must be considered: (1) chronic infection at the insertion sites of percutaneous leads or cannulas; (2) preexisting and iatrogenic infections; (3) bacteremic seeding of the blood–device interface; and (4) potential immunosuppression due to chronic blood pumping. The relative importance of each has changed drastically over the last 8 years.

Temporary/permanent percutaneous leads or cannulas in the setting of impending heart transplantation and subsequent immunosuppression seemed to provide a particularly good opportunity for chronic infection that might migrate into the mediastinum or contaminate the operative field at the time of transplantation. Particular concern focused on the paracorporeal placement of biventricular VADs with four transcutaneous cannulas. This requirement of the Thoratec system could lead to an increased incidence of wound infection and death. Surprisingly no such scenario has occurred, despite the fact that the duration of support has increased from days to weeks to months.

One of the most important findings of the Thoratec technology is the strength of the tissue–cannula surface adhesive bond, which makes it resistant to infection. Among over 300 paracorporeal implants to date, involving over 1000 percutaneous blood cannulas, superficial infections of percutaneous sites are not uncommon, but no instances of ascending infection and mediastinitis have occurred. In fact, once a device is implanted for 21 days, the adhesive bond is so strong that it resists forces of over 50 lbs of tension and must be removed by sharp dissection at the time of heart transplantation.

The presence of preexisting and iatrogenic infections, such as pneumonia, cystitis, or line sepsis, are still a major concern after 8 years of clinical experience. The looming prospect of an associated bacteremia necessitates early, accurate, and thorough initiation of antibiotic therapy. If a secondary organ infection is not controlled, the outlook for the patient is poor. Patients cannot have a device implanted in the presence of infection, and they cannot undergo transplantation in the presence of any but a minor infection. The interaction of infection and thrombosis is an important area of investigation in all chronic blood-pumping devices. The apparently synergistic relationship between infection and thrombosis is seriously detrimental to the patient.

Bacteremic seeding of the blood–device interface of chronically implanted VADs is the third major concern. Prophylactic antibiotic regimens are not yet clearly defined, although most centers do not use chronic prophylactic antibiotic therapy. Usually seeding cannot be treated successfully, and patients cannot undergo transplantation.

Finally, the role of chronic blood pumping on the body's natural immunity remains an area of concern. Although acute extracorporeal circulation temporarily suppresses the immune response, this suppression does not appear to have serious effects on the patient. However, the effect of chronic blood pumping on the immunologic system is not well understood, and apprehension over a possible negative relationship between the two remains.

Because duration of support is uncertain and infection is one of the major late complications, patient management should emphasize infection prevention and control from the outset. Monitoring lines should be pulled and the patient extubated as soon as possible. Ambulation and exercise should be encouraged.[17]

Bleeding

Bleeding (related to surgery and coagulopathy) and the need for early reoperation have been consistent problems in bridge to transplant.[10] Not only is bleeding a major complication in itself, but reoperations to control bleeding also increase the risk of late infection. The reasons for the relatively high incidence of bleeding are not completely understood, but two observations are worth noting: (1) a learning curve associated with device implantation is reflected in the early incidence of bleeding after insertion, and (2) the incidence of bleeding varies sharply among the different centers.

Patient Selection

Proper selection of patients and early implantation continue to be the principal factors influencing survival. Restoration of blood flow with VAD support may be too late to reverse preexisting conditions, as in patients who die from multi-organ failure and pre-VAD neurologic hypoxia. Unfortunately, it is often clear only in retrospect that the window of opportunity was missed; making the decision to proceed with early intervention remains a challenge. Debate continues over the best criteria for the timing of VAD insertion. The ideal candidate is in imminent risk of dying from irreversible myocardial damage but without end-organ involvement or contraindications to heart transplantation. The hemodynamic criteria used in the clinical investigation (cardiac index <1.8 L/min/m^2 and pulmonary capillary wedge pressure >20 mmHg) have been useful for study purposes, but sometimes they are inappropriate indicators in patients who deteriorate clinically at earlier points.

CONCLUSIONS

Preparation and team training are absolutely mandatory for a successful circulatory support program with the Thoratec VAD or any other device. The roles of hospital support staff should be clearly defined and the team organized and trained.[4,18] Nursing protocols and continuing education are necessary to meet the needs of circulatory support patients.[14]

The principal advantage of the Thoratec VAD system is its versatility. Left-heart cannulation can be accomplished via the left atrium or the left ventricular apex, and the paracorporeal approach allows it to be used in a wide range of body sizes; the smallest patient in this series was an 11-year-old with a body surface area of 1.06 m². The device can be used for support pending recovery of the natural heart[12,15] and for univentricular or biventricular support as a bridge to cardiac transplantation in critically ill patients. Posttransplant survival rates are comparable to those of conventional heart transplantation.

REFERENCES

1. Annas GJ: No cheers for temporary artificial hearts. Hastings Cent Rep 15:644–645, 1985.
2. Carpentier A, Brugger JP, Berthier B, et al: Heterotopic artificial heart as bridge to cardiac transplantation. Lancet 2:97–98, 1986.
3. Cooley DA, Liotta D, Hallman GL, et al: Orthotopic cardiac prosthesis for two-staged cardiac replacement. Am J Cardiol 24:723–730, 1969.
4. Elsesser CC, Smith BJ: Implementing a ventricular assist device program: A partnership between nursing and clinical engineering. Focus Crit Care AACN 18:14–22, 1991.
5. Farrar DJ, Compton PG, Lawson JH, et al: In vivo evaluations of a new thromboresistant polyurethane for artificial heart blood pumps. J Thorac Cardiovasc Surg 95:191–200, 1988.
6. Farrar DJ, Compton PG, Lawson JH, et al: Control modes of a clinical ventricular assist device. IEEE Eng Med Biol 5:19–25, 1986.
7. Farrar DJ, Hill JD, Gray LA Jr, et al: Heterotopic prosthetic ventricles as a bridge to cardiac transplantation: A multicenter study in 29 patients. N Engl J Med 318:333–340, 1988.
8. Farrar DJ, Lawson JH, Litwak P, Cederwall D: Thoratec VAD system as a bridge to heart transplantation. J Heart Transplant 415–423, 1990.
9. Ganzel BL, Gray LA Jr, Slater AD, Mavroudis C: Surgical techniques for the implantation of heterotopic prosthetic ventricles. Ann Thorac Surg 47:113–120, 1989.
10. Gray LA, Ganzel BL, Mavroudis C, Slater AD: The Pierce-Donachy ventricular assist device as a bridge to cardiac transplantation. Ann Thorac Surg 48:222–227, 1989.
11. Hill JD, Farrar DJ, Hershon JJ, et al: Use of a prosthetic ventricle as a bridge to cardiac transplantation for postinfarction cardiogenic shock. N Engl J Med 314:626–628, 1986.
12. Holman WL, Bourge RC, Kirklin JK: Case report: Circulatory support for seventy days with resolution of acute heart failure. J Thorac Cardiovasc Surg 102:932–934, 1991.
13. Kriett JM, Kaye MP: The registry of the International Society for Heart and Lung Transplantation: Eighth official report—1991. J Heart Transplant 10:491–498, 1991.
14. Ley SJ: The Thoratec Ventricular Assist Device: Nursing Guidelines. AACN Clin Issues Crit Care Nurs 2:529–544, 1991.
15. Pennington DG, McBride LR, Swartz MT, et al: Use of the Pierce-Donachy ventricular assist device in patients with cardiogenic shock after cardiac operations. Ann Thorac Surg 47:130–135, 1989.
16. Pennington DG, Swartz MT: Assisted circulation and the mechanical heart. In Braunwald E (ed): Heart Disease: A Textbook of Cardiovascular Medicine. Philadelphia, W.B. Saunders, 1991, pp 535–550.
17. Reedy J, Swartz M, Lohmann D, et al: The importance of patient mobility with ventricular assist device (VAD) support. ASAIO J 38:M151–153, 1992.
18. Swartz MT, Ruzevich SA, Reedy SE, et al: Team approach to circulatory support. Crit Care Nurs Clin North Am 1:479–484, 1989.

SCOTT LICK, MD
JACK G. COPELAND, MD
RICHARD G. SMITH, MSEE, CCE
MARILYN CLEAVINGER, MSBME

SYMBION ACUTE VENTRICULAR ASSIST DEVICE: THE UNIVERSITY OF ARIZONA EXPERIENCE

From the University of Arizona
 Health Sciences Center
Tucson, Arizona

Reprint requests to:
Jack G. Copeland, MD
Department of Surgery
University of Arizona Health
 Sciences Center
1501 N. Campbell Ave.
Tucson, AZ 85724

Since the pioneering work of Pierce and colleagues in postcardiotomy recovery with paracorporeal pulsatile univentricular assist,[5] a modest experience with several types of devices in both postcardiotomy recovery and bridge to transplant has been reported. Our experience with such devices has been limited to the Symbion acute ventricular assist device (AVAD), which we have found useful in many situations and in patients of various sizes. Currently the fate of the Symbion AVAD is under discussion with the Food and Drug Administration (FDA). We hope that soon it will again be available for further clinical investigation.

MATERIALS AND METHODS

The Symbion AVAD is a pneumatic, pulsatile, paracorporeal ventricular assist device. Compressed air alternated with vacuum displaces a Biomer (Ethicon Inc., Somerville, NJ) diaphragm to drive the pump. Modified Medtronic-Hall valves (Medtronic, Minneapolis, MN) are used in the inflow and outflow positions. The AVAD, placed in parallel with the native circulation, is capable of augmenting cardiac output up to 5 L/min.

Since February 1987, 18 patients have been supported with the device at the University of Arizona Health Sciences Center. In 5 patients the Symbion was used to provide left ventricular support only, and in 13 patients biventricular

CARDIAC SURGERY: State of the Art Reviews—Vol. 7, No. 2, 1993
Philadelphia, Hanley & Belfus, Inc.

327

assist devices (BVADs) were placed. The early implants of our series were primarily left ventricular assist devices (LVADs); the later implants were exclusively BVADs. This preference reflects the observation that LVAD output rose from 2.5–3.5 to 3.5–5 L/min when both ventricles were supported. Moreover, morbidity associated with routine addition of a second device appeared to be minimal, and the BVAD provided protection against potential right-heart failure as well as poor output due to cardiac dysrhythmias. The AVAD was used in patients who remained in cardiogenic shock despite adequate filling pressure, optimal inotropic support, and, when appropriate, an intraaortic balloon pump (IABP).

Implantation was accomplished without the use of cardiopulmonary bypass in 3 of the 18 patients (nos. 13, 14, 18). For left-heart support, inflow is accomplished by insertion of a right-angle 51-Fr cannula into the left atrium immediately posterior to the interatrial groove through the area between the right superior and inferior pulmonary veins. Blood returns to the patient through a graft sutured to the ascending aorta. For right-heart support, inflow is achieved via a 51-Fr cannula in the body of the right atrium; the outflow graft is sutured to the pulmonary artery. The cannulas are tunneled beneath the rectus sheath and exit through the upper abdominal skin. Several distinct orientations of the device were used before an optimal orientation was adopted. The objective was to minimize mediastinal dead space and driveline crossing as well as to reduce skin trauma. Our current technique is to orient the deairing ports posteriorly and to place the LVAD on the right epigastrium, with the RVAD on the left epigastrium. The device rate is adjusted to provide a stroke volume between 45 and 65 cc (maximal stroke volume: 70 cc). Complete washout at device systole minimizes thrombus formation. Maximal vacuum applied is 20 mmHg; we use as little vacuum as possible. The devices were run in the asynchronous mode at approximately 80 pulsations/minute, thus allowing for optimal filling of the artificial ventricle. Hemolysis correlates directly with drive pressure and usually can be maintained at <10 mg/dl plasma free hemoglobin with drive pressures <180 mmHg.

Anticoagulation measures were used in all patients. Dextran 40 was started at 25 cc/hr immediately after operation unless bleeding was excessive. When postoperative chest-tube output became clear, heparin was initiated to maintain the partial thromboplastin time (PTT) at twice control value, and the dextran was stopped. Dipyridamole (50–200 mg) was administered orally every 6 hours soon after surgery. Patients in whom prolonged assist was anticipated were converted from heparin to Coumadin anticoagulation.

Physical therapy was initiated in the early postoperative period. Moving the patient prevents areas of stasis in the artificial ventricle, and an upright posture results in a more symmetrical diastolic excursion of the VAD diaphragms than a supine position. Only after resolution of nutritional deficiencies and end-organ function, particularly renal function, were patients considered candidates for transplantation.

Prophylactic antibiotics directed particularly at staphylococcal organisms were given to all patients. After removal of the devices the mediastinum was assumed to be contaminated, and antibiotics were given for at least 7 postoperative days. After transplant a closed irrigation system with dilute betadine was used for the first 2–3 days, followed by saline irrigation for 1–2 days. The irrigation system and chest tubes were not removed until the culture of the chest-tube drainage was negative.

RESULTS

Profiles of the AVAD patients are summarized in Tables 1 and 2. The devices were used in 8 patients in the postcardiotomy state. One patient (no. 3) deteriorated precipitously in the intensive care unit (ICU) shortly after coronary artery bypass grafting and was emergently placed on portable femorofemoral cardiopulmonary bypass (Bard CPS system). After transport to the operating room he was placed first on the Symbion LVAD and then on a Centrimed RVAD. He died in the operating room of intraabdominal hemorrhage from an undetected iliac vein laceration sustained during difficult placement of the CPS system. Seven patients (nos. 1, 4, 5, 7, 9, 10, 14) were placed on the devices after failure to wean from cardiopulmonary bypass. Three of these patients were operated at our institution and placed on the Symbion at the end of the procedure. One patient (no. 5) suffered immediate failure of the transplanted heart. The allograft recovered function, and she was successfully weaned after 10 days of biventricular support. The patient has survived 5 years after removal of the VAD. Another patient (no. 1) was placed on the Symbion after coronary grafting and was weaned after 9 days of support, but died of multiple organ failure the next day. A third patient (no. 7) died of emboli and multiple organ failure after 11 days of left ventricular support. The other 4 patients (nos. 4, 9, 10, 14) were brought to our hospital after 2–8 days of centrifugal support with IABP after cardiotomy in anticipation of prolonged need for mechanical assistance and possible need for transplantation. None recovered function to the point of becoming a transplant candidate; all died of multiple organ failure.

The other 10 patients placed on the AVAD had not undergone cardiotomy. Two patients (nos. 2, 12) suffered from viral myocarditis and died of multiple organ failure after 21 and 5 days of support. Both were anuric and in poor physiologic condition before VAD placement. A third patient (no. 15) was placed on biventricular support because of acute rejection of his 48-day-old cardiac allograft. He succumbed to cytomegalovirus sepsis 21 days later. The other 7 patients (nos. 6, 8, 11, 13, 16–18) were placed on BVADs because of an acute myocardial infarction (3) or a postpartum (1) or idiopathic (3) cardiomyopathy. Six of the 7 underwent successful transplantation after 23, 65, 53, 164, 39, and 33 days of support, respectively, and survived to discharge. After discharge one (no. 11) died of rejection 48 days after transplantation. The mean survival is 3.3 years; the longest survival is 4.8 years. The seventh patient (no. 18) was removed from the transplant list after suffering multiple emboli and died of multiple organ failure. Three patients (nos. 11, 16, 17) were placed on the Symbion emergently after stabilization with the Bard CPS system. All 3 underwent successful transplantation.

COMPLICATIONS

Blood cultures from 8 patients on the device grew bacteria. Three of these patients had isolated positive blood cultures with minimal growth (<1 colony/ml) that may have been due to contamination and was not clinically significant. In the remaining 5 patients, 2 infections (patients 13, 18) were due to intravenous catheter sepsis, which resolved with catheter removal and appropriate antibiotics. Blood drawn from a third patient (no. 2) the day before implantation grew enterococcus, which may have been due to acalculous cholecystitis, for which she was treated with antibiotics and then cholecystectomy on VAD day 5. Bile cultures taken at cholecystectomy were negative. *Pseudomonas aeruginosa* later grew in her blood,

TABLE 1. Patient Profile

Patient No.	Age/Sex	Weight (kg)	BSA (M2)	Device	Implant Duration	Hemodialysis on VAD	Indication for Implant	Support Before Implant	Outcome	Years Alive	Preoperative BUN
1	69M	87	1.96	L	9 d	Y	After CABG	IABP	W→D	0	24
2	34F	78	1.90	L	21 d	Y	Ifluenza B myocarditis	IABP	D	0	62
3	63M	67	1.78	L + CR	2 hr	N	After CABG	IABP + BARD CPS	D	0	14
4	41F	100	2.16	L	11 d	Y	After CABG	IABP + CLVAD	D	0	NA (preop dialysis)
5	56F	65	1.72	B	10 d	N	Immediate Tx failure	CPB	W	4.9	17
6	40M	59	1.65	B	23 d	N	Acute MI	IABP	T	4.8	54
7	42M	81	2.00	L	11 d	N	After CABG	IABP	D	0	26
8	40F	54	1.55	B	65 d	Y	Postpartum CM	IABP + CBVAD	T	4.7	16
9	46M	102	2.27	B	1 d	N	Acute MI, CABG	IABP + CBVAD	D	0	30
10	56M	100	2.22	B	15 d	Y	After CABG	IABP + CLVAD	D	0	17
11	46M	64	1.74	B	53 d	N	Idiopathic CM	CPS	T → D	0.3	21
12	42F	80	1.93	B	5 d	Y	Influenza B myocarditis	IABP	D	0	18
13	48M	110	2.36	B	164 d	N	Acute MI	IABP	T	3.0	65
14	45M	80	1.99	B	6d	Y	After MVR/CABG	IABP + CBVAD	D	0	32
15	65M	82	2.02	B	21 d	Y	Acute rejection	IABP	D	0	79
16	49M	70	1.82	B	39 d	Y	Acute MI	CPS	T	2.3	19
17	56F	73	1.82	B	33 d	N	Idiopathic CM	CPS	T	1.9	23
18	54M	59	1.69	B	35 d	N	Idiopathic CM	0	D	0	15
Total					522 d						
Average	49.6	78.4	1.92		29 d						31.3
Average Survivors	47.8	70.7	1.81		55.3 d						30.7
Average Non-survivors	50.6	83.3	1.99		12.3 d						31.7

BSA = body surface area; L = left ventricular assist device; B = biventricular assist device; C = Centrimed right ventricular assist device; CR = Centrimed right ventricular assist device; W = weaned, T = transplanted, BUN = blood urea nitrogen, CABG = coronary artery bypass graft; MI = myocardial infarction, MVR = mitral valve replacement, IABP = intraaortic balloon pump, NA = not available, CM = cardiomyopathy.

TABLE 2. Morbidity and Mortality

Patient No.	Embolism	Reexplore	Viral and Blood Cultures No. Positive/No. Done	Mediastinal Infection No. Positive/No. Done	Driveline Infection	Cause of Death
1	Kidneys, spleen	0	0/5	Explant: 0/3	0	MOF
2	0	0	2/24 Enterococcus day 1 1/24 Pseudomona day 8	Pericardial fluid Day 14 → pseudomonas	0	Sepsis/MOF*
3	0	0	NA	No cultures	0	Bleeding into pelvis
4	0	0	NPS Ab. influenza B 0/8	No cultures	Day 7 Diphtheroids	MOF/sepsis
5	0	0	1/10 S. Epi day 9	Explant: S. Epi., diphtheroids, candida, strep	0	NA
6	0	0	4/19 S. aureus 0/9	Explant 3/3 S. aureus	0	NA
7	Kidneys, spleen, right brain	Day 1 bleed Day 6? debridement	0/9	Day 6 (reop) 1/3 S. Epi	0	Emboli/MOF
8	Cerebellar CVA day 57	Day 26 decorticate left thorax	1/80 Strep 1/80 S. Epi day 12	Decortication: Bacteroides Explant: 2/11 S. Epi	RVAD S. Epi day 17	NA
9	0	0	NA	No cultures	0	Low cardiac output/ coagulopathy MOF/emboli
10	Splenic infarct, necrotic toes	0	0/13	Implant: 1/1 Strep, bacillus Explant: no cultures	0	Acute rejection after discharge
11	0	0	0/36	Explant: 0/4	0	Sepsis/MOF
12	0	Day 1: bleeding	Influenza B Myocardial FA.	No cultures	0	Sepsis/MOF
13	Amaurosis day 7	0	5/27 S. aureus days 19-22	Explant: 1/7 S. epi	0	NA
14	Kidneys, spleen	0	0/5	Implant: 1/2 S. Epi Explant: no cultures	0	Emboli*
15	Spleen, right kidney	0	PAN + CMV	CMV	0	CMV sepsis
16	Pontine lesion day 29	0	1/16 E. coli day 28	Explant: 0/3	E. coli day 26	NA
17	0	Day 13 mediastinal clot	1/5 diptheroids	Day 13 clot enterobactercloacae Explant: 0/4	Enterobacter day 15	NA
18	Cerebral × 2, spleen, kidneys	0	2/21 S. aureus, 1/21 S. epi.	Negative at postmortem	0	Emboli/MOF*

* Clots in left heart at postmortem.
MOF = multiorgan failure, NA = not available, CVA = cerebrovascular accident, CMV = cytomegalovirus, NPS = nasopharyngeal swab, FA = fluorescent antibody.

sputum, and pericardial fluid; she died of sepsis and multiple organ failure. A fourth patient (no. 16) developed *E. coli* bacteremia, apparently due to a driveline infection, which resolved with local wound care and intravenous antibiotic therapy. Patient 6 developed bacteremia due to a mediastinal staphylococcus infection. Of these 5 patients with clinically significant bacteremias, 3 (nos. 6, 13, 16) underwent transplantation; all 3 made uneventful recoveries.

In 8 patients some bacterial growth was found in mediastinal cultures taken during reoperation (nos. 7, 17), conversion from centrifugal VAD to Symbion (no. 10), pericardial aspiration (no. 2), or explantation (nos. 5, 6, 8, 13). Only 1 patient had a clinically significant mediastinal infection (no. 2). All other VAD conduits were well incorporated, without clinical signs of infection at explantation. All conduit material was completely removed before transplantation, and each anastomotic site was closed primarily. No postoperative infections were due to the devices, and perigraft infection did not cause major morbidity in survivors to transplantation.

Two patients (nos. 7, 12) required early reoperation for bleeding. A third (no. 17) needed late reoperation (day 14) for a slowly progressing hematoma that obstructed device inflow. A fourth patient (no. 8) required evacuation and decortication of a clotted left hemothorax on day 26.

Tiny clots and plaques ≤ 1 mm in diameter could be seen inside the VADs through the clear housing. These appeared most frequently at the diaphragm-housing junction, but also on the housing near the outflow valve and at the deairing port. The clots and plaques appeared and disappeared from day to day. Disappearance did not correlate with clinical emboli. This phenomenon has been reported in detail.[2,4] Nine patients (nos. 1, 7, 8, 10, 13–16, 18) developed thromboembolic complications. Two (nos. 8, 16) suffered strokes, but their deficits almost completely resolved. A third (no. 13) had a 3-minute episode of amaurosis fugax 7 days after implant, apparently due to the accidental discontinuation of the heparin infusion. All 3 patients with isolated cerebral embolic phenomena underwent successful transplantation. The other 6 patients had multisystem emboli; none were long-term survivors. Three (nos. 7, 14, 18) had clots in the left heart at postmortem examination.

Nine patients (nos. 1, 2, 4, 8, 10, 12, 14–16) underwent hemodialysis while on the VADs. Their dialysis runs were generally uneventful, but often goals of fluid removal were not met because of intolerance of diminished VAD inflow. Two patients (nos. 8, 16) recovered renal function while on the VADs and underwent transplantation. Of the 5 survivors not requiring dialysis, 3 experienced progressive renal compromise, with rising blood urea nitrogen/serum creatinine ratios. In 1 patient (no. 17), the problem resolved with evacuation of a mediastinal hematoma. In another (no. 5), pump output had always been low, running around 2.7 L/min. We have no good explanation for the third patient (no. 11), who at 64 kg was well below the average in weight and had a cardiac output between 3.5 and 5 L/min. His prerenal condition resolved after transplantation. Preoperative BUN levels did not correlate with survival, in contrast with registry data.[1] Weight did correlate weakly with survival (p = 0.11); however, for many of the patients, especially the nonsurvivors, the first accurate weight was taken in the postoperative state, which is acutely edematous. Smaller body surface area also correlated weakly with survival (p = 0.09).

DISCUSSION

We have used biventricular support almost routinely since February 1988. Improved LVAD output with RVAD support, as well as frustration with dysrhythmias and right-heart failure, led to this approach.

Our postcardiotomy experience includes 8 patients. However, 4 were placed on the device after a delay of 2–8 days, during which they were on a centrifugal VAD. Of the 4 placed on the device shortly after cardiotomy, 2 were weaned and 1 is a long-term survivor.

Ten patients fall into the category of bridge to transplantation. All but 1 (no. 2) were given biventricular assist. Six of the 10 patients underwent transplantation, and 5 remain alive after an average follow-up of 3.3 years. The sixth patient succumbed to acute rejection 48 days after receiving his allograft. Of the 3 bridged patients who did not survive to transplant, 2 suffered from viral myocarditis. Both were anuric before VAD placement and died of multiple organ failure. Our bridge-to-transplant data may be summarized as follows:

Total number of patients = 10
Number of patients undergoing transplantation = 6 (60%)
Number of patients surviving >30 days = 6 (60%)

These data can be compared with a recent summary of world data on bridge to transplant with pulsatile ventricular assist devices:[6]

Total number of patients = 74
Number of patients undergoing transplantation = 54 (72%)
Number of survivors = 38 (52%)

Data from a recent worldwide summary of the Thoratec bridge to transplant may be summarized as follows:[3]

Total number of patients = 68
Number of patients undergoing transplantation = 50 (73%)
Number of survivors = 53 (63%)

Of note is that the cytotoxic antibody crossmatch of 1 patient (no. 13) rose to 97% positive shortly after placement on the AVAD, presumably because of multiple transfusions. After several weeks with minimal blood draws and no further transfusions, the antibody screen fell to <10% positive, and the patient underwent successful transplantation after 164 days on the device.

Our preference for the asynchronous drive mode may be a reflection of our success in the bridge-to-transplant setting. Whereas the synchronous mode may give better decompression of the native ventricle, the device rate is slave to the native heart rate, which is often too fast or too irregular for optimal filling and thus limits VAD output. Moreover, the higher drive pressures needed to overcome the shortened ejection periods result in increased hemolysis. Thus we prefer the asynchronous mode. Our aim is not so much to optimize decompression of the heart as to optimize end-organ perfusion.

Emergent use of the AVAD has not been a risk factor in properly selected patients. Three patients awaiting transplantation were placed emergently on the Symbion after bedside stabilization with the Bard CPS portable cardiopulmonary bypass system. All 3 underwent successful transplantation. On the other hand, of the 4 patients who arrived from outside institutions on centrifugal devices after cardiotomy, none survived.

The Symbion AVAD is an obligatory atrial cannulation system with device output limited to around 5 L/min. We have tended not to use the device in patients weighing over 80 kg. In larger patients we prefer a total artificial heart. However, our longest supported survivor (164 days) weighed the most (110 kg).

The Symbion AVAD has proved reliable and durable in our experience. Results improved after routine use of biventricular support, which we believe is superior to single left ventricular support with this device. Proper patient selection requires the exclusion of patients with preexisting multiple organ failure (but not necessarily isolated renal and cardiac failure), left-heart clots, and possibly large body size.

REFERENCES

1. Hill JD: Bridging to cardiac transplantation. Ann Thorac Surg 47:167–171, 1989.
2. Icenogle TB, Smith RG, Cleavinger M, et al: Thromboembolic complications of the Symbion AVAD system. Artif Organs 13:532–538, 1989.
3. Lawson JH, Cederwall G: Clinical experience with the Thoratec ventricular assist device. In Unger F (ed): Assisted Circulation III. Berlin, Springer Verlag, 1989.
4. Lick S, Copeland JG, Rosado LJ, et al: Long-term bridge to transplantation with the Symbion Acute Ventricular Assist Device System. Ann Thorac Surg 52:308–309, 1991.
5. Pierce WS, Par GVS, Myers JL, et al: Ventricular assist pumping in patients with cardiogenic shock after cardiac operations. N Engl J Med 305:1606–1610, 1981.
6. Unger F: Ventricular assist devices: Possibilities and limits. In Unger F (ed): Assisted Circulation III. Berlin, Springer Verlag, 1989.

VALLUVAN JEEVANANDAM, MD
ERIC A. ROSE, MD

TCI HEARTMATE LEFT VENTRICULAR ASSIST SYSTEM: RESULTS WITH BRIDGE TO TRANSPLANT AND CHRONIC SUPPORT

Valluvan Jeevanandam, MD
Assistant Professor
Cardiothoracic Surgery
Surgical Director
Heart Failure and Transplantation
   Program
Temple University Hospital
Philadelphia, Pennsylvania

Eric A. Rose, MD
Chief
Cardiothoracic Surgery
Columbia–Presbyterian Medical
   Center
New York, New York

Reprint requests to:
Valluvan Jeevanandam, MD
Cardiothoracic Surgery
Temple University Hospital
Parkinson Pavilion, Suite 300
Broad and Ontario Streets
Philadelphia, PA 19140

The Institute of Medicine estimates that 35,000–70,000 patients require some form of circulatory support annually in the United States. Cardiac transplantation, the preferred treatment for endstage heart disease, has moved from research to clinical reality. Although the indications for transplant and the number of selected patients have increased, the number of transplants performed has reached a plateau of approximately 2,000/year because of the limited number of donors. The average wait before transplant is currently 10 months; it is estimated that 10–30% of the candidates die while awaiting transplant.[8] Many patients who survive require inotropic support or intraaortic balloon pumps (IABPs) before transplant, and the morbidity and mortality from multisystem organ failure (MSOF) are high during the period of aggressive support. However, their survival, once a transplant is performed, is similar to that of elective candidates.[6,9]

Temporary mechanical circulatory support for patients awaiting donor organs was introduced by Cooley and coworkers in 1969. Since 1985, mechanical circulatory support devices have gained acceptance as a bridge to transplantation. The initial device, with the goal of long-term support, was the Jarvik-7 total artificial heart, which allowed biventricular support. But morbidity, primarily due to infection (50–70%) and thromboembolism (10%), was

CARDIAC SURGERY: State of the Art Reviews—Vol. 7, No. 2, 1993
Philadelphia, Hanley & Belfus, Inc.

335

high.[4] A left ventricular assist device (LVAD) is a potential alternative to TAH. Because it does not require excision of the native heart, infectious and bleeding complications may be fewer. In 1984 the first successful use of a ventricular assist device (VAD) as a bridge to transplant was accomplished with a Novacor LVAD. A number of groups have reported success with these and other LVADs as a bridge to transplantation. Successful bridging has occurred in up to 75% of patients receiving mechanical devices, with the rate of success depending on the device and criteria for patient selection. Once transplantation has been performed, survival is nearly equal to that in patients undergoing transplantation without bridging.[7,10,17]

Among the currently available LVADs, two are specifically designed for long-term mechanical circulatory support. Thermo Cardiosystems Inc. (TCI, Woburn, MA) and Novacor (Oakland, CA) have developed implantable, pusher-plate LVADs that are undergoing clinical evaluation under FDA-approved investigational device exemptions. Both devices have been successfully used as a bridge to transplantation for durations exceeding 11 months in patients with endstage cardiomyopathy (ischemic and dilated). This chapter summarizes results with the TCI HeartMate 1000 LVAD and discusses management of patients during the pre-, peri-, and postoperative phases.

HEARTMATE SPECIFICS

The HeartMate blood pump is a pulsatile device positioned in the left upper quadrant of the abdominal cavity (Fig. 1). The pump inlet tube is placed into the left ventricular apex through an incision in the diaphragm. Blood enters the pump from the patient's native left ventricle and is pumped into the ascending aorta. The LVAD is a pusher-plate blood pump driven through a percutaneous driveline by a portable external console. The pump consists of a titanium housing that measures 11.2 cm in diameter and 4.0 cm in thickness.

Inside the pump, a flexible polyurethane diaphragm is bonded to a rigid pusher plate. The diaphragm divides the pump into two halves: a blood chamber and an air chamber. Programmed pulses of air are delivered from the console to the air chamber behind the pusher-plate diaphragm. As the air accumulates, the diaphragm is displaced, propelling the blood through the outflow graft into the ascending aorta.[14] The pump fills passively during diastole; i.e., negative pressure is not created to suck blood from the heart. This minimizes the potential for entrapping air in the system. However, the pump can decompress the left ventricle (LV), lower the cardiac filling pressures, and allow maximal reduction in right ventricular afterload.

The short inlet cannula is inserted into the cored apex of the LV and secured with a silicone cuff. The smooth angle created by the LV, cannula, and device allows for nonturbulent flow and reduces stasis with potential for thromboembolism. The cannula is made of sintered titanium and can be placed in areas of scar or myocardium. Some investigators report ventricular rupture with placement of the cannula in areas of fresh infarct and necrosis. Bleeding from the inlet cannula is rare because the device makes the ventricle into basically an extension of the left atrium and hence into a low-pressure system. The outflow from the device is through a 20 mm, woven Dacron graft that is anastomosed end-to-side to the ascending aorta. The outflow graft traverses the diaphragm at the midline and may be placed into the right pleural cavity if closing the sternum after LVAD insertion is difficult.

Air-Driven VAD System

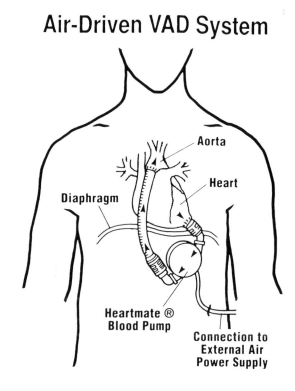

Aorta

Heart

Diaphragm

Heartmate ®
Blood Pump

Connection to
External Air
Power Supply

TCI
Thermo Cardiosystems Inc.

FIGURE 1.   Implant position for the HeartMate pneumatic assist device.

Porcine xenograft valves (25 mm, Medtronic-Hancock) are placed in the inlet and outlet conduits to ensure unidirectional blood flow. They are preassembled and attached to the device by threaded connectors. In clinical studies bioprosthetic valves do not have the same long-term durability of mechanical valves. This difference may be magnified during support since the dp/dt generated across the valves in a pulsatile mechanical device may be greater than across native heart valves. However, the incidence of thromboembolic events is significantly increased with mechanical prostheses, even with a higher level of anticoagulation. An advantage of the bioprosthetic valve for the HeartMate LVAD is the lack of requirement for long-term anticoagulation.[3] The incidence of hemolysis, a major consideration in the overall long-term safety of an implantable assist device, also appears to be less with bioprosthetic valves. During the relatively short duration of an LVAD implant the valves perform well, but their durability needs to be tested and may become the limiting factor in duration of support before the need for reoperation when the device is used as an alternative to transplantation.

A unique feature of the HeartMate LVAD is the use of textured instead of smooth biomaterials for the blood-contacting surfaces. Embolic episodes due to the release of loosely adherent biologic material from smooth-surface blood pumps is a major complication of circulatory support. Thromboembolic events from smooth-surface pumps are thought to occur for several reasons: (1) Although Biomer (Ethicon, Inc., Somerville, NJ) is an excellent mechanical and biocompatible surface, it still demonstrates thrombogenic properties. (2) A microscopically smooth surface is difficult to fabricate, and minor imperfections serve as a nidus for thrombus. The thrombi cannot adhere to the surface and escape as emboli. Seams and junctions have presented a greater problem, especially at the juncture between the pump chamber and valves. (3) It has been difficult to balance thrombus formation with effective anticoagulation therapy in each unique clinical setting.[2,13,15,16]

An alternative approach for controlling thromboembolic events involves the use of textured surfaces.[13,16] The textured polyurethane (ITP) (Fig. 2) used on the diaphragm and the sintered titanium microspheres (STM) (Fig. 3) used on the inlet cannula and on the housing are designed to encourage the formation and adherence of a pseudoneointimal (PNI) biologic lining. The PNI functions as the permanent biocompatible blood-contacting surface and may contain cells active in creating a nonthrombogenic interface. PNI development on textured surfaces was originally investigated in animals using adhesively bonded polyester fibrils on a polyurethane pump diaphragm.[1,12] These studies demonstrated the feasibility of the approach, but the individual fibers dislodged and created a nidus for thrombus accumulation. The ITP diaphragm surface was designed to eliminate the adhesive previously used to fabricate the flocked surface. The polyurethane fibrils are integral with the underlying diaphragm, thus eliminating the possibility of fibril detachment.[5]

The STM surface also reflects an attempt to create an attractive substrate for PNI development. Titanium microspheres are deposited on the pump housing and fittings to form a continuous layer. The pump is then heated to sinter the balls to each other as well as to the pump housing.

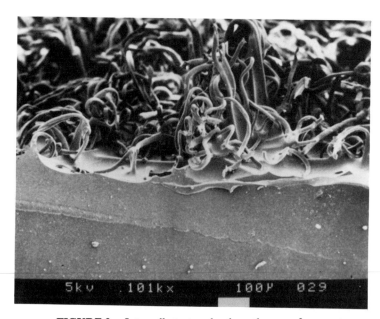

FIGURE 2. Integrally textured polyurethane surface.

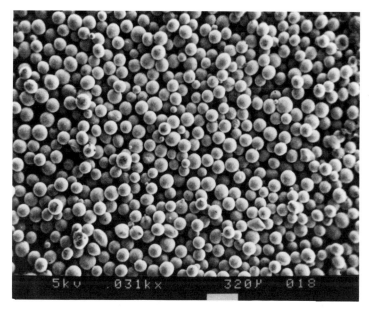

FIGURE 3. Textured titanium surface.

The ITP and STM surfaces are manufactured with a specific pattern and density of texture to produce an optimal pseudointima. For further reduction of thromboembolic events, the inlet and outlet ports of the HeartMate are contoured. This allows for a vortex during filling and emptying, with complete circulation of blood elements, and prevents stasis of blood with the potential for clot formation.

The HeartMate blood pump may be implanted in a subfascial position; however, the recommended site is intraperitoneal. This placement allows a short, straight inlet cannula and reduces the bleeding complications seen with the subfascial position. In addition, infection around the device has not been a problem, probably because of elimination of dead space by abdominal contents around the device and because of the immunologic status of the peritoneal cavity. The disadvantages include a potential for bowel obstruction, the relative contraindication of major previous bowel surgery, and the difficult dissection encountered at time of device explant.

The blood pump is driven directly without the need for tanks of compressed air by a portable console (Fig. 4), which operates on batteries or standard alternating current. It was designed primarily for ease of operation and mobility. A stroke sensor in the pump housing is precalibrated and can precisely measure and display the amount of blood at the end of pump diastole and systole. The console uses information from the stroke sensor to determine the stroke volume and displays the VAD output by multiplying that value by the LVAD rate. The asynchronous modes include fixed-rate and pump-on-full (auto) options. If set to operate in the auto mode, the device automatically ejects when the pump is 90% full (75 cc stroke volume). Therefore, when flow into the LVAD increases, the rate also increases to maintain the 75 cc stroke volume. Conversely, with decreased filling, the LVAD slows to permit more time for filling.

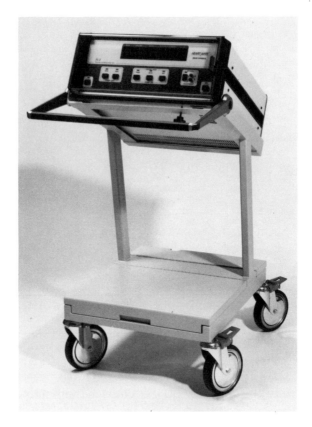

FIGURE 4. A portable pneumatic drive console for the HeartMate blood pump.

Synchronization of the pump is also possible with an external QRS detector. Clinical experience has shown that synchronization is not necessary and that the auto mode allows optimal decompression of the LV and hemodynamics. The only other parameters that can be adjusted are eject duration and volume of the alarms. The internal battery supplies adequate power to allow the patient to ambulate and exercise. Patients are encouraged to begin an exercise program of walking and stationary bicycling as soon as possible after device implantation to improve their general physiologic status before transplantation. A mobile driver (10 lbs in weight, with a battery life of 6–8 hours) that allows even more patient mobility is currently under development.

INCLUSION AND EXCLUSION CRITERIA

The device is currently limited for use as a bridge to transplant in approved transplant candidates with nonreversible LV failure. This group includes patients with endstage cardiomyopathy or subacute myocardial infarction [>7 days since onset of myocardial infarction (MI)] and excludes patients after cardiotomy or with acute MI. Hemodynamic criteria must also be met, including failure of maximal inotropic support, insertion of an IABP if possible, and either (1) pulmonary capillary pressure ≥ 20 mmHg with either systolic blood pressure ≤ 80 mmHg or cardiac index ≤ 2.0 L/min/m^2 or (2) cardiac arrest with systolic pressure ≤ 60 mmHg.

The exclusionary criteria avoid use of the LVAD in patients who would not benefit because of other significant systemic illness, including irreversible hepatic, renal, or respiratory failure; severe blood dyscrasia; sepsis; and fixed pulmonary hypertension with right-sided failure. The last condition is particularly important because right failure is a significant predictor of adverse outcome after LVAD insertion. Right-sided VADs in this population have high rates of morbidity and mortality. Patient selection is critical to success of assist devices. If the patient has deteriorated to the point of irreversible endstage disease, the LVAD only prolongs an unsalvageable situation.

MANAGEMENT

Once a patient has met the inclusion criteria and has consented to insertion of an LVAD, it is prudent to proceed with the implant at the earliest possible time. The patients are fragile and can deteriorate rapidly with arrhythmias, worsening heart failure, or respiratory decompensation. To avoid line sepsis, we remove indwelling catheters and replace all monitoring lines. Coagulopathy is corrected with fresh frozen plasma (FFP), and we avoid operating on patients with prothrombin times >25% of control. Platelets are administered after the implant. Intraoperative aprotinin may also reduce bleeding.

In the operating room the patient is prepped and draped widely. A mark is made in the left lower quadrant 2-3 cm above the anterior superior iliac spine for the exiting driveline. The incision is made from the sternal notch to the umbilicus. Meticulous hemostasis is important because neglected surfaces can bleed from the coagulopathy that follows the procedure. The peritoneal cavity is entered, and the falciform ligament is divided to allow placement of the device above the stomach and right lobe of the liver. The device is placed into the left upper quadrant and positioned with regard to three sites: (1) position for the diaphragmatic penetration of the apical cannula; (2) area for the outlet cannula, which may require dividing the diaphragm over the right lobe of the liver; and (3) peritoneal exit site for the driveline. The amount of driveline exposed to the abdominal cavity should be minimized to prevent adhesions and secondary bowel obstruction. A tunnel is created from the previous cutaneous mark in the left lower quadrant to the peritoneal exit site. The pump is removed to the back table, where it is calibrated, de-aired, and assembled with inlet and outlet conduits. The valved conduits are made of Dacron. The inlet conduit is preclotted with whole blood, whereas the outlet valve assembly is not. Therefore, the saline used to fill the device oozes out of the outlet valve assembly. The pump can be completely de-aired only in the process of separation from cardiopulmonary bypass (CPB).

After heparinization, standard ascending aortic and single right atrial cannulation is used. The aortic cannulation should be as high as feasible so that the outflow conduit can be anastomosed without a cross-clamp. CPB is initiated. The LV apical cannula may be placed with either a hypothermic, arrested heart or a warm beating heart. The patient is placed in Trendelenburg position, and the LV apex is cored. The core should allow direction of the inlet cannula toward the mitral valve and not against the septum. A plastic stent similar in size to the inlet cannula is partially placed into the LV, and the inlet cuff (reinforced silastic with a Teflon sewing cuff) is placed over the stent. The apical cuff is secured with 2-0 pledgeted, nonabsorbable sutures through the epicardium. Although this connection is low pressure, hemostasis is essential because it is inaccessible after implantation. The stent is removed, and the inlet cannula of the device is placed into the apical graft through the diaphragm. Resistance may make placement of the inlet cannula difficult; the procedure is facilitated by distal countertraction and a twisting motion. Once the inlet cannula is palpated in the LV, it is secured to the apical graft with tie bands.

The outlet graft is anastomosed end-to-side to the ascending aorta. It is cut to length and placed to the right of the midline for ease of future reentry. The right pleura may be opened for good positioning. The graft is back bled to evacuate air and reclamped near the aorta. Saline is used to fill the pump and the outlet graft, and the graft is attached to the pump. Active suction is applied to a needle in the graft, and the LVAD function is initiated with manual cranking. The entire field (thorax and abdomen) may be flooded with saline to avoid the possibility of entraining air. Volume is slowly returned to the patient, and the device is completely de-aired. After de-airing is complete, the bypass flow is reduced to 1–2 L/min before the HeartMate is activated, the outlet graft is unclamped, and the patient is slowly weaned from bypass. This procedure reduces the possibility of entraining air when the device is initially started.

Volume is infused to allow adequate LVAD filling. As the LVAD fills, the rate is increased progressively from 20 beats/min to the maximal attainable rate that permits adequate filling. LVAD flow is determined by right-heart function, which may be augmented by inotropes and/or vasodilators, such as sodium nitroprusside or prostaglandin E_1. Transesophageal ultrasound is important to determine right ventricular (RV) function and to assess the ability of the LVAD to decompress the LV. If the LV is distended, poor drainage into the LVAD, secondary to inflow cannula obstruction or inadequate LVAD function, needs to be considered and corrected. Because electrocautery interferes with the auto mode, fixed mode is used until the patient leaves the operating room. Protamine is administered along with exogenous factors, as necessary. After satisfactory hemostasis is obtained, first the abdomen and then the sternum are closed. Intestinal distention may hinder abdominal closing, in which case intraoperative colonoscopy can be used to decompress the large and small intestines up to the ligament of Treitz. Chest tubes are placed as indicated. A Gore-Tex pericardial membrane may be used to decrease the difficulty of reentry during transplantation.

The two primary complications after insertion are bleeding and right heart failure (RHF). Because the LVAD pumps the blood that fills the right heart, right heart function and pulmonary vascular resistance (PVR) are the main determinants of cardiac output. Methods to treat RHF include (1) fluid loading to an adequate central venous pressure (CVP); (2) inotropes to increase RV function; (3) correction of rhythm disturbances with restoration of sinus rhythm; (4) vasodilators; (5) avoidance of high peak end-expiratory pressure (PEEP); (6) early extubation if possible; (7) prevention of abdominal distention, which can decrease blood return to the heart via the inferior vena cava; (8) elevation of the lower extremities to increase venous return; (9) rhythmic inflation and deflation of pneumatic trousers to act as a venous pump, thus increasing venous return; and (10) if necessary, insertion of a RVAD.

Postoperative bleeding is a problem caused by preimplant Coumadin therapy or coagulopathy from hepatic congestion. Liberal amounts of FFP and platelets are administered, and heparin is fully reversed. Pressures may not equalize because of the LVAD, and any decrease in flow with elevated CVP is highly suspicious for tamponade. Dextran and low-dose heparin may be used if indicated.

As the patient recovers, the balloon pump, if present, is removed and the inotropes are slowly weaned. Because of RHF, the procedure should be gradual over several days, and the threshold for increasing inotropic support (if indicated) should be very low. The Swan-Ganz catheter is removed once the right-sided pressures are satisfactory.

Patients are extubated at the earliest possible time. Epidural anesthesia is used to help in management of incisional pain from the sternotomy as well as the laparotomy. Pulmonary care is essential. The chest tubes can be removed as indicated. Patients are started on clear diet and advanced as tolerated. Some have early satiety, which resolves over time. They may prefer frequent lighter meals to larger meals. Antibiotics are continued for the perioperative period or for treatment of a specific source.

Rehabilitation is started at the earliest possible time. Although most patients are severely deconditioned before insertion of the LVAD, they recover quickly and adapt to the portability of the device. Any activity that may cause moisture in the junction of the console and pump driveline is limited, because moisture can disturb the electronic circuits.

Chronic care is simple and usually supplied by the patient. Antiplatelet therapy with aspirin (100 mg/day orally) and dipyridamole (75 mg orally tid) are suggested, but both have been omitted in several patients without sequelae. Some patients have required antihypertensive medication, especially if they were on an ACE inhibitor before implantation. The pump requires venting every 6 hours, usually by the patients themselves. Venting can cause dizziness and should be performed with patients sitting or recumbent. Moisture accumulates in the driveline over 7–14 days, depending on the temperature in the room. This water is removed by disconnecting the driveline from the LVAD, temporarily stopping the device by pressing the vent button, emptying the water, reconnecting, and releasing the vent button. Some patients may be symptomatic during the procedure. Twice a day the patient cleans the driveline site and applies silver sulfadiazine ointment. Complications once the patient is stabilized are uncommon, and the patient is autonomous with minimal nursing care.

The transplant surgery to end the period of mechanical support may be difficult. Once the abdominal cavity is entered, enterolysis is performed carefully to avoid overt spillage of bowel contents or to create an occult enterotomy. Once the pocket of the device is entered, explantation can proceed more easily. Femoral cannulation may be required if the outflow graft does not allow sufficient length of aorta to be cross-clamped. The pericardial space and the heart shrink with chronic support; it may be necessary to undersize the heart or to leave the sternum open if closure is not tolerated.

EXPERIENCE AT THE COLUMBIA-PRESBYTERIAN MEDICAL CENTER

We used the TCI HeartMate LVAD as a bridge to transplantation in 4 patients from August 1990 to February 1992. Inclusion and exclusion criteria are described above. Patient profiles (expressed respectively as patient A, B, C, D) were as follows:

1. Age (sex): 36 (F), 57 (M), 28 (M), 62 (M)
2. Cardiomyopathy: idiopathic in A and C, ischemic (coronary artery bypass graft 5 years ago) in B, and ischemic (anterior MI with LV aneurysm) in D
3. Preoperative IABP in all

4. Creatinine (mg/dl): 1.0, 1.4, 1.5, 1.8
5. Normal liver enzymes
6. Echocardiogram: RV function moderately depressed in A and D, severely depressed in B and C
7. PVR (Woods units) and cardiac index (L/min/M^2) immediately preceding LVAD insertion: A, 2 and 1.9; B, 5 and 1.7; C, 5.8 and 1.7; D, 3.2 and 1.8
8. B, C, and D were on respirators

Patients A, B, and C had the LVAD placed intraabdominally under hypothermic CPB and an arrested heart with left apex and ascending aorta cannulation. Patient D had the implantation under normothermic bypass in a beating heart. Heparinization was completely reversed after bypass, and patients B, C, and D received aprotinin for further reduction of intraoperative bleeding.

Patient A required inotropes for RHF and blood products for postoperative bleeding. She was extubated on postoperative day 2, and all lines and inotropes were removed on postoperative day 3. Following a smooth support period, she survived to transplantation 324 days after LVAD insertion. She had a high plasma renin activity and required 5 crossmatches before undergoing successful transplantation. Until that time she was ambulatory and did not require nursing care. Her only device-associated complication was a loosening of the driveline from the console, leading to air loss in the system and low output. This was attributed to excessive twisting of the driveline when she got out of bed. The connecting nut was tightened, and there were no further difficulties. She did not tolerate dipyridamole and took only aspirin (100 mg/day). At LVAD explant, the surfaces had developed a smooth neointima without thrombus.

Reoperation for transplantation was difficult. The RV was lacerated on reentry, and because of previous IABP, femoral cannulation was difficult. Femoral arterial and venous cannulation was eventually accomplished with long Biomedicus (Minneapolis, MN) cannulas over dilators. A fibrous nonadherent capsule around the VAD facilitated explantation. Significant bleeding and mechanical tamponade occurred after transplantation because the size of the pericardial space had decreased over the 324 days of support and the donor heart was large. The patient required reexploration and pectoralis major musculocutaneous flap, but eventually recovered and is thriving. The sternum was left open.

Patient B had persistent hypoxia and progressive RHF after LVAD insertion. Attempts to increase right-sided cardiac output included pneumatic trousers and intraoperative colonoscopy to decrease abdominal distention. A Biomedicus RVAD was eventually inserted, but the patient died from multiorgan failure.

Patient C died intraoperatively from high PVR and inability to fill the LVAD. The LVAD sucked in air from the inlet cannula and complicated successful clearing. An RVAD was not used. To prevent air entrapment at the inlet cannula, we suggest submerging the LVAD with saline during weaning from CPB.

Patient D was febrile without an infectious source, had an IABP, and was intubated for 6 weeks before implantation. He had a large, thin-walled LV aneurysm; the VAD was placed with a beating heart. The aorta was fragile and required reinstitution of CPB to refashion the aortic outflow graft anastomosis. In addition, with the sternum open, LVAD output acutely dropped. On transesophageal echocardiogram the inlet cannula was obstructed by a mass that turned out to be intussecception of the aneurysm. Plication of the LV aneurysm resolved the problem. Gore-Tex pericardial membrane was used during sternal closing to decrease the problems of reentry encountered in the first patient. Patient D required inotropic support for RVF but did well and was eventually extubated. Upper gastrointestinal bleeding from a chronic gastric ulcer required abdominal exploration, gastrotomy, and oversewing of the ulcer. Because of his debilitated state, a long period of rehabilitation followed, but he became quite vigorous and mobile. Support continued for 90 days without anticoagulation or antiplatelet medication. Reentry at transplantation was simplified by the pericardial membrane. His transplant period was complicated by donor heart dysfunction that required IABP. He recovered and is doing well after transplant.

OVERALL RESULTS

Between August 1985 and February 1992, the U.S. clinical experience with the pneumatic TCI HeartMate LVAD as a bridge to transplantation included 60 implants. Five are ongoing; 55 patients were supported from 1–324 days. Thirty-four patients survived to transplantation, of whom 29 were discharged from the hospital. Five died after transplantation: 2 from donor heart failure, 1 from liver failure present before LVAD implant, and 2 from MSOF, again present before LVAD implant. The latter 3 patients were operated in the early experience (before 1988) when criteria for patient selection were not precisely established; certain patients perhaps had irreversible end-organ dysfunction.

Twenty-one patients died before transplantation. Reasons for death included RHF, bleeding, MSOF, and encephalopathy. Only 2 patients who survived beyond 14 days of implant died. One patient developed Candida sepsis and died from a cerebrovascular accident (CVA) and renal failure. The other patient continued on a downward course because of systemic lupus erythmatosus; although the device functioned well, it was turned off after 72 days.

The HeartMate has been shown to be reliable and capable of generating adequate pressures and flows. The average pump index for all patients was 2.86 L/min/m^2, which was approximately 30% greater than the average cardiac index at the time of implant. The systolic, diastolic, and mean pressures were 119 mmHg, 71 mmHg, and 95 mmHg, respectively (Fig. 5). In the auto mode, flow adjusted appropriately to normal activity, exercise, and increased metabolic requirements, such as sepsis.

The average plasma free hemoglobin level was 8.7 mg/dl, suggesting a mild but clinically acceptable level of hemolysis. One patient had a plasma free hemoglobin value of 40 mg/dl before LVAD implant and continued with this high level during support. He remained on the device for 66 days and was successfully transplanted. The average hemoglobin was 11.0 mg/dl, hematocrit was 34%, and platelet counts were 249,000/μl. These values reflect adequate support without significant damage to blood elements.

Most LVAD patients had elevated values of total bilirubin ($\geq$1.4 mg/dl) or serum glutamate oxaloacetate transaminase and/or serum glutamate pyruvate transaminase ($\geq$50 mg/dl) before or during device support. All three parameters tended to increase during the first month, then returned to normal after approximately 60 days of augmented perfusion. The values remained normal for the remaining period of support. Reversibility of hepatic function correlated with favorable outcome during LVAD support. When the preimplant values of total bilirubin are compared with the final values obtained just before transplant or time of death, total bilirubin values decreased in all survivors, whereas the values either failed to decrease or increased in all nonsurvivors. These data show that LVAD support is not deleterious to hepatic function and leads to improvement in patients

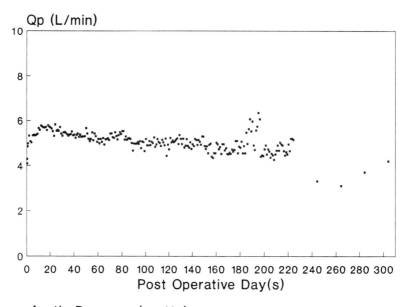

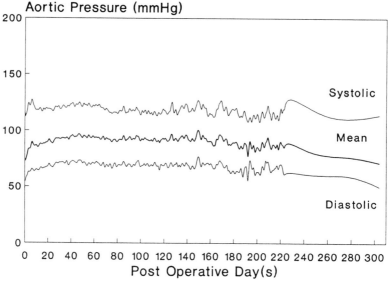

FIGURE 5. *A,* Average pump flow (Qp) for 60 patients. *B,* Average aortic pressure for 60 patients.

with reversible hepatic dysfunction. Renal function was not adversely affected by support. Levels of serum creatinine and blood urea nitrogen were stable during support. In contrast to the hepatic response, the renal parameters did not transiently increase after implantation and stabilized within a shorter period of time (Fig. 6).

The principal risks associated with ventricular assist technology include RHF, bleeding, hemolysis, and thromboembolism. Criteria for patient selection

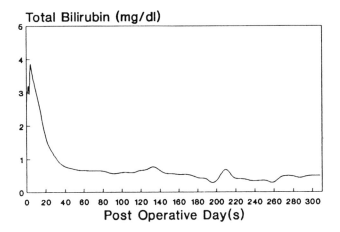

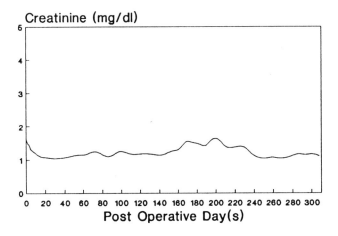

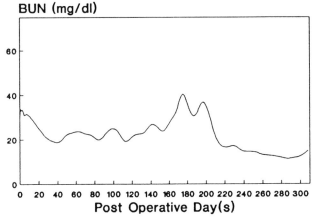

FIGURE 6. Hepatic and renal response for survivors.

play an important role in the success of LVAD implantation. In the earlier experiences, the LVAD corrected the hemodynamics of moribund patients, but irreversible liver, renal, and other end-organ dysfunction led to death from MSOF. RHF remains the primary complication in the perioperative period. Despite hemodynamic exclusion criteria (i.e., PVR >6 Wood units, RVEDP ≥25 mmHg, CVP ≥20 mmHg), it is difficult to predict the patient population that will exhibit significant RHF. It is not known whether RHF was due to the direct effects of aggressive LV support or to the unmasking of preexisting RV failure and pulmonary hypertension.[11] Earlier insertion of the device may obviate this problem. The patient catheterization data may become invalid during the period of decompensation immediately preceding implant. Large fluid requirements to maintain circulatory stability, respiratory decompensation, and congestive heart failure (CHF) can lead to a higher PVR than previously calculated. This should be reversible, as reflected by the observation that once the patients survive the initial perioperative period, they generally do not exhibit progression of right heart dysfunction. Among the adverse effects of the LVAD, RHF was shown to have a significant negative correlation with outcome; the transplantation and survival rate in these patients was significantly decreased.

Although the HeartMate allows for full reversal of heparin without need for systemic anticoagulation, bleeding remains a problem after implant. Before implantation patients generally have a history of anticoagulation with warfarin, coagulopathies resulting from hepatic congestion, or long-term use of inotropes, such as amrinone. Furthermore, implantation is a major operation that exposes raw surfaces in the abdomen and diaphragm, especially in patients with previous cardiac operations.

Anastomoses are required for LVAD implantation. Because it is a low-pressure connection, the LV apex has a low incidence of bleeding. The outlfow anastomosis is treated like an aortic graft. Although preclotted, the valved Dacron conduits and the Dacron outflow graft may ooze until the patient's coagulopathy is resolved. Blood products are administered for hemostasis, but one should be cautious because these patients eventually require a transplant and sensitization to histocompatibility leukocyte antigens may occur.

Other complications include systemic infections, such as respiratory, urinary, or line sepsis. Infection involving the device itself is less common. The percutaneous driveline is covered with Dacron and becomes incorporated into the skin; therefore, infection at this site is rare. The LVAD was never explanted as a result of an uncontrollable infection. In previous implants the driveline coursed through the abdomen to the right lower quadrant. Bowel obstruction and adhesion were reported in 2 cases, with subsequent perforation in 1. With the current implant technique, the driveline is minimally exposed in the peritoneal cavity, and intestinal obstruction has not been a problem. Some patients have early satiety, but with modification of diet all patients have been adequately nourished.

Thromboembolism, the main complication of mechanical assist devices, is remarkably decreased with the HeartMate. Patients are treated with dipyridamole and aspirin, and with increasing experience even that regimen may prove to be unnecessary. Despite the lack of anticoagulation, only 2 thromboembolic events have occurred in patients on the device. One patient had a malaligned inlet cannula coupled with a Candida infection. He had a CVA while on heparin and died. Another patient had a prosthetic mechanical aortic valve in the native heart, and when his native ventricle ejected, he had an embolic CVA. He was eventually transplanted and has fared well. Other than these 2 patients, no other episodes of thromboembolism are known in this group of supported patients, probably because of textured surface and the prevention of stasis by the vortex pattern of blood flow in the pump.

The textured Biomer surface has been studied in detail in all supported patients. The mild thrombogenic nature of the material induces initial events on the surface that lead to controlled development of PNI. The materials later become masked by blood components that evolve into the ultimate blood-contacting surface (Fig. 7). By day 4, a well-adherent, smooth, fibrin-cellular lining is observed on the surface of the material. Mononucleated cells, composed of macrophages and myofibroblasts, appear by day 14 and increase in number up to day 41. RNA hybridization techniques demonstrate that for the first 30 days the primary protein synthesized is type III collagen; after 90 days there is a shift to type I collagen. Endothelial cells are present on the surface after 120 days of implantation. Endothelial cells, however, have not been observed at earlier periods. The thin heterogenous NI continues to evolve throughout support, remaining firmly adherent.

Random white islands of tissue, composed of 30% collagen, may be seen on the surface. Whether with increasing support the PNI will grow or collagen deposits will increase needs to be evaluated after longer periods of support. Calcification was an initial concern because of its high incidence in the bovine model. However, energy dispersive x-ray spectroscopy has not demonstrated calcium deposits in any of the surfaces after explant.

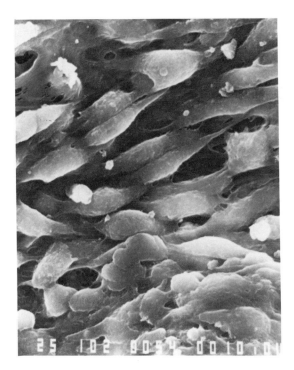

FIGURE 7. Scanning electron photomicrograph of the blood contacting surface of the neointima.

FUTURE DIRECTIONS

The TCI LVAD investigational system currently consists of three models: the pneumatic, the vented electric, and the totally implantable. The pneumatic device has completed phase II trials, and a premarket approval application has been submitted to the FDA. A portable driver that weighs 10 lbs should be available in the near future, allowing patients even greater mobility to rehabilitate and to maintain a reasonable quality of life before transplantation.

The vented electrical system (Fig. 8) consists of the same pump described above, with the actuator positioned within the nonblood side of the pump housing. The electromechanical driver consists of an electronically commutated, low-speed torque motor that drives the pusher plate by means of a pair of nested helical cams. The motor makes one revolution for each pump ejection. Control and power to the electrically actuated LVAD are provided by a small, external control module and batteries that are worn by the patient. The portable controller weighs 120 gm and provides power conditioning to the motor, rate control, feedback of operating parameters, diagnostic information, and alarms. Two electrical leads connect the controller to a pair of gel-cell lead acid batteries (used for video camcorders). The controller is connected to the LVAD via a percutaneous lead. Another small tube is exteriorized to provide transfer of air in and out of the actuator compartment on the nonblood side of the pusher plate. For every beat, a volume of air equal to the amount of blood pumped must be exchanged with the atmosphere outside the body. To reduce the risks of infection, each of the two percutaneous lines is incorporated within a special access device implanted at the skin level.

Patients can connect themselves to a battery charger console at night and then to the batteries placed in shoulder holsters during the day. Battery charge ranges from 6–9 hours, depending on the device rate. The vent port is open to air, and the only limitation is to avoid submerging the port under water. This device

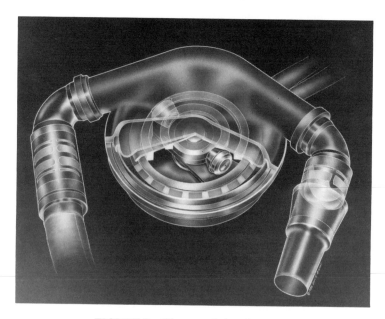

FIGURE 8.   The vented electric system.

is currently under phase I clinical trials in the Texas Heart Institute (THI). The device performed satisfactorily in the first patient, but he died from hemorrhage on postoperative day 15. The next patient has been supported for 220 days and is enjoying a good quality of life. He is independent, fully ambulatory, and untethered. The study will be expanded to other centers after 5 are implanted at THI. This device allows enough freedom to be either a long-term bridge to transplant or, in selected patients, an alternative to transplant.

The third model is a totally implanted device similar to the vented electric model but with no ports exiting the skin. The compliance chamber is placed in the left thoracic cavity and exchanges air with the lung. The controller and back-up battery source are internal; power is supplied by transcutaneous power leads. This model is under animal investigation and is several years from clinical testing. Ultimately this device is considered an alternative to transplantation.

COMMENTS

With the increasing incidence of death from CHF, the demand for definitive treatment of endstage heart disease will be higher. Because the donor heart pool is not expanding and transplantation has limitations such as rejection, infection, and graft atherosclerosis, the need for mechanical alternatives is increasing. The first attempts at orthotopically positioned TAHs have met with major obstacles and have been withdrawn by the FDA in the United States. In a majority of patients, LV support alone can provide sufficient circulatory support in the setting of normal pulmonary artery pressures and unloading of the left heart. The TCI HeartMate pneumatic device is a forerunner of the more self-contained vented electrical and totally implantable LVADs and in an FDA-controlled study proved to be safe and efficacious in bridging patients to transplantation. The most impressive aspect of the TCI devices is the low incidence of thromboembolic events without anticoagulation and the paucity of complications once the immediate 2-week perioperative period is crossed. The patients become New York Heart Association class I, are rehabilitated, and, other than being in the hospital, have few complaints. Better patient selection, especially in reference to right-heart function and reversibility of end-organ dysfunction, will lead to improved results and to the progression of mechanical assist devices from bridges to transplant to alternatives to transplantation.

REFERENCES

1. Clark R, Boyd J, Moran J: New principles governing the tissue reactivity of prosthetic materials. J Surg Res 16:510–512, 1974.
2. Dasse KA, Chipman S, Sherman C, et al: Clinical experience with textured blood contacting surfaces in ventricular assist devices (VADs). ASAIO Trans 33:418–425, 1987.
3. Graham TR, Marrinan MT, Frazier OH, et al: Current clinical experience with Medtronic porcine xenograft valves in the Thermo Cardiosystems (TCI) implantable left ventricular assist device (LVAD). International Seminar on Surgery for Valvular Diseases, June 12, 1989.
4. Griffith BP, Kormos RL, Hardesty RL, et al: The artificial heart: Infection-related morbidity and its effect on transplantation. Ann Thorac Surg 45:409–414, 1988.
5. Harasaki H, Field A, Sato N, et al: Polyester fibril flocked surface for blood pumps. ASAIO Trans 29:563–568, 1983.
6. Hardesty RL, Griffith BP, Trento A, et al: Mortally ill patients and excellent survival following cardiac transplantation. Ann Thorac Surg 41:126–129, 1986.
7. Hill JD: Bridging to cardiac transplantation. Ann Thorac Surg 47:167–171, 1989.
8. Hogness JR, Malin VA: The artificial heart: Prototypes, policies and patients. Washington, DC, National Academy Press, 1991, p 75.
9. Hsu J, Griffith BP, Dowling RD, et al: Infections in mortally ill cardiac transplant recipients. J Thorac Cardiovasc Surg 98:506–509, 1989.

10. Joyce LD, Emery RW, Eales F, et al: Mechanical circulatory support as a bridge to transplantation. J Thorac Cardiovasc Surg 98:935–941, 1989.
11. Kormos RL, Harvey SB, Gasior T, et al: Experience with univentricular support in mortally ill cardiac transplant candidates. Ann Thorac Surg 49:261–272, 1990.
12. Lelah MD, Lambrecht LK, Young B, Cooper S: Physiochemical characterization and in vivo blood tolerability of cast and extruded biomer. J Biomed Mater Res 17:1–22, 1983.
13. Levinson MM, Smith R, Cork R, et al: Thromboembolic complications of the Jarvik-7 total artificial heart: Case report. Artif Organs 10:236–244, 1986.
14. McGee M, Parnis S, Nakatani T, et al: Extended clinical support with an implantable left ventricular assist device. ASAIO Trans 35:614–616, 1989.
15. Nakatani T, Frazier OH, McGee M, et al: Extended support prior to cardiac transplant using a left ventricular assist device with textured blood contacting surfaces. ISAIO, Sapporo, Japan, October 1–4, 1989.
16. Olsen DB, Unger F, Oster H, et al: Thrombus generation within the artificial heart. J Thorac Cardiovasc Surg 70:248–255, 1975.
17. Phillips WS, Burton NA, Macmanus Q, Lefrak EA: Surgical complications in bridging to transplantation: The Thermo Cardiosystems LVAD. Ann Thorac Surg 53:482–486, 1992.

O.H. FRAZIER, MD

LONG-TERM VENTRICULAR SUPPORT WITH THE HEARTMATE IN PATIENTS UNDERGOING BRIDGE-TO-TRANSPLANT OPERATIONS

Director
Cardiopulmonary Transplant
    Service
Texas Heart Institute/St. Luke's
    Episcopal Hospital
        and
Co-director
Cullen Cardiovascular Research
    Laboratories
Texas Heart Institute
Houston, Texas

Reprint requests to:
O.H. Frazier, MD
Texas Heart Institute
PO Box 20345
Houston, TX 77225-0345

More than 20 years ago, researchers at the Texas Heart Institute (THI) began work with the total artificial heart (TAH) and the ventricular assist device (VAD). Cooley, who performed the first successful heart transplant in the United States in 1968,[1] a year later became the first surgeon in the world to bridge a seriously ill patient to heart transplant with a TAH.[2] At that time, however, the promise of heart transplantation as a treatment for endstage heart disease was yet to be realized. The heart transplant program at THI was curtailed in the early 1970s because of inadequate immunosuppressive regimens, which resulted in high rates of rejection, infection, and mortality.

Mechanical circulatory support research, on the other hand, continued to be a primary focus in our surgical research laboratories. The laboratories were founded in 1972 with the goal of developing a tether-free, permanently implantable device to treat patients with endstage heart disease and to return them to active, productive lives.

Since 1986, we have been conducting clinical trials of the HeartMate (Thermo Cardiosystems, Inc., Woburn, MA) left ventricular assist device (LVAD), an implantable blood pump capable of fulfilling the function of the natural left ventricle.[3,4] This device has already proved effective in patients who are suffering from endstage heart failure and require a bridge to transplantation.

CARDIAC SURGERY: State of the Art Reviews—Vol. 7, No. 2, 1993
Philadelphia, Hanley & Belfus, Inc.

Our most extensive experience has been with the pneumatically powered version of the HeartMate, but in January 1991, the Food and Drug Administration (FDA) granted approval for testing of the vented-electric model. This model allows the greatest degree of mobility and should allow patients to be discharged from the hospital. Our experience has shown that the risk of thromboembolic complications has been greatly reduced by uniquely textured blood-contacting surfaces as well as by the favorable flow characteristics of the pump. This chapter chronicles our involvement in the research of this promising technology.

RESEARCH AND DEVELOPMENT

In 1970 construction began on the surgical research laboratories at THI. They were conceived, designed, and built in collaboration with the National Heart and Lung Institute, with the goal of testing and evaluating LVADs in an experimental model and transferring this knowledge to the clinical setting.

Our goal, however, was not just to prolong the lives of patients with heart disease, but to restore them to normal or near-normal activities. We wanted to develop an LVAD that would work with the natural heart to provide full cardiac output and that would function for years. Whereas external or partially implantable support devices have merit in short-term clinical settings in which the left ventricle has the potential to recover within days or weeks, these systems restrict mobility and require that the patient be hospitalized. The only choice for a long-term LVAD was one that would be fully implantable. Thus, the major considerations in designing such a system were efficacy, biocompatibility, reliability, and safety.

Major problems associated with mechanical circulatory support devices had to be addressed. The risk of thromboembolic complications and hemolysis, as well as infections, had to be greatly reduced; a suitable implantation site had to be found; and an efficient, dependable power system had to be developed.

Preventing thromboembolic complications and hemolysis depends partially on development of more biocompatible materials. To avoid destruction of elements within the blood, the blood-contacting surfaces of the pump and the conduits must promote formation of a smooth biologic lining. Thus, specially textured surfaces were created for the blood-contacting surfaces of the blood pump so that fibrin and other cellular components could be captured from the circulating blood. This action would result in a gradual, natural healing process, like that in injured blood vessels, and a smooth, stable biologic lining would be formed.

A totally implantable LVAD with an internal power source would not only yield freedom of mobility but also minimize complications. A compact, nontoxic power source would have to be found, and it would have to be reliable to delay, for as long as possible, the need for reoperation to replace it. While a transcutaneously powered, electric blood pump was undergoing development, a pneumatic drive system was used in the initial clinical studies.

As for an appropriate site to place the LVAD, the abdomen was chosen because it eliminated dealing with the space constraints within the chest. In addition, the integrity of the native heart is maintained, so that the left ventricle can continue to provide circulatory support in the event of mechanical failure.

Two prototype LVADs made of a titanium alloy and with textured blood-contacting surfaces were investigated in our laboratories during the 1970s. An implantable, pneumatically powered system designed for temporary support periods went through animal and clinical testing in the mid 1970s (Fig. 1). This

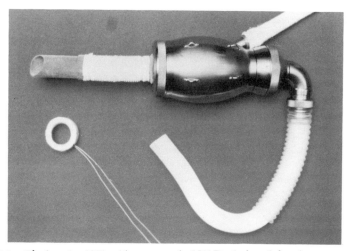

FIGURE 1. During the 1970s this pneumatic LVAD, designed for short-term support, was tested in 22 patients.

LVAD was used to treat 22 patients with either cardiogenic shock after myocardial infarction or postcardiotomy shock and failure to wean from cardiopulmonary bypass.[5] In all cases, the LVAD was used on an emergent basis, and the duration of support ranged from 1 day to 1 week. The device was removed after ventricular recovery in 3 patients, and 1 patient was successfully bridged to transplantation.[6] That patient, a 47-year-old man with postcardiotomy "stone heart" syndrome, required LVAD support for 5 days until a donor heart became available. This case proved that profound left and right ventricular failure unresponsive to conventional therapy can be treated without total heart replacement in the presence of normal or low pulmonary vascular resistance.

In these first clinical studies, long-term survival was not achieved. The patients were treated after irreversible, end-organ damage had occurred, and bleeding complications and multiorgan failure were observed. Persistent renal failure resulted in plasma hemoglobin levels that remained high or increased. Our clinical experience, however, showed that the LVAD can provide adequate systemic perfusion, that the failing left and right ventricles can recover when the total circulatory requirements of the body are provided by the LVAD, and that LVAD support works best when it is implemented early in patients in whom conventional support, including the intraaortic balloon pump (IABP), had failed. In addition, we observed that the LVAD continued to provide adequate circulation during periods of ventricular fibrillation and asystole.

Studies on the long-term implantable LVAD, the precursor to the electrically activated HeartMate, were conducted in calves in the late 1970s and in the early 1980s to determine the safety and effectiveness of the pump.[7] Minimal-to-moderate degrees of calcification were noted at the areas of the pump subjected to mechanical stress, but this phenomenon was thought to be age-related and species-specific.[8] Another problem in the animal model was the development of pannus occlusion within the long Dacron inlet conduit. This problem was addressed by shortening the Dacron portion of the conduit, leaving only the segment containing the porcine valve.[9]

Overall, the animal studies showed excellent pump function. The animals were able to exercise, and the pump could respond to the increased demands for cardiac output. Moreover, the pump proved capable of functioning safely and reliably for more than 1 year after implant.

As laboratory studies were conducted to perfect the LVAD, the THI transplant program was resumed in 1982, when effective immunosuppression with cyclosporine became possible. Since then, we have performed more than 450 heart transplants, and the 1-year survival rate now approaches 90%. Despite this positive experience and improved immunosuppressive regimens, we cannot provide a heart transplant for every patient whom it could potentially benefit because of the severe shortage of donor hearts. Currently in the U.S. approximately 2,500 patients are on the active waiting list for a heart transplant, but on the average only 6 donor hearts become available each day.[10] This discrepancy underscores the importance of finding alternative treatments.

THE HEARTMATE

In 1986 FDA approval was granted to test the pneumatic version of the HeartMate LVAD, but only as a bridge to heart transplantation.

The HeartMate is a pulsatile blood pump that improves hemodynamic parameters.[11] Cardiac output is captured within the blood pump, which propels the blood into the ascending aorta. The pump can be operated in a synchronous or asynchronous mode, independent of heart function. The maximal stroke volume of the pump is 85 ml; it is capable of providing flows up to 12 L/min.

The blood pump housing, measuring 11.2 cm in diameter and 4.0 cm in thickness, is made of a smooth, rigid titanium alloy (Fig. 2). Within the pump

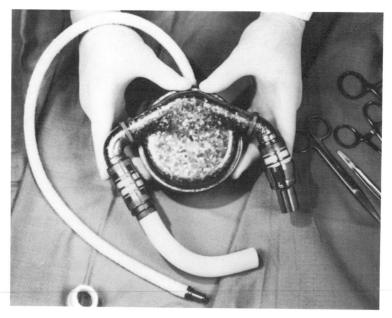

FIGURE 2.   The pneumatic HeartMate LVAD that has undergone clinical testing at the Texas Heart Institute.

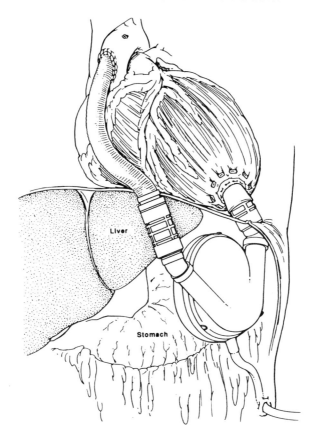

FIGURE 3. Placement of the HeartMate LVAD. The inlet conduit is sutured at the left ventricular apex, and the outflow graft is anastomosed to the ascending aorta. (From Radovancevic B, Frazier OH: Implantation technique for the HeartMate left ventricular assist device. J Card Surg 7:203, 1992, with permission.)

housing, a flexible, pusher-plate diaphragm separates the blood chamber from the air chamber. Pulsatile flow is created by pumping air into the chamber behind the diaphragm, thus forcing the diaphragm to move forward and to expel blood.

The blood-contacting surfaces of the pump are uniquely textured: the metallic surfaces are covered with sintered-titanium microspheres and the diaphragm with polyurethane fibrils. These surfaces capture fibrin and cellular components as blood flows across them. This process creates a stable biologic lining that reduces the risk of thromboembolic complications and hemolysis.

The LVAD is placed in the left upper quadrant, below the diaphragm (Fig. 3). The inlet and outflow conduits are made of low-porosity Dacron, and each one contains a 25-mm bioprosthetic porcine valve (Medtronic Blood Systems, Irvine, CA), which creates unidirectional flow (Fig. 2). The conduits are joined to the pump with rotatable joints so that anatomic variations can be accommodated.

The pneumatic pump is powered through a percutaneous driveline connected to a portable control console (Fig. 2). The electric pump is powered through a transcutaneous driveline connected to a light-weight, rechargeable battery pack that is worn in a shoulder holster.

Patient Selection

Only patients approved for heart transplant are eligible to undergo HeartMate support. In the event that endstage heart failure progresses to the point that aggressive medical support, IABP support, or both do not work, HeartMate support can be instituted. The specific indications are pulmonary capillary wedge pressure ≥ 20 mmHg and a cardiac index ≤ 2.0 L/min/m^2 or a systolic blood pressure ≤ 80 mmHg. Because success depends on reversing end-organ dysfunction, if present, support must be instituted before end-organ function deteriorates to the point that it cannot be reversed. Indices of kidney and liver function are therefore helpful in assessing when to institute LVAD support. Kidney dysfunction is defined as a blood urea nitrogen level ≥ 40 mg/dl, with or without a serum creatinine level ≥ 2 mg/dl. A urine output < 0.5 cc/kg/hr despite treatment with diuretics is also considered a sign of kidney dysfunction. The protocol restricts use of the HeartMate in the presence of chronic kidney failure requiring hemodialysis within 1 month of operation. Liver dysfunction is defined as a total bilirubin concentration ≥ 2.5 mg/dl, with or without a serum glutamic oxaloacetic transaminase concentration ≥ 500 U/L. Again, the protocol restricts use of the HeartMate in the presence of severe liver disease, evidenced by a total bilirubin value > 10 mg/dl.

In addition to chronic, irreversible end-organ failure, severe blood dyscrasia and right heart failure preclude treatment with the HeartMate. The presence of any condition that contraindicates heart transplantation also precludes LVAD treatment because clinical trials are conducted solely in bridge-to-transplant operations. Finally, because of the size of the pump, use in patients whose body surface area is < 1.5 m^2 is not recommended.

Surgical Technique

IMPLANT OPERATION

Prostaglandin E1, if tolerated by the patient, is administered before implantation and continued throughout the LVAD implant operation. We have found this treatment helpful in decreasing pulmonary vascular resistance and in improving right ventricular function. The implant operation is accomplished through a midline sternotomy incision that is extended almost to the umbilicus.[12] Heparin is administered, and preparations are made to institute total cardiopulmonary bypass. A single-bore cannula is carefully placed in the aorta so that enough room remains for the outflow conduit anastomosis. After cardiopulmonary bypass is begun and the aorta is cross-clamped, the left ventricular apex is cored with a special circular knife to create an opening for the inlet conduit. Mural thrombus and redundant myocardial tissue are removed from the left ventricle, and the apical opening is reinforced with a Teflon sewing ring using interrupted horizontal mattress sutures.

The HeartMate pump is then placed intraperitoneally in the left upper quadrant of the abdomen, below the diaphragm. (Extraperitoneal placement, which was used in our early experience, resulted in a large hematoma in the pocket and excessive angulation of the inlet conduit.) The inlet conduit is passed through an incision in the diaphragm and then connected to the apical opening. The outflow conduit is measured to obtain an appropriate length, then secured to the pump. The conduit is positioned over the diaphragm to the right of the midline incision and cross-clamped before end-to-side anastomosis to the ascending aorta with a running 4-0 polypropylene suture. Finally, a stab incision is made in the left lateral abdominal wall, above the iliac crest, through which the driveline is passed in the pneumatic model and the vent tube in the electric model.

The patient is placed in the Trendelenburg position, and a 19-G needle is inserted into the Dacron outflow conduit to remove air from the heart and the pump. Pumping with the LVAD is then initiated, and the patient is weaned from cardiopulmonary bypass as LVAD flow is gradually increased. After the patient is weaned from bypass, the arterial and venous cannulas are removed, and protamine sulfate is administered to reverse heparinization. The sternotomy is then closed.

EXPLANT OPERATION

At the time of the heart transplant operation, femoral and caval cannulas are placed for total cardiopulmonary bypass. The aorta is cross-clamped and the heart arrested. After bypass has been initiated, LVAD support is stopped, and the outflow conduit is removed from the aorta. The inlet conduit is dissected free, and the pump is removed. An orthotopic transplant is performed in routine fashion, as is a heterotopic transplant. In the latter case, however, the apical opening in the native heart must be repaired, either by oversewing it with pledgeted sutures or by applying a Dacron patch.

Patient Management

After implantation of the LVAD, patients are treated with low-molecular-weight dextran for 7 days to reduce the risk of thromboembolic complications.[3] Patients are carefully monitored for signs of postoperative bleeding that can result from cardiopulmonary bypass and from administration of anticoagulants during the operation. During support, patients do not require aggressive anticoagulation because of the biologic lining that forms on the textured blood-contacting surfaces, usually beginning within 5 days of implant. Minimal anticoagulation with aspirin (80 mg once a day) and dipyridamole (75 mg 3 times daily) has proved adequate in most cases. Patients with a mechanical heart valve in place, known pulmonary emboli, or other indications for more aggressive anticoagulation may be treated with Coumadin.

Preexisting conditions, such as kidney and liver dysfunction, are continually assessed to determine the efficacy of LVAD treatment. Another consideration in treating patients during support is the need to prevent high pulmonary vascular resistance and resultant right ventricular failure. In the event of right ventricular failure and normal pulmonary vascular resistance, the HeartMate is capable of providing total circulatory requirements.

LONG-TERM HEARTMATE SUPPORT

The HeartMate has worked exceptionally well in patients requiring prolonged support as a bridge to heart transplantation. Of the first 18 patients to undergo treatment with the pneumatically powered HeartMate at THI, 15 were successfully supported to the time of transplantation, and 12 received support for 1 month or longer.[3] The cumulative duration of LVAD support was 1,400 days, with the average being 80 ± 74 days (range: 5–233 days).

Based on our experience, proper patient selection is the key to a successful clinical outcome with use of the HeartMate. When permanent end-organ damage secondary to severe multiorgan dysfunction is present before HeartMate support is instituted, the patient's chances of surviving are lessened. In contrast, instituting LVAD support before permanent end-organ damage occurs increases the patient's chances of a good clinical outcome.

The capacity of the blood pump to produce high flow rates helps to promote hemodynamic stability and thus adequate end-organ perfusion. Patients in New York Heart Association functional class III or class IV can be returned to class I, especially when LVAD support is continued longer than 1 month. Moreover, the portable control console has allowed patients to take part in cardiac rehabilitation programs, including exercise on an incline treadmill and stationary bicycle. As our experience has grown with the HeartMate, we have gained confidence in prolonging the support period until end-organ function recovers. Patients do not require urgent transplantation and therefore can be optimally matched with a donor heart.

The HeartMate has proved reliable and safe. Prolonged periods of support have been achieved without mechanical failures. The titanium alloy blood pump does not cause adverse reactions within the body. A fibrous tissue capsule forms around the pump, such as that with implanted pacemakers, and this pocket may afford protection against infections.[13,14]

Within the blood pump, a thin, fibrin-cellular coagulum covers the texturized surfaces and helps to prevent thromboembolic complications, even in the presence of nonaggressive anticoagulative therapy with antiplatelet agents. Examination of explanted blood pumps has revealed no evidence of thrombus formation on the internal pump surfaces, within the conduits, or around the valves. Mild hemolysis has been noted immediately after the implant operation, but this can be attributed to the cardiopulmonary bypass procedure. The level of plasma free hemoglobin usually returns to normal in patients who are supported longer than 2 weeks.

Superficial wound infections have occurred at the exit site of the driveline, but they have resolved with appropriate treatment. No evidence of infection has been found on the internal pump surfaces or within the conduits.

The occurrence of right ventricular failure during LVAD support appears to be the only factor that has an adverse effect on survival, especially when pulmonary vascular resistance is high.[4] Further investigation of this problem is necessary to determine what preexisting conditions induce right ventricular failure and what can be done to prevent it during LVAD support.

Effect of HeartMate Support on Results of Heart Transplantation

To assess the effects of pretransplant LVAD support on the results of transplantation, we compared a group of patients who received LVAD support as a bridge to transplantation with a group of patients who received conventional medical support and with a second group of patients who received IABP treatment as a bridge to transplantation.[15] We found that the HeartMate patients were at no greater risk of postoperative complications, rejection, infection, or mortality than the other patients, nor did they require longer periods of hospitalization after the transplant. The episodes of rejection and infection among the LVAD patients were no more severe than those among the other patients. Thus HeartMate support had a positive effect on the outcome of heart transplantation in these severely ill patients, particularly those who were supported for more than 30 days and who had returned to class I cardiac status. In our experience with 15 patients receiving support for more than 30 days, 1-year survival was 100%, compared with 67% in 60 patients who were on IABP support at the time of transplant.

THE FUTURE

In May 1991, the first step toward a permanently implantable LVAD was made, when a 52-year-old man became the first patient to receive treatment with the vented-electric HeartMate. Although the electric device worked as well as the pneumatic device, the patient died of multiorgan failure and sepsis after 2 weeks of support. Currently, support with the vented-electric HeartMate is ongoing in 2 men. One of the patients, a 33-year-old man, has been on the device for 9 months. The large body stature of the patient and the need for a type O donor heart have necessitated prolonged LVAD support. Whereas current policy requires that the patient remain hospitalized while undergoing LVAD support, he is well enough to return home and to work. During hospitalization, this patient has been serving as a volunteer in the Network Services department. The other patient, a 49-year-old man, has been on LVAD support for 3 months, and his condition continues to improve.

As our experience with the HeartMate increases, we should be able to specify criteria for determining which patients will benefit from LVAD support and at what point support should be instituted. For example, the IABP or more advanced circulatory support devices may be used to treat patients suffering from postcardiotomy cardiogenic shock. When left ventricular dysfunction is potentially irreversible, however, it may be more appropriate to bypass temporary treatment measures and to initiate LVAD support to avoid permanent end-organ damage.

Finally, the opportunity to study the potential for permanent left ventricular support is likely to grow as the shortage of donor hearts intensifies. The number of patients who will require a bridge to transplantation can be expected to rise significantly as the waiting time for a donor heart increases. As of April 1991, the median waiting time for a transplant in the United States was 51 days.[15] A large number of the patients were in the intensive care unit at the time of transplantation, at a cost of $4,000/day, including physician and laboratory fees. Even after a successful heart transplant, the potential for long-term survival (>5 years) is still hampered by complications such as accelerated coronary allograft atherosclerosis. Such patients could be inexpensively supported by devices like the HeartMate. In some patients, this technology may also be a suitable long-term alternative to heart transplantation, and it should allow patients to return to a productive role in society.

REFERENCES

1. Cooley DA, Bloodwell RD, Hallman GL, Nora JJ: Transplantation of the human heart: Report of four cases. JAMA 205:479, 1968.
2. Cooley DA, Liotta D, Hallman GL, et al: Orthotopic cardiac prosthesis for two-staged cardiac replacement. Am J Cardiol 24:723, 1969.
3. Frazier OH, Duncan JM, Radovancevic B, et al: Successful bridge to heart transplantation with a new left ventricular assist device. J Heart Lung Transplant 11:530, 1992.
4. Frazier OH, Rose EA, Macmanus Q, et al: Multicenter clinical evaluation of the HeartMate 1000 IP left ventricular assist device. Ann Thorac Surg 53:1080, 1992.
5. Norman JC, Duncan JM, Frazier OH, et al: Intracorporeal (abdominal) left ventricular assist devices or partial artificial hearts: A five-year clinical experience. Arch Surg 116:1441, 1981.
6. Norman JC, Brook MI, Cooley DA, et al: Total support of the circulation of a patient with postcardiotomy stone-heart syndrome by a partial artificial heart (ALVAD) for 5 days followed by heart and kidney transplantation. Lancet 1:1125, 1978.

7. Fuqua JM Jr, Igo SR, Hibbs CW, et al: Development and evaluation of electrically actuated abdominal left ventricular assist systems for long-term use. J Thorac Cardiovasc Surg 81:718, 1981.
8. Turner SA, Bossart MI, Milam JD, et al: Calcification in chronically implanted blood pumps: Experimental results and review of the literature. Tex Heart Inst J 9:195, 1982.
9. Pool GE, Parnis SM, Creager GJ, et al: Evaluation of occlusive inlet pannus formation: Comparison of conduit designs. Trans Am Soc Artif Intern Organs 31:408, 1985.
10. UNOS Update 8:27, 1992.
11. Frazier OH, Radovancevic B: Ventricular assist devices. Card Surg State Art Rev 4:335, 1990.
12. Radovancevic B, Frazier OH: Implantation technique for the HeartMate left ventricular assist device. J Card Surg 7:203, 1992..
13. Myers TJ, McGee MG, Zeluff B, et al: Frequency and significance of infections in patients receiving prolonged LVAD support. ASAIO Trans 37:M425, 1991.
14. Capek P, Kadipasaoglu KA, Radovancevic B, et al: Human intraperitoneal response to left ventricular assist devices with Ti-6A1-4V alloy surface. ASAIO J 38:M543, 1992.
15. UNOS statistics, 1991.

NARAYANAN RAMASAMY, PhD
PEER M. PORTNER, PhD

NOVACOR LVAS: RESULTS WITH BRIDGE TO TRANSPLANT AND CHRONIC SUPPORT

From Baxter Healthcare
    Corporation
Novacor Division
Oakland, California

Reprint requests to:
Narayanan Ramasamy, PhD
Baxter Healthcare Corporation
Novacor Division
7799 Pardee Lane
Oakland, CA 94621

Cardiac transplantation is the only recognized treatment for endstage heart failure. Of the >19,000 procedures performed worldwide since the first heart transplant in 1967, >85% have occurred since 1985. The number of heart transplants has leveled over the last 4 years, however, because of limited donor availability.[10] Consequently, the waiting period for donor organs has increased significantly; 25% of candidates wait 6–12 months for a suitable donor organ.[21] Many of these patients will die while waiting. An estimated 17,000–35,000 people <70 years old who develop endstage heart failure annually could benefit from heart replacement.[22] Thus, the need for an alternate mode of therapy is urgent, not only for those awaiting donor organs, but also for a majority of the patients who cannot have a transplant because of chronic organ shortage or ineligibility.[14,21,22] A recent epidemiologic study conducted by the Institute of Medicine concludes that 30,000–60,000 people per year in the United States may be eligible for long-term mechanical cardiac support systems (MCSSs).[7]

A number of MCSSs have been developed and tested over the last two decades, including nonpulsatile and pulsatile artificial ventricles (extracorporeal and implantable) and total artificial hearts (TAHs). Considerable progress has been made in the use of pulsatile artificial ventricles since the first clinical success in 1971 for salvage of patients in heart failure refractory to medical treatment.[5] In the 1980s, with a chronic donor shortage, the focus of circulatory

CARDIAC SURGERY: State of the Art Reviews—Vol. 7, No. 2, 1993
Philadelphia, Hanley & Belfus, Inc.

363

support shifted to the treatment of irreversible, terminal, myocardial failure. Two approaches have been pursued: replacement of the native heart by a TAH and assist of the native heart by a ventricular assist device (VAD). After experience with 5 patients, heart replacement was discontinued because of multiple complications.[6,9] TAHs have also been used as a temporary bridge to transplant (BTT) for candidates who cannot be maintained by conventional pharmacotherapy or intraaortic balloon pump (IABP). The first such attempt to use a mechanical VAD as a bridge was made in 1978, but the patient died of infection within days after cardiac transplantation.[12]

The first successful bridging was accomplished in 1984 at Stanford University Medical Center with the Novacor electrically powered left ventricular assist system (LVAS) in a patient with endstage ischemic heart disease (IHD).[17] The first successful bridging with a TAH was achieved 1 year later.[3] The use of the artificial heart as a BTT, however, has been discontinued in the U.S. Since the initial BTT experience, VADs have been used extensively at many clinical centers. As of January 1990, about 300 patients worldwide have been supported by VADs (right, left, and biventricular).[13] Of the currently available pulsatile VADs, one (Novacor Division, Baxter Healthcare Corporation, Oakland, CA) was originally designed as an electrically driven implantable device for chronic use.[18]

Since 1984, the Novacor LVAS has been used clinically as a BTT at 16 U.S. and 3 European centers for durations to 370 days. This chapter reviews the results of an 8-year, 126-patient, multicenter BTT experience with the Novacor system with emphasis on chronic (>30 d) support.

DESCRIPTION OF THE NOVACOR LVAS

The three configurations of the Novacor LVAS are illustrated in Figure 1. The implanted pump/drive unit is common to all configurations; the differences

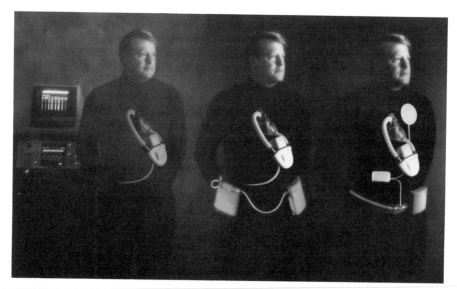

FIGURE 1. The Novacor left ventricular assist system in three configurations: the temporary BTT application with a console-based ECP *(left panel)*, with a wearable ECP and battery pack and separate monitor unit *(center panel)*, and the totally implantable system *(right panel)*.

are only in the electronic control and power subsystem (ECP). The current clinical configuration uses a console-based external ECP, coupled via a percutaneous power line/vent tube to the implanted pump (left panel). In the second configuration, a wearable compact controller with an attached battery serves as the ECP, providing a tether-free device (center panel). Monitoring and reprogramming functions are also miniaturized and computer-controlled (monitor unit) for use in the immediate postoperative phase or for diagnostic purposes. The third configuration is the totally implantable system with no percutaneous connection (right panel). Designed for multiyear use, this system provides a viable long-term therapy for patients with endstage heart failure. The tether-free, nonvented LVAS configuration successfully completed a 12-system, 2-year testing program, sponsored by the NIH, for device readiness.[8] It has also been used for chronic support for up to 9 months in the ovine model.[20]

The Novacor LVAS has a nominal maximal stroke volume of 70 ml, can provide pump outputs in excess of 10 L/min, and can operate in synchronous counterpulsation at high cardiac rates (to 240 beats per minute). The Novacor blood pump consists of a seamless sac, with a smooth blood-contacting surface made of polyurethane (Biomer, Ethicon, NJ) bonded to dual, symmetrically opposed pusher plates and to a lightweight housing that incorporates valve fittings (Fig. 2). The pump uses bovine pericardial valves (Edwards CVS Division, Baxter Healthcare Corporation, Irvine, CA). The pump geometry was designed to ensure symmetric sac deformation for optimal flow patterns without stasis sites, flow separation, or turbulence. The electromechanically activated drive unit—a unique spring-decoupled, pulsed solenoid energy converter with only 2 moving parts—provides efficient, durable, and reliable pump operation.[19] The pump/drive unit is encapsulated by a fiberglass-reinforced polyester resin shell (Fig. 3). Externally reinforced, low porosity, woven Dacron (Meadox Medical Corporation, NJ) inflow and outflow conduits connect the pump to the left ventricular apex and ascending aorta, respectively.

The pump/drive unit is positioned in the anterior abdominal wall of the left upper quadrant, anterior to the posterior rectus sheath between the left iliac crest and the costal margin. The inflow conduit cannulates the left ventricle, and the

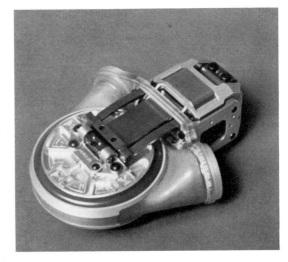

FIGURE 2. The unencapsulated pump/drive unit with seamless polyurethane sac/dual pusher-plate pump integrally coupled to pulsed solenoid energy converter.

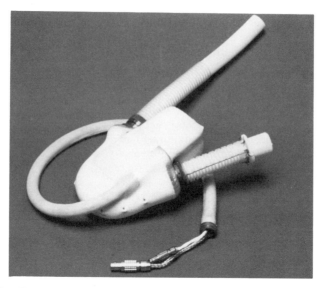

FIGURE 3.   The pump/drive unit encapsulated in a fiberglass-reinforced polyester shell with inflow and outflow conduits.

outflow conduit is anastomosed to the ascending aorta. Both conduits are externally reinforced and traverse the diaphragm. The pump is connected to the console via leads contained within a percutaneous vent tube (Fig. 1, left panel). Details of the implant procedure have been described previously.[16]

PATIENT SELECTION AND MANAGEMENT

After extensive in vitro and in vivo testing, clinical protocols and consent forms were developed and approved by the Food and Drug Administration (FDA). An investigational device exemption (IDE) was granted for the first clinical trial at Stanford University Medical Center in 1984. Supplemental approvals were obtained for additional U.S. investigational centers, and the Novacor LVAS is undergoing a multicenter clinical trial in the U.S. and Europe.

Inclusion and exclusion criteria that apply to cardiac transplantation are also applicable to LVAS candidates. The Medicare guidelines for acceptance as a transplant candidate provide an initial set of criteria for patient selection in the LVAS study.[4] Because the LVAS is approved for use only in patients not sustained by conventional therapy (IABP and/or inotropes), only a subset of patients under UNOS category I are eligible. Additional criteria for inclusion/exclusion include hemodynamic and other parameters (Table 1).

In addition to the standard postsurgical care of cardiothoracic patients, postoperative management of LVAS patients includes an anticoagulant regimen (initially intravenous heparin, then oral Coumadin); platelet antiaggregating agents (initially low-molecular-weight dextran, then aspirin or dipyridamole); prophylactic antibiotics (perioperatively); percutaneous tube exit-site care; and gradual weaning from inotropic support. In addition to pump output and stroke volume, central venous, pulmonary arterial and radial artery pressures are monitored during the immediate postoperative period.

TABLE 1.   Bridge to Transplant: Novacor Study Entry Criteria

Accepted or acceptable transplant candidate

Male or female, $\geq$15 years and $\leq$65 years old

Body surface area $\geq$1.5 m^2 but $\leq$2.5 m^2

Hemodynamic deterioration (Swan-Ganz catheter placed to document hemodynamics) within a
48-hour period and either A or B:
  A. Cardiac index <2.0 L/min/m^2, with either mean systemic pressure <65 mmHg or LAP
     (PCWP) or mean RAP >18 mmHg
  B. Increasing inotropic support and/or need for IABP (within 48 h preimplant) to include
     any two of the following:
       Dopamine $\geq$10 μg/kg/min
       Dobutamine $\geq$10 μg/kg/min
       Epinephrine $\geq$0.02 μg/kg/min
       Isoproterenol $\geq$0.05 μg/kg/min
       Amrinone $\geq$10 μg/kg/min
       Other equivalent drug (specify drug and dose)
       IABP support

Absence of pulmonary parenchymal disease and/or fixed pulmonary hypertension with PVR
$\geq$6 Wood units or pulmonary artery systolic pressure $\geq$65 mmHg

Absence of renal and/or hepatic function not explained by underlying heart failure and deemed
reversible

Absence of systemic infection unresponsive to treatment

Absence of documented cerebrovascular or peripheral vascular disease

Absence of cancer with metastases

Absence of blood dyscrasia that would dispose to uncontrollable postoperative bleeding

Absence of prosthetic aortic valve

LAP = left arterial pressure; PCWP = pulmonary capillary wedge pressure; RAP = right arterial
pressure; IABP = intraaortic balloon pump.

At transplantation, the pump/drive unit is explanted after institution of
cardiopulmonary bypass. The inflow and outflow conduits are cross-clamped
and transected. The vent tube is also transected and the exposed ends covered
with povidone-iodine-filled silicone caps to prevent contamination. The pump/
drive unit is removed from the sterile field. Orthotopic transplantation is then
carried out in the usual manner. Posttransplant patient management is unchanged
for this subset of bridged patients.[16]

RESULTS AND DISCUSSION

Since the first Novacor implant in September 1984, 126 patients have been
enrolled in the study, including 3 who are currently supported (123 completed
cases). Seventy-four of these patients have been successfully bridged; the longest
posttransplant survival is 8 years (Table 2).

Patient Demographics: Age, Sex, Size.   The youngest patient was 15 years
old and the oldest was 67, with a mean age of 45 years. For purposes of analysis, patients were divided into 4 age groups: <20, 20–39, 40–59, and $\geq$60 years
of age (Fig. 4). The single largest age group was 40–59 years, representing 61%
of the patients admitted to the study.

Thirteen patients (10%) were women. In contrast, women constitute 20% of
transplant patients (difference not significant, p >0.35) in the registry of the
International Society for Heart and Lung Transplantation (ISHLT).[10] Women
treated with the Novacor were significantly younger than men (women, 36 yr;

TABLE 2. Novacor LVAS Bridge to Transplant: Current Status

Number of patients	126 (113 M, 13 F)
Average age (yr)	45 (range: 15–67)
Average weight (kg)	79 (range: 49–142)
Average size (m²)	2.0 (range: 1.5–2.8)
Average support duration (d)*	42 (range: 1–370)
Currently supported	3 (2%)
Transplanted (excluding currently supported patients)	74 (60%)
Transplant survivors	66 (89%)
Average follow-up (yr)	2.1 (range: 0.003–8)
Late deaths	5 (7%)
Cumulative experience (yr)	13.1

* Operative survivors.

men, 46 yr; p <0.0005). The median ages of women and men were 38 and 47 years, respectively. The mean body surface area (BSA) was 1.90 m². The smallest patient was 1.54 m² and the largest was 2.78 m², with a median of 1.90 m².

Admitting Etiology. Cardiomyopathy (CM) and coronary artery disease (CAD) were the major admitting etiologies for Novacor LVAS recipients (58 patients, or 46%, and 65 patients, or 51%, respectively). By comparison, the etiology distribution reported for transplant patients is 49% CM and 41% CAD (difference not significant, p >0.10).[10] Two cases involved acute viral myocarditis and 1 acute rejection. Figure 5 illustrates the proportion of patients with acute myocardial infarction (AMI), IHD, and CM. CM was the admitting etiology for most women (8 patients, or 62%), but not for men (50 patients, or 44%). On the other hand, CAD accounts for 56% (63 patients) of men and only 23% (3 patients) of women. The number of women in these subcategories is too small for comparison with ISHLT data.

Duration of LVAS Support. The duration of Novacor LVAS support has ranged from 1–370 days. For analysis, the duration of LVAS support was divided into 3 periods: acute (<3 d), short-term (3–30 d), and chronic (>30 d). Whereas

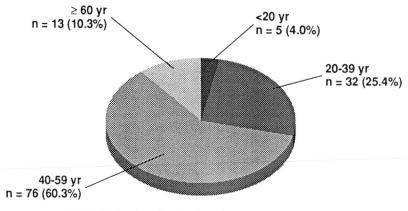

FIGURE 4. Age distribution of Novacor BTT patients.

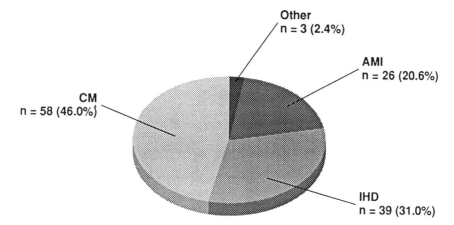

FIGURE 5. Etiology distribution of Novacor BTT patients. AMI = acute myocardial infarction, IHD = ischemic heart disease, CM = cardiomyopathy, and other, including 1 with acute rejection and 2 with acute viral myocarditis.

23 patients (19%) fall into the category of acute support, an approximately equal number had short-term (51 patients, or 41%) and chronic (49 patients, 40%) support (Fig. 6). The cumulative duration of LVAS support for chronic patients accounts for 85% (11 yr) of total LVAS support, and the mean duration of support for this group was 82 days (longest 370 days, successfully transplanted and discharged). Fifteen chronic patients (12%) were supported for more than 3 months.

Outcome in Acute, Short-term, and Chronic Patients. Duration of LVAS support had a direct correlation with patient survival to transplant (Fig. 6). Whereas overall survival to transplant was 60%, chronic patient survival was >80%, about 4 times the survival rate of acute patients.

Of the 23 acute patients, 9 (39%) died at operation. The operative mortality rate, although a consequence of the critical preimplant condition, also reflects a

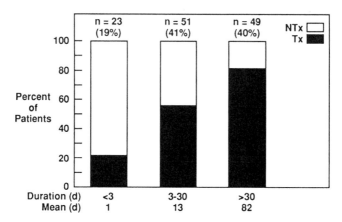

FIGURE 6. Duration of LVAS support: acute support (<3 d); short-term support (3–30 d), and chronic support (>30 d).

learning curve for patient selection. Another 9 patients died during the postoperative acute period. The data show that patients with highly impaired vital organ function declare themselves early. Of the 5 acute patients (22%) who survived to transplant, 2 (40%) died early after transplant (<3 d). The high mortality rate of acute patients early after transplant may also reflect the effect of 2 major cardiac procedures within a few days.

Twenty-eight short-term patients (56%) were successfully bridged. Twelve (55%) of the nonsurvivors developed progressive multiorgan failure despite LVAS-restored normal cardiac output; this rate highlights the issue of patient selection. The impossibility of predicting when a patient has developed irreversible organ failure presents one of the major challenges in patient selection. Late LVAS intervention cannot restore organ function despite the restoration of normal systemic blood circulation.

Chronic patients (>30 d) represented 40% of the study population with an 82% survival rate. Posttransplant survival for this group appears better than that for nonstaged transplants, although the number of patients is too small for statistical significance. This increase in survival rate with duration of implant supports device safety, because device-related complications might be expected to result in a progressive decrease in survival with increasing duration.

Hemodynamics, Pre- and Postimplant. Mean ($\pm$ SD) preimplant cardiac index (CI) and pulmonary artery diastolic pressure (PAD) for the patient population were 1.89 ± 0.47 L/min/m^2 (n = 112) and 28.0 ± 8.4 mmHg (n = 104), respectively. At 24 hours after implant, the corresponding values were CI 3.02 ± 0.62 L/min/m^2 and PAD 19.3 ± 6.1 mmHg (n = 69). The increase in CI and the decrease in PAD are both statistically significant ($p < 0.005$). The improvement in hemodynamics—a 60% mean increase in CI and a 45% mean decrease in PAD—clearly demonstrate LVAS efficacy. The restored cardiac output is sustained for the duration of LVAS implant.

After the first 24 hours following implant, no significant difference in mean CI or PAD ($p > 0.3$) is found between transplanted and nontransplanted groups. Trends in CI and PAD for the first 96 hours in both transplanted and nontransplanted groups show that a plateau is reached within about 24 hours after implant (Figs. 7 and 8). The lack of a statistically significant difference between the two

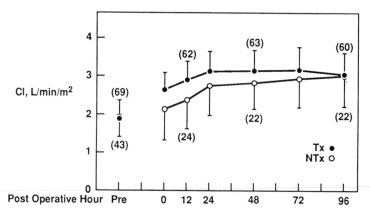

FIGURE 7. Comparison of pre- and postimplant cardiac index (CI) for transplanted and nontransplanted patients.

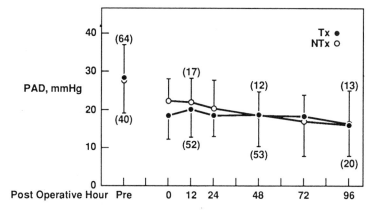

FIGURE 8. Comparison of pre- and postimplant pulmonary artery diastolic pressure (PAD) for transplanted and nontransplanted patients.

subgroups shows that hemodynamic improvement (or the lack thereof) is not a predictor of patient survivability to transplant. Other, presumably preexisting, patient-related factors such as vital organ function are important, and patient selection appears to be the primary determinant of survival to transplant.

Right Ventricular Function. Adequate right ventricular (RV) function was sustained for a majority (81%) of LVAS patients with some inotropic support during the first few days after implant. Twenty-three patients (19%) required concomitant RVAD support instituted intraoperatively or within a few hours after implant. No cases required late (>3 d) institution of RV mechanical assist. RVAD support, usually transient, was provided by an extracorporeal centrifugal pump. Eighteen patients (78%) with an RVAD did not survive to transplant, including 11 who died in the acute period (<3 d after implant). An RVAD was employed in 5 (56%) of the 9 operative deaths in the series. Five patients were weaned from the RVAD after a short period of support and then maintained on univentricular support to successful transplant. Of these, 3 patients were long-term (>24 mo) survivors. In many instances, RVAD insertion was a final, fruitless attempt at patient salvage.

Renal, Hepatic, and Pulmonary Function. All vital organ functions significantly improved with chronic LVAS support: bilirubin, creatinine, and blood urea nitrogen were at normal levels for patients who survived to transplant. In those who did not survive to transplant, renal and hepatic functions continued to deteriorate despite adequate pump output. Preimplant laboratory values were not predictive of organ recovery. For example, 6 patients who had a preimplant bilirubin level >4.0 mg/dl progressively improved and were successfully bridged. Five other patients with a similarly high bilirubin level, however, exhibited progressive deterioration in hepatic (multiorgan) function and did not survive to transplant.

Hematology. All hematologic parameters were within normal limits except for those patients with severe bleeding diatheses. Hemolysis was not clinically significant, typically with low plasma free hemoglobin levels (<5 mg/dl). Platelet counts remained generally within the normal range after a transient reduction (consumption) during the immediate postoperative period.

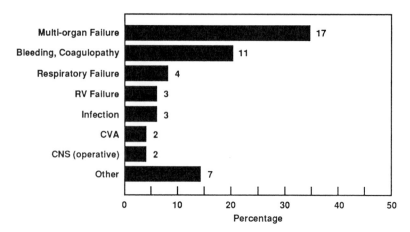

FIGURE 9. Cause of death in nontransplanted patients. [CNS = patients who succumbed following operative, iatrogenic cerebrovascular accidents (air embolus, LV mural thrombus embolization[19])].

Complications in LVAS Nonsurvivors. Forty-nine patients (40%) did not survive to transplant. Eighteen (37%) were acute patients (<3 d support), 22 (45%) were short-term patients (3–30 d support), and 9 (18%) were chronic patients (>30 d support). The causes of death are presented in Figure 9. Eight (44%) of the 18 acute patients died because of bleeding complications, whereas 13 (59%) of the 22 short-term patients developed multiorgan failure. Among chronic support nonsurvivors, bleeding, cerebrovascular accident (hemorrhagic), and infection resulted in 2 deaths each; support was withdrawn in 2 other cases; and 1 patient developed multiorgan failure.

Bleeding/coagulopathy was, therefore, the most frequent cause of death during the acute support period, whereas multi-organ failure was the primary cause of death in the short-term support patients. Although no primary cause of death was evident in chronic support patients, their complications usually developed within the earlier periods.

Posttransplant Survival. Among the 74 patients successfully bridged, 8 (11%) "operative deaths" occurred after transplant (deaths ≤30 d after transplant; ISHLT registry definition of operative mortality). This rate compares favorably with the outcome of transplantation without bridging.[10] An actuarial comparison of Novacor BTT patients with routine transplant patients is illustrated in Figure 10. Long-term posttransplant survival of Novacor BTT patients appears better than that for routine transplant patients. Other published data comparing patient survival after routine and staged cardiac transplants have demonstrated similar results.[2,15]

Causes of early deaths after transplant were donor graft failure (4), sepsis or presumed sepsis (3), and acute rejection (1). Five late deaths were due to viral infection (1; 5 mo), rejection (2; 10, 37 mo), presumed arrhythmia (1; 15 mo), and noncardiac causes (1; 10 mo, cancer). Sixty patients (82%) are long-term survivors, with the longest survivor (the first LVAS recipient) at 8 years post-transplant.

COMMENT

Patients with Chronic LVAS Support (>30 d). The results suggest that duration of support has a direct positive effect on outcome, both in overall survival

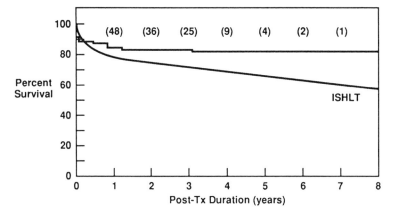

FIGURE 10. Kaplan-Meier posttransplant actuarial survival of Novacor LVAS patients compared with ISHLT registry data for routine transplants.

to transplant (Fig. 6) and in survival after transplant. This increased survival rate among chronic patients is observed for the 3 major admitting etiologies (AMI, IHD, and CM) as well as for patients in all age groups. Thus, although the overall survival to transplant is <46% for patients with AMI and 70% for patients with CM, a stratification based on duration of LVAS support presents a different picture. Patients with chronic LVAS support consistently demonstrated better rates of survival to transplant (AMI, 70%; IHD, 82%; and CM, 86%) (Fig. 11).

Of the 126 patients admitted into the study, 25% were in the 20–39-year group and 60% were in the 40–59-year group (Fig. 4). The overall patient survival rates for these two groups were 65% and 61%, respectively. For the subset of chronic patients, however, the survival rate for the two age ranges is >80% (Fig. 12). Although the ≥60-year group, as one might expect, experienced a lower overall survival rate (38%), the chronic patient subgroup still showed a marked increase (60%) (Fig. 13).

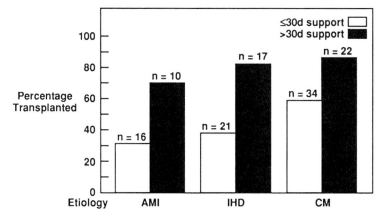

FIGURE 11. Admitting etiology and patient survival to transplant as a function of LVAS support duration.

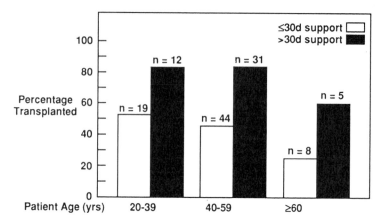

FIGURE 12. Patient age and survival to transplant as a function of LVAS support duration.

Suitability for Long-term Use.   The implantable pump/drive unit of the Novacor LVAS was designed for multiyear chronic use. A totally implantable LVAS with a slightly larger (90 ml stroke volume) pump/drive unit has proved its reliability in an NIH-sponsored, preclinical readiness testing in vitro study.[8] Clinical experience with the console-based LVAS has also demonstrated high reliability and capability for chronic patient support with full rehabilitation, providing a therapeutic alternative to cardiac transplantation in the treatment of terminal heart disease.

Reversal of Vital Organ Dysfunction with Prolonged LVAS Support.   In the majority of cases, chronic LVAS support has resulted in restoration of vital organ function. The data on patients who died of multiorgan failure despite adequate pump output also suggest that irreversible vital organ dysfunction secondary to terminal heart failure usually declares itself early. Death in the operative or early

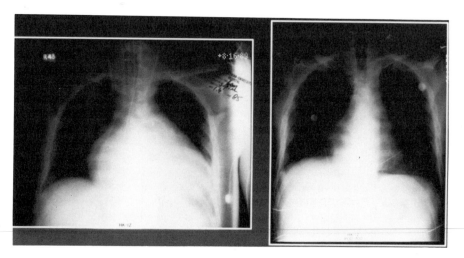

FIGURE 13.   Chest x-ray of an LVAS patient before and 100 days after implant (courtesy of Presbyterian–University Hospital, Pittsburgh).

postoperative period, despite significant improvement in hemodynamics, highlights the difficulty of patient selection and timing of LVAS implant to avoid multiorgan failure.

Adequacy of Univentricular Support. The current experience in >100 patients has shown adequacy of univentricular assist to support the circulation in patients with terminal (often biventricular) failure. Continued inotropic support was needed only during the first few days after implant to sustain adequate RV function. RV function in some patients, however, cannot be managed by pharmacotherapy and may require transient RVAD support. No need for chronic RVAD support was demonstrated.

Long-term LVAS Support: Absence of Cardiac Muscle Atrophy. A concern with continued and chronic decompression of the left ventricle is the possibility of atrophy of the cardiac muscle. A limited study of Novacor patients has shown that, although myocyte dimension decreased, there was no evidence of atrophy.[1] The observed decrease could be due to restoration to normal size of the substantially enlarged heart secondary to preimplant chronic heart failure. Chest x-rays of a Novacor BTT patient before implant and 100 days after implant show clearly the reduction in cardiac size as a result of LV decompression and reduction of RV afterload, both produced by the LVAS (Fig. 13).

Chronic Support. Patients with chronic Novacor LVAS support show restoration of normal vital organ function within 3–4 weeks after implant. Typically, all inotropic support is withdrawn within 1 week to 10 days. Patients are free of IV medication/nutrition in 1–2 weeks and able to exercise on a stationary bicycle by the second or third week after implant. Thereafter, they can lead an essentially normal life.

Out-of-hospital Experience of Chronic LVAS Patients. Although the patient is physically rehabilitated, emotional and social needs, such as privacy and living with the family, are not met by a continued hospital stay. In an effort to improve quality of life, selected LVAS patients at Presbyterian-University Hospital in Pittsburgh have been discharged from the hospital to an apartment building where they can live with family members while awaiting a transplant.[11] FDA approval for the first out-of-hospital living arrangement for ventricular assist recipients was obtained in 1990.

To date, 3 LVAS recipients have lived outside the hospital. The longest stay has been nearly 5 months (a 57-year-old man with cardiomyopathy was supported for a total of 169 days, underwent successful transplantation, and was then discharged). No clinical or device-related emergencies have been reported among the 3 patients. In addition to the many benefits to the LVAS recipient and his or her family, living outside the hospital reduces unnecessary costs and releases a hospital bed.

Wearable System. Since the first 8-day Novacor experience in 1984, the duration of support has been steadily increasing because of a progressively increasing donor shortage. Because the control console was originally conceived as a bedside unit, a wearable system has been developed (Fig. 1, center panel) in which the ECP (incorporating primary console functions) and its battery packs are worn by the recipient. This provides tether-free mobility and moves one step closer to the totally implantable system.

Novacor BTT Summary. The Novacor LVAS BTT experience has demonstrated safety and efficacy for extended circulatory support. The major findings from this multiyear experience are summarized in Table 3. The results of chronic

TABLE 3. Novacor BTT Experience: Observations

Patients fully rehabilitated	High device reliability
Univentricular support adequate	Out-of-hospital experience
Implant well tolerated	Chronic feasibility demonstrated

use with the console configuration provide a promising view of the applicability of the totally implantable system as an alternative therapy for endstage heart disease.

REFERENCES

1. Aerbe JL, Stein KL, Kormos RL, et al: Evolution of human cardiac myocyte dimension during prolonged mechanical support. J Thorac Cardiovasc Surg 101:256–259, 1991.
2. Birovljev S, Radovancevic B, Burnett CM, et al: Heart transplantation after mechanical circulatory support: Four years' experience. J Heart Lung Transplant 11:240–245, 1992.
3. Copeland JG, Levinson MM, Smith R, et al: The total artificial heart as a bridge to transplantation: A report of two cases. JAMA 256:2991, 1986.
4. Criteria for Medicare coverage of heart transplants: Medicare program. Federal Register 51:201; 37164–37170, 1986.
5. DeBakey ME: Left ventricular bypass pump for cardiac assistance: Clinical experience. Am J Cardiol 27:3–11, 1971.
6. DeVries WC: The permanent artificial heart: Four case reports. JAMA 259:849–859, 1988.
7. Hogness JR, Antwerp MV (eds): The Artificial Heart: Prototypes, Policies and Patients. Washington, DC, National Academy Press, 1991.
8. Jassawalla JS, Daniel MA, Chen H, et al: In vitro and in vivo testing of a totally implantable left ventricular assist system. ASAIO Trans 34:470–475, 1988.
9. Joyce LD, Johnson KE, Pierce WS, et al: Summary of the world experience with clinical use of total artificial hearts as heart support devices. J Heart Transplant 5:229–235, 1986.
10. Kaye MP: The registry of the International Society for Heart Transplantation: Ninth Official Report, 1992. J Heart Transplant 11:599–606, 1992.
11. Kormos RL, Borovetz HS, Pristas JM, et al: Out of hospital facility for the Novacor bridge to transplant patient: The Pittsburgh family house experience. Abstracts of the 37th Annual Meeting of the Am Soc Artif Intern Organs, p 113, 1991.
12. Norman JC, Cooley DA, Kahan BD, et al: Total support of the circulation of a patient with postcardiotomy stone-heart syndrome by a partial artificial heart (ALVAS) for five days followed by heart and kidney transplantation. Lancet 1:1125, 1978.
13. Oaks TE, Pae WE, Miller CA, et al: Combined registry for the clinical use of mechanical left ventricular assist pump and the total artificial heart in conjunction with heart transplant: Fifth official report, 1990. J Heart Transplant 9:621–625, 1991.
14. Pennington DG: Circulatory support at the turn of the decade: A clinician's view. ASAIO Trans 36:126–131, 1990.
15. Pifarre R, Sullivan H, Montoya A, et al: Comparison of results after heart transplantation: Mechanically supported versus nonsupported patients. J Heart Lung Transplant 11:235–239, 1992.
16. Portner PM: The Novacor heart assist system: Development, testing and initial clinical evaluation. In Akutsu T (ed): Artificial Heart 2. Tokyo, Springer Verlag, 1988, pp 89–97.
17. Portner PM, Oyer PE, McGregor CGA, et al: First human use of an electrically powered implantable ventricular assist system. Artif Organs 9A:36, 1985.
18. Portner PM, Oyer PE, Miller PJ, et al: Evolution of the solenoid actuated left ventricular assist system: Integration with a pusher-plate pump for intra-abdominal implantation in the calf. Artif Organs 2:402, 1978.
19. Portner PM, Oyer PE, Pennington DG, et al: Implantable left ventricular assist system: Bridge to transplantation and the future. Ann Thorac Surg 47:142–150, 1989.
20. Ramasamy N, Chen H, Miller PJ, et al: Chronic ovine evaluation of a totally implantable electrical left ventricular assist system. ASAIO Trans 35:401–404, 1989.
21. Report to the Chairman, Subcommittee on Health, Committee on Ways and Means, House of Representatives. Heart Transplants: Concerns about Cost, Access and Availability of Donor Organs. Washington, DC, U.S. General Accounting Office, 1989.
22. The Working Group on Mechanical Circulatory Support, National Heart Lung and Blood Institute. Artificial Heart and Assist Devices: Directions, Needs, Costs, Societal and Ethical Issues. U.S. Department of Health and Human Services publ no. (NIH) 85-2723, Public Health Service, 1985.

ROBERT W. EMERY, MD
MARC R. PRITZKER, MD
IRVIN F. GOLDENBERG, MD

USES OF MECHANICAL CIRCULATORY ASSIST DEVICES AT THE MINNEAPOLIS HEART INSTITUTE

From the Minneapolis Heart
Institute
Minneapolis, Minnesota

Reprint requests to:
Robert W. Emery, MD
920 East 28th Street
Suite 420
Minneapolis, MN 55407

Beginning in January of 1985, the Minneapolis Heart Institute (MHI) embarked on a formal program for the management of acute and chronic endstage heart disease, including structured programs in mechanical circulatory support, cardiac transplantation, and pharmacologic treatment of congestive heart failure. Over the past 7 years, a variety of devices have been used to provide partial or total support to patients with cardiogenic shock in the early postoperative period, while awaiting transplantation, or for fulminant cardiac failure associated with acute myocarditis. Patients were supported to functional recovery or transplantation or until multisystem failure precluded recovery.

Over the past 2 years, the use of ventricular assist devices (VADs) has declined (5 VADs/ 3301 cardiopulmonary bypass [CPB] cases, 0.15%). The reasons are complex, centering on issues of more precise patient categorization, improved myocardial preservation, enhanced pharmacologic support for congestive heart failure, Food and Drug Administration restrictions on use of devices, and the problem of obtaining timely donors in our tristate UNOS region.[5,6,20,25] Additionally, advances in the management of congestive heart failure have altered the natural history of endstage heart disease, reducing the incidence of progressive congestive heart failure without affecting the incidence of sudden death. Thus, endstage heart patients in the 1990s are more likely to die suddenly outside the hospital

CARDIAC SURGERY: State of the Art Reviews—Vol. 7, No. 2, 1993
Philadelphia, Hanley & Belfus, Inc.

377

without an opportunity to receive mechanical support.[3,25] In spite of these changes, an interest in circulatory support persists, with efforts focused on the limited number of available devices. This review of the MHI experience focuses on each of the devices that we have used, including indications and results.

OVERVIEW

Initially the rotary pump was used to support the left ventricle in cases of postcardiotomy shock. With the subsequent introduction of Vortex technology, postcardiotomy support with centrifugal pumps expanded the use of VADs. Over the last decade, more sophisticated devices have been developed that allow enhanced support, greater patient mobility during the period of support, and extended duration of support. In our experience a tiered strategy of mechanical support, beginning with the simplest and most economic devices and proceeding, as necessary, toward more complex and expensive therapies, allows critical early organ support and maximal flexibility in decision-making.[5]

In the majority of cases in which mechanical circulatory support is instituted, the extent of the injury and therefore the prognosis for recovery are not easily and immediately assessable. Thus, the choice of support device should favor ease and immediacy of insertion, preservation of options, and satisfactory support of circulation. The selected device should be capable of providing adequate cardiac output while completely draining and "resting" the heart. The efficiency of most devices is drainage-dependent, and data indicate that the extent of diversion away from the ventricle correlates with the probability of recovery, given the appropriateness and completeness of the operation and the absence of irreversible myocardial damage.[18,21,23] The expectation is that duration of support will be limited because myocardial recovery will be sufficient to allow autonomous circulatory function.

The importance of establishing adequate preload diversion to facilitate myocardial recovery cannot be overstated. Preload reduction diminishes myocardial oxygen consumption and work by reducing ventricular cavity dimensions and wall stress as well as by enhancing subendocardial perfusion. Assuming adequate preload reduction and constant cardiac output supplied by the device, alterations in systemic pressure are the results of changes in resistance. Pharmacologic emphasis should be shifted away from inotropic agents and concentrated on agents to titrate systemic vascular resistance and arterial pressure toward optimal values. Nitroglycerin and nitroprusside are used for arterial and venous dilution, whereas phenylephrine, dopamine, and norepinephrine are used to augment resistance and/or blood pressures to provide critical perfusion pressure in secondary organs.

When possible, we have found it useful to contemplate, at the outset, whether the patient is a candidate for transplantation. The enhanced needs for mobility over this longer duration of support and the absolute need for surgical techniques that potentially preserve intrathoracic sterility dictate cannula choices, cannula-exiting strategies, and in some cases device selection.

Previous articles have reviewed the availability of devices and their use as bridges to transplantation or recovery.[6,8,23] At the MHI we have used the centrifugal and axial flow pumps as bridges to myocardial recovery, with the intraaortic balloon pump (IABP) as a common adjunct. A percutaneous CPB system is available in the catheterization laboratory to initiate timely support in unstable patients, including those awaiting operation, undergoing supported angioplasty, or with extreme hemodynamic instability. Centrifugal flow VADs, the Novacor left VAD, and the Jarvik total artificial heart (TAH) have been used for the more extended support associated with bridge to transplantation.

INTRAAORTIC BALLOON PUMP

The IABP is the most commonly used device for mechanical circulatory support in cardiovascular surgery today. The balloon pump reduces afterload, improving the ratio of oxygen delivery to oxygen use, and augments diastolic coronary blood flow, although this second factor has been questioned in the face of coronary disease.[1] The IABP has also been successful in the treatment of cardiogenic shock secondary to idiopathic dilated cardiomyopathy, as support in acute rejection of the transplanted heart, and occasionally as adjunctive treatment in septic shock.[8] The use of this device is the first line of attack in the treatment of low cardiac output states that are unresponsive to inotropic medications and adequate volume loading.[6]

Often, prophylactic insertion of an IABP obviates later problems when used in prospectively identified patients at high risk for cardiovascular surgery and angioplasty. IABP placement alone may improve cardiogenic shock in up to 71% of patients suffering acute myocardial infarction.[17] In addition, cardiovascular surgical procedures are more safely performed with preoperative IABP insertion in certain patients, including those with high-grade left main coronary disease and either left ventricular (LV) dysfunction or systemic hypotension; those undergoing elective coronary bypass surgery with moderate-to-severe LV dysfunction (ejection fraction < 35%) and elevated end-diastolic pressures at the time of catheterization (end-diastolic pressure > 20); those with angina coupled with hypotension after myocardial infarction; and those with severe LV dysfunction. The IABP is also useful to assist myocardial recovery after acute infarction and as preoperative support in the presence of severe acute mitral regurgitation or ventricular septal defect.[26]

Over the past several years, improvements in the sizing of the balloon pump sheath have facilitated ease of percutaneous insertion, and the smaller external diameter chord obviates obstructive arterial symptoms in all patients but those with severe peripheral vascular disease. Contraindications to IABP insertion include a severely diseased atherosclerotic aorta, absence of femoral pulses, abdominal aortic aneurysm, and moderate or severe aortic insufficiency. The use of the IABP has thus been both prophylactic and therapeutic. In 1991 Cardiac Surgical Associates performed 1,765 open-heart surgical procedures. In 214 (12%) the IABP was used. The IABP was placed preoperatively in 145 (68%), intraoperatively in 58 (28%), and postoperatively in 3 (1%); timing is unknown in 8 (4%).

Review of 1,000 consecutive IABP insertions conducted at the MHI revealed a 7% incidence of serious complications, including but not limited to exploration for bleeding, thrombosis, or infection. Transient symptoms, such as ischemia or neurologic symptoms that resolved after removal of the balloon, were not considered as major complications in this review.[19] Even smaller balloons are being developed, and the use of the IABP will continue to increase over time as the ease of insertion and safety of the device become more apparent. Our indications for IABP are liberal and the threshold for insertion low.

PERCUTANEOUS CARDIOPULMONARY BYPASS

A system for percutaneous access to CPB was devised by our perfusion group for use by the catheterization laboratory. This system was not applied on a hospitalwide basis because of other reported overall poor results.[9,16] We used the emergent bypass system to obtain rapid percutaneous access in the catheterization laboratory for patients in whom anatomic diagnoses had been, or could be, rapidly undertaken. We found that patients with defined anatomic lesions could be brought urgently to surgery and undergo CPB procedures with excellent survival, using either the emergent system or a standard CPB circuit.[16] Patients without anatomically correctable lesions did not fare as well, although some were salvageable. In addition to use in patients with circulatory collapse in catheterization, this system has also been used for CPB-supported angioplasty in patients either with poor ventricular function or with the entire coronary circulation provided by a single vessel with critical stenosis. In the latter patients, with inflation of the angioplasty balloon and occlusion of the coronary circulation, pulsatile aortic pressure completely disappeared, but cardiac decompression and nonpulsatile circulatory support were maintained by bypass. With deflation of the angioplasty balloon, cardiac function with pulsatile pressure in the face of CPB immediately returned.

Among the patients brought to emergent surgery for coronary bypass because of hemodynamic compromise in the catheterization laboratory, 7 over 3 years have been operated, with an operative mortality of 14%. Six of 7 patients are long-term survivors. In the supported angioplasty group, 35 of 40 (88%) angioplasties were successful; 5 were unsuccessful, or the lesion could not be passed with a wire. None of these patients went to coronary bypass grafting. There were no myocardial infarctions and no mortality. At 6 months, 34 of these 35 successfully dilated patients were alive.[15] After experience was gained with supported angioplasty, the indications for the use of bypass-supported angioplasty diminished. Currently, most supported angioplasties are scheduled for standby, and cannulation is undertaken only if hemodynamic deterioration occurs. This device represents a valuable backup to our cardiac catheterization laboratory with excellent results, in both the emergent patient with hemodynamic collapse and the high-risk angioplasty patient.

CENTRIFUGAL VENTRICULAR ASSIST

Both for patients in cardiogenic shock from an etiology that does not require operation (less common) and for patients in the postcardiotomy period with failure to wean from CPB, circulatory support is initiated with VADs when a judicious and expeditious trial of IABP support, volume loading, and inotropic support fail to stabilize the patient. Indications are similar to those described by Pennington, as modified by inotropic support (Tables 1 and 2).[6,20] The only absolute contraindication to the use of the VAD for cardiogenic shock in the postcardiotomy period is neurologic injury, but factors listed in Table 3 constitute relative contraindications. The centrifugal flow pumps are used in association with an IABP almost universally. Currently, cannulation is undertaken for inflow via the standard aortic cannula and for outflow via the right superior pulmonary vein

TABLE 1.   Criteria for Mechanical Ventricular Support

Cardiac index <2.0 L/m^2/min	Urine output <20 ml/hr with:
Systemic vascular resistance >2100 dynes/s/cm^5	Optimal preload
Atrial pressure >20 mmHg	Maximal drug therapy
	Corrected metabolism
	Intraaortic balloon pump

TABLE 2.   Maximal Inotropic Support*

Dopamine	10 mg/kg/min
Dobutamine	10 mg/kg/min
Epinephrine	0.02 mg/kg/min
Isoproterenol	0.05 mg/kg/min
Amrinone	10 mg/kg/min

* Dosage of any 2 constitutes maximal support except when dopamine is used in renal doses as a third agent.

for LVAD and right atrium to pulmonary artery for RVAD. All cannulas exit the chest via separate stab wounds, and the surgical incision is completely closed whenever feasible. Occasionally, the sternum may need to be left open and the skin closed, but most commonly the operation can be completed. With effective circulatory support using centrifugal devices of both the Sarns (Sarns, Ann Arbor, MI) and BioMedicus (Medtronic, Minneapolis, MN) types, the patients are allowed to awaken during the postoperative period and are not kept paralyzed or intubated, except when indicated. In fact, on rare occasions patients with centrifugal ventricular assist in place have been able to be out of bed.

As noted previously, adequate chamber drainage is most important in obtaining appropriate ventricular decompression and support. In our experience, early use of ventricular assistance has lessened the need for biventricular support and the incidence of secondary organ system damage resulting from prolonged low output/high inotropic states. Criteria developed by Pennington et al.[22] are useful in this assessment. Via the right superior pulmonary vein, a right-angle, metal-tip cannula is often effective for outflow drainage. If it is not effective, a right-angle tube (Central Medical, Inc., Minneapolis, MN) placed through the pulmonary vein and across the mitral valve is effective and nonobstructive for left heart assist (Fig. 1), with flows of 5 or 6 L obtainable. Postoperatively, patients are managed without heparin until flows diminish to <2 L, at which time systemic heparinization is instituted with an activated clotting time (ACT) maintained at >200 seconds for flows of 1–2 L; full heparinization with an ACT >400 seconds is the target level for flows of 1 L or during formal weaning. Ventricular function is followed closely by serial transesophageal echocardiographic examinations, which allow determination of regional wall motion and global cardiac function to ascertain the timing of weaning, the effectiveness of weaning, and the timing of transplantation, should the need arise.[2] Effective recovery, if likely, is observable by 72 hours. In our experience, the longest duration of support on an RVAD has been 14 days and on LVAD, 8 days.

Over the past 5 years (1 January 1987–31 December 1991), ventricular assistance has been used in 21 postcardiotomy patients and in 1 patient who suffered cardiovascular collapse while awaiting transplantation. Over this 5-year period, Cardiac Surgical Associates performed 6,826 open-heart surgical procedures. The incidence of VAD use was 0.3%, or 1 usage for every 297 CPB cases. Configurations included 3 RVADs, 12 LVADs, and 7 BVADs. Two of these 22 patients were bridged to transplant and survived; 3 others were supported after

TABLE 3.   Risk Factors for Insertion of Ventricular Assist Device

Unsuccessful or incomplete operation	Age >65 years
Perioperative myocardial infarction	Bleeding on cardiopulmonary bypass
Biventricular failure	Delayed insertion of ventricular assist device

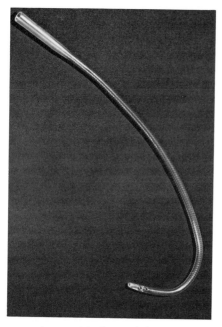

FIGURE 1. Example of an effective drainage cannula that can be inserted via the right superior pulmonary vein into the left ventricular chamber without obstruction of the upper lobe pulmonary drainage. Flows of 4/6 L/min can be obtained.

transplant, with 2 surviving. The remaining 17 patients were supported after cardiotomy. Seven of these patients (38%) died on the device. Ten patients were weaned (62%), and 2 died after device removal. The remaining 8 (44%) were discharged from the hospital.

NIMBUS HEMOPUMP

For a brief period during the clinical trials, the Nimbus Hemopump (Johnson and Johnson, Inc., Warren, NJ) was used at the MHI in patients with postinfarction cardiogenic shock (n = 6) and in patients unable to be weaned from CPB (n = 2). The device was inserted via a 10-mm graft sewn to the femoral artery. Insertion was performed in both the cardiac catheterization laboratory and the operating room. This approximately 10-mm device is based on the Archimedean screw principle, rotating at more than 25,000 rpm to generate flow (Fig. 2). Inability to place the catheter has occurred in approximately 20% of cases (a rate consistent with our experience), most commonly as a result of small peripheral vessels or arteriosclerotic plaques. Once placed intraarterially, the device is threaded across the aortic valve into the ventricular chamber, and support is achieved by varying the speed of the pump to obtain flow. A maximal support of approximately 3.5 L/min has limited the use of this device in large patients, in whom the device alone was not adequate to support the entire circulatory function and residual underlying ventricular function was necessary. We also found the device to be critically afterload-dependent, with high peripheral vascular resistance limiting pump flow despite maximal rpm setting. The device is currently unavailable by FDA regulation. The Johnson and Johnson company is formulating protocols for further clinical trials and designing a 13-Fr model to facilitate insertion. The Nimbus Hemopump, based on preliminary experience, has a bright future as a mechanical support device. The next generation will facilitate percutaneous

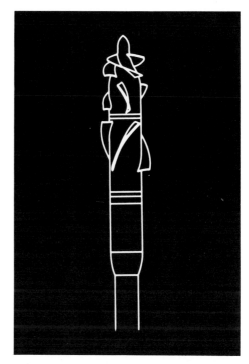

FIGURE 2.   Flow-generating head of the Hemopump rotates more than 25,000 rpm to generate nonpulsatile systemic flow.

insertion, allowing the device to be used in much the same fashion as an IABP, but also allowing substantially more circulatory support. A shorter Nimbus Hemopump that can be inserted via the ascending aorta has also been developed and used in limited circumstances.[4]

TOTAL ARTIFICIAL HEART

The Jarvik-7-70 was first used at the MHI in October of 1986. The patient, a 40-year-old woman with acute myocarditis, constituted the first-ever use of the "mini-Jarvik." Although the patient survived bridging to transplantation, she died after a hospitalization of 236 days of multiorgan failure.[11] This experience led to the placement of 8 more Jarvik devices.[7] The indication for use was cardiogenic shock in patients who were otherwise candidates for bridging to transplantation; it was not used as a resuscitative device. Patients had to be of adequate size to accept the Jarvik and to have no known neurologic injury. All patients in whom the Jarvik device was used were effectively bridged to transplantation with no failures of the unit. Seven of these patients survived transplantation. Two patients died later. We found the Jarvik to be an effective circulatory support device and noted that the better the preoperative condition of the patient, the easier the transition through total circulatory support to transplantation.[2] Complications occurring in the pretransplant period were often carried through the posttransplant period and became the limiting factor in the success of transplantation (Tables 4–6). Our data confirmed those previously reported for the artificial heart.[12,24] The Symbion 7-70 and 7-100 devices have been withdrawn from use since April of 1990 by the FDA but may have investigative availability in the near future from initiatives provided by Cardiowest, Inc. (Tucson, AZ). Limited activity has occurred worldwide.[10]

TABLE 4. Patient Demographics

	ML	NC	CL	PT	SG	DM	BV	BK	PL
Age	40	28	15	50	45	19	16	19	52
Sex	F	F	M	M	F	M	M	M	F
Height (cm)	154	161	163	182	152	170	180	187	162
Weight (kg)	55	63	46	94	48	69	66	86	57
Etiology	Postviral	Giant cell myocarditis	IDC	Ischemic CM	RHD	Congenital hypertrophic myopathy	Postviral	IDC	IDC
Indication	Cardiogenic shock	Cardiogenic shock	Cardiogenic shock	Failure to wean CPB	Failure to wean VAD	Donor organ failure	Cardiogenic shock	Cardiogenic shock	Cardiogenic shock
Pre-J-7-70 support	Inotropic IABP	Inotropic	Emergent CPB	Inotropic IABP	Inotropic IABP; BVAD	Inotropic BVAD; IABP	Inotropic	Inotropic	Inotropic IABP
Pre-J-7-70 organ dysfunction	Renal	(−)	Renal CVA	(−)	Respiratory	(−)	(−)	(−)	LLL infiltrate

RHD = rheumatic heart disease; IDC = idiopathic dilated cardiomyopathy; CM = cardiomyopathy; CPB = cardiopulmonary bypass; VAD = ventricular assist device; IABP = intraaortic balloon pump; BVAD = biventricular assist device; CVA = cerebrovascular accident; LLL = left lower lobe.
From Emery RW, Joyce LD, Prieto M, et al: Experience with the Symbion Total Artificial Heart as a bridge to transplantation. Ann Thorac Surg 53:282–288, 1992, with permission.

TABLE 5. Complications on Jarvik-7-70 Support

	ML	NC	CL	PT	SG	DM	BV	BK	PL
Implant duration (days)	44	4	25	17	5	18	15	25	7
Ventilator (days)	20	1	21	1	4	1	1	1	1
Blood loss 48 hr (U)	19	5	11	8	2	3	2	2	9
Surgical wound infection	(-)	(-)	(-)	(-)	(-)	(-)	(-)	(-)	(-)
Other infection	Driveline	(-)	(-)	(-)	Blood; CVP driveline; urine; mediastinum	(-)	(-)	Driveline	Blood pneumonia
Dialysis	+	(-)	(-)	(-)	(-)	(-)	(-)	(-)	(-)
Stroke	(-)	(-)	(-)	TIA	(-)	(-)	(-)	Confusion TIA	(-)
Hemolysis	(-)	(-)	(-)	(-)	(-)	(-)	(-)	(-)	(-)
Reoperative bleeding	Early	(-)	(-)	(-)	(-)	Late	Late	(-)	(-)
Device malfunction	(-)	(-)	(-)	(-)	(-)	(-)	(-)	(-)	(-)
Other	PVD Pancreatic Pseudocyst	(-)	Prolonged ventilatory support	(-)	(-)	(-)	(-)	Catatonia Sacral decubitus	Pneumonia

CVP = central venous pressure; TIA = transient ischemic attack; PVD = peripheral vascular disease.
From Emery RW, Joyce LD, Prieto M, et al: Experience with the Symbion Total Artificial Heart as a bridge to transplantation. Ann Thorac Surg 53:282–288, 1992, with permission.

TABLE 6. Posttransplant Course

	ML	NC	CL	PT	SG	DM	BV	BK	PL
Survival 1 mo	+	+	+	+	(−)	+	+	(−)	(−)
Survival 3 mos	+	+	+	+	NA	+	+	+	NA
Survival 1 yr	(−)	+	+	+	NA	+	+	+	NA
Posttransplant survival (mos)	(9*)	(29*)	(46)	44	(1*)	34	33	26	(0*)
Rejection 1 yr (days post-transplant)	(−)	6, 38, 854	367	(−)	(23)	(−)	(−)	(−)	NA
Infections 1 yr	CMV Pneumonitis Pneumocystitis Pseudomonas Sepsis	(−)	Mumps	(−)	NA	(−)	(−)	Sacral ulcer Confusion	NA
Other complications	Leg ischemia Multiorgan failure	(−)	Ganciclovir Leukopenia	(−)	NA	(−)	(−)	BVAD support of donor heart	NA
Current steroids	NA	NA	(−)	(−)	NA	(−)	(−)	(−)	NA
Posttransplant hospitalization	226*	11	139	17	28*	17	15	63	1*

* Died during hospitalization.
NA = not applicable; CMV = cytomegalovirus; BVAD = biventricular assist device.
From Emery RW, Joyce LD, Prieto M, et al: Experience with the Symbion Total Artificial Heart as a bridge to transplantation. Ann Thorac Surg 53:282–288, 1992, with permission.

NOVACOR LEFT VENTRICULAR ASSIST SYSTEM

The Novacor left ventricular assist system (LVAS) (Baxter Healthcare, Novacor Division, Oakland, CA) has been used for bridge to transplantation since 1984.[14] The Novacor LVAS is a univentricular device that is useful for bridging to transplantation. Right ventricular support is not available with this device, and occasionally a separate right ventricular centrifugal VAD system may be necessary after surgical implantation, particularly if pulmonary vascular resistance is elevated.[13] Although we have limited the use of the Novacor to patients with purely LV failure, we have used it 3 times. One patient is alive and well after transplantation; 1 patient died at surgery during the insertion; and 1 patient died of right ventricular failure in the immediate postoperative period. By itself, the Novacor device is probably not an adequate support system if high pulmonary resistance and right ventricular dysfunction intervene. The device has been shown to provide adequate circulatory support and has become useful in experimental bridges to transplantation, with excellent results.[6] A permanently implantable device is currently under laboratory investigation.

COMMENT

Limitations to the use of mechanical circulatory assistance have arisen over the past several years. Following the rush of interest in support devices in the 1980s, an indolence that developed in the 1990s has limited the introduction of new devices in broad application. Reasons include the tremendous expense of caring for device-supported patients, strict FDA restrictions on the use of certain support devices, and a changing population of patients eligible for mechanical bridging. Devices that can be used for limited time frames, such as the centrifugal VAD, are most commonly used because of availability, cost considerations, and absence of federal restrictions. Continued interest in their use, coupled with appropriate rather than limiting indications for further application, is necessary to allow the development of a permanently implantable system in the foreseeable future. Current data indicate that the most important aspect in the use of devices is not the device itself but patient selection.[6] The use of VADs as resuscitation devices, whether for myocardial recovery or bridge to transplantation, has had poor results; in spite of occasional spectacular successes, careful patient selection is imperative. Overall results from multiple devices are similar in wean rates, survival rates, and bridge-to-transplantation rates.[6,8] Centers interested in the use of VADs must select the device most appropriate to their need.

REFERENCES

1. Balooki H: Physiology of Balloon Pumping in Clinical Applications of Internal Aortic Balloon Pump, 2nd ed. Mount Kisco, NY, Futura, 1984, pp 57–90.
2. Brack M, Olsen JD, Pedersen WR, et al: Transesophageal echocardiography in patients with mechanical circulatory assistance. Ann Thorac Surg 52:1306–1309, 1991.
3. Defibrillator Study Group: Actuarial risk of sudden death while awaiting cardiac transplantation in patients with atherosclerotic heart disease. Am J Cardiol 68:545–546, 1991.
4. Duncan JM, Frazier OH, Radovanervic B, Velebit V: Implantation techniques for the Hemopump. Ann Thorac Surg 48:733–735, 1989.
5. Emery RW, Eales F, Joyce LD, et al: Mechanical circulatory assistance after heart transplantation. Ann Thorac Surg 51:43–47, 1991.
6. Emery RW, Joyce LD: Directions in cardiac assistance. J Card Surg 6:400–414, 1991.
7. Emery RW, Joyce LD, Prieto M, et al: Experience with the Symbion Total Artificial Heart as a bridge to transplantation. Ann Thorac Surg 53:282–288, 1992.
8. Goldenberg IF: Nonpharmacologic treatment of cardiogenic shock. Chest (in press).

9. Hill JG, Bruhn PS, Cohen SE, et al: Emergent applications of cardiopulmonary support: A multi-institutional experience. Ann Thorac Surg 54:699–704, 1992.

10. Johnson KE, Prieto M, Joyce LD, et al: Summary of the clinical use of the Symbion Total Artificial Heart: A registry report. J Heart Lung Transplant 11:103–116, 1992.

11. Joyce LD, Pritzker MR, Kiser JL, et al: Use of the Mini-Jarvik 7 total artificial heart as a bridge to transplantation. J Heart Transplant 5:203–209, 1986.

12. Kawaguchi AT, Gandjbalich I, Pavig A, et al: Liver and kidney function in patients undergoing mechanical circulatory support with Jarvik 7 artificial heart as a bridge to transplantation. J Heart Transplant 9:631–637, 1990.

13. Kormos RL, Borovetz HS, Gasior T, et al: Experience with univentricular support in mortally ill cardiac transplant candidates. Ann Thorac Surg 49:261–272, 1990.

14. McCarthy PM, Portner PM, Tobler HG, et al: Clinical experience with the Novacor ventricular assist system: Bridge to transplantation and the transition to permanent application. J Thorac Cardiovasc Surg 102:570–587, 1991.

15. Mooney JF: MHI Angioplasty Registry. Personal communication.

16. Mooney MR, Arom KV, Joyce LD, et al: Emergency cardiopulmonary bypass support in patients with cardiac arrest. J Thorac Cardiovasc Surg 101:450–454, 1991.

17. Mundth ED: Mechanical and surgical interventions for the reduction of myocardial ischemia. Circulation 53(Suppl I):176–183, 1975.

18. Ott RA, Eugene J, Moore-Jefferies F, et al: Left atrial-to-aortic assistance with in-line left ventricular venting. ASAIO Trans 24:580–585, 1983.

19. Pedersen W: Personal communication.

20. Pennington DG (McBride LR), Joyce LD, Pae WE, Burckholder JA: Patient selection for ventricular assistance: A panel discussion. Ann Thorac Surg 47:77–81, 1989.

21. Pennington DG, McBrion LR, Kanter KR, et al: Effect of peri-operative myocardial infarction on survival of post-cardiotomy patients supported with ventricular assist devices. Circulation 78(Suppl III):110–115, 1988.

22. Pennington DG, Reedy JE, Swartz MT, et al: Univentricular versus biventricular assist device support. J Heart Lung Transplant 10:258–263, 1991.

23. Pennington DG, Termuhlen DF: Mechanical circulatory support: Device selection. Card Surg State Art Rev 3:507–519, 1989.

24. Reedy JE, Schwartz MT, Termuhlen DF, et al: Bridge to transplantation: Importance of patient selection. J Heart Transplant 9:473–481, 1990.

25. Stevenson LW, Hamilton MA, Tillisch IH, et al: Decreasing surgical benefit from cardiac transplantation for outpatients as the waiting list lengthens. J Am Coll Cardiol 18:915–925, 1991.

26. Weber KT, Janicki JS: Intra-aortic balloon counterpulsation: A review of physiological principles, clinical results and device safety. Ann Thorac Surg 17:60–66, 1974.

LAWRENCE R. McBRIDE, MD
MARC T. SWARTZ

ANTICOAGULATION IN PATIENTS WITH VENTRICULAR ASSIST DEVICES

From the Department of Surgery
St. Louis University Medical
Center
St. Louis, Missouri

Reprint requests to:
Lawrence R. McBride, MD
Department of Surgery
St. Louis University Medical
Center
3635 Vista Ave. at Grand Blvd.
PO Box 15250
St. Louis, MO 63110-0250

In 1937 Gibbons reported the first successful use of cardiopulmonary bypass (CPB) in animals.[7] Since that time a wide range of devices has been used in both experimental animals and humans for temporary support of the circulation. Because of the artificial surface/blood interface inherent to the design of circulatory support systems, thrombus formation and complications resulting from embolization have been viewed as primary drawbacks to long-term support. Short-term CPB with systemic heparinization has proved to be safe. By the late 1970s improved biomaterials and design led to a generation of devices that required lower levels of anticoagulation.[2,4,13,15] Until the early 1980s the duration of mechanical circulatory support seldom exceeded 3–4 days. For perfusions of this interval, intravenous heparin at reduced levels (activated clotting time [ACT] of 200–250 sec) proved to be relatively safe. By the mid 1980s patients were supported for longer durations as a bridge to cardiac transplantation. Optimal support for extended durations required the replacement of continuous intravenous heparinization with oral regimens of anticoagulation.[17] Durations of support >30 days are now commonplace, and many patients are maintained on oral anticoagulant protocols, ranging from dipyridamole alone to a combination of warfarin and aspirin. Despite the ability to support patients longer over the last decade, the reported incidence of thromboembolism has increased in both recovery and bridge-to-transplant patients (Figs. 1 and 2).

CARDIAC SURGERY: State of the Art Reviews—Vol. 7, No. 2, 1993
Philadelphia, Hanley & Belfus, Inc.

389

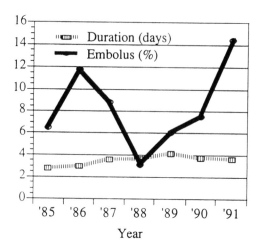

FIGURE 1.   Incidence of thromboembolism vs. duration of support per year in postcardiotomy patients (ASAIO-ISHLT Registry).

The information in this chapter is based on data obtained from a literature review, our clinical experience at St. Louis University, and the Registry for Mechanical Assist Devices and Total Artificial Hearts, which is maintained at Pennsylvania State University and jointly sponsored by the American Society of Artificial Internal Organs and the International Society of Heart and Lung Transplantation (ASAIO-ISHLT Registry).

PATHOPHYSIOLOGY

Mechanical circulatory support devices are associated with significant and often detrimental effects on many body systems.[3,5,6,19] Bleeding and thromboembolism are recognized as major complications, along with transient ischemic attacks and cerebrovascular accidents.[6,18]

The etiology of thrombus formation within a mechanical circulatory support device is just beginning to be understood. When blood comes in contact with an artificial surface, a complex series of events results in activation of platelets and white blood cells, the blood coagulation/fibrinolytic system, and the complement system.[1,15,16] Theoretically these initial responses are followed by a progressive passivation of the device surfaces, probably as a result of protein absorption and protein/protein interaction.[9,10] The exact mechanism of passivation is not known, and it is unclear whether passivation always occurs. Current theory states that passivation is a process in which layers of protein accumulate on the artificial surface of the device. Thus the circulation sees protein rather than an artificial surface; as a result, less platelet/surface interaction occurs and the risk of thrombus formation is reduced. The initial interactions before passivation may lead to thrombus formation, thromboembolic complications, consumption coagulopathy, or excessive bleeding.

Platelets become refractory and dysfunctional as a result of interaction with artificial surfaces.[9] This transient platelet dysfunction is related to selective alpha granule release. The hemostatic function of platelets is related to the duration of their contact with an artificial surface. Platelet activation also results in platelet-platelet

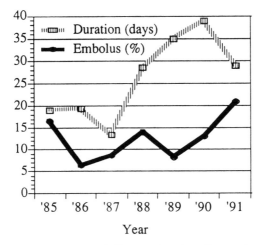

FIGURE 2.   Incidence of thromboembolism vs. duration of support per year in bridge to transplant patients (ASAIO-ISHLT Registry).

interaction or platelet aggregation. When platelets come in contact with a foreign surface, especially at high sheer rates, they undergo conformational changes associated with pseudopod formation; this reaction is called platelet spreading. Platelet adherence, which includes contact and spreading, leads to the release of adenosine diphosphate, which attracts other platelets streaming close to the adherent platelet. Patients with mechanical circulatory support devices probably undergo a continuous activation of platelets until the artificial surface is pacified. Platelet activation is associated with thrombocytopenia, which can persist for several days after device implantation. During this interval platelet transfusions may be necessary.

DEVICE-SPECIFIC ANTICOAGULATION REGIMENS

Laboratory and clinical experiences have now determined that anticoagulant protocols must be tailored specifically for a particular type of device. Table 1 shows the mechanical circulatory support devices presently available and the generally recognized anticoagulant regimen for each.

TABLE 1.   Recommended Anticoagulant Protocols for Available Devices

Device	Anticoagulation Required	Preferred Application	Duration
Biomedicus	Moderate–heparin	P, B-Tx	Short–intermediate-term
ECMO	Full–heparin	R	Short-term
Sarns/Centrimed	Moderate–heparin	P, B-Tx	Short–intermediate-term
Abiomed BVS	Moderate–heparin	P, B-Tx	Short–intermediate-term
Pierce-Donachy VAD	Low–heparin or oral	P, B-Tx	Intermediate–long-term
Sarns Pulsatile VAD	Low–heparin or oral	P, B-Tx	Intermediate–long-term
Hemopump	Moderate–heparin	R, P	Short-term
Novacor LVAS	Low–heparin or oral	B-Tx	Intermediate–long-term
Thermocardiosystems LVAS	Low–oral	B-Tx	Intermediate–long-term

BVS = biventricular support system; ECMO = extracorporeal membrane oxygenation; LVAS = left ventricular assist system; VAD = ventricular assist device; R = resuscitative; P = postcardiotomy; B-Tx = bridge to transplantation.

TABLE 2.   Anticoagulant Protocol (St. Louis University) for Postcardiotomy Shock

Centrifugal pump	1. Implant—full heparinization
	2. Reverse heparin with protamine
	3. Wait until <75 cc/hr bleeding for 3 consecutive hours and no apparent coagulopathy, then start heparin drip to maintain ACT at 150–175 sec.
	4. Increase heparin to raise ACT to 200–225 sec when weaning
Pulsatile pump	1. Implant—full heparinization
	2. Reverse heparin with protamine
	3. Wait until <75 cc/hr bleeding for 3 consecutive hours, then start dextran drip at 25 cc/hr
	4. Start heparin to raise ACT to 175–200 sec at 5–7 days or when weaning; discontinue dextran

ACT = activated clotting time.

Several factors influence which anticoagulant regimen is used in a particular patient. The expected duration of support as well as the type of device can influence the maintenance anticoagulant regimen. By general consensus, anticoagulation should not be initiated until bleeding after device insertion has subsided.

Centrifugal pumps are the most commonly used type of ventricular assist device (VAD). This family of devices is used primarily in patients with postcardiotomy shock. They are usually inserted with full systemic heparinization and ACTs > 400 seconds. If centrifugal devices are inserted after cardiac repair and long CPB times, the systemic heparin should be reversed with protamine (Table 2). The patient should be observed for a period of time (approximately 12–24 hours), and once postoperative bleeding has diminished to <75 cc/hr for 3 consecutive hours, then intravenous infusion of heparin should be initiated to maintain the ACT at 150–175 seconds. If the patient is to be weaned from the centrifugal pump, the continuous infusion of heparin should be increased proportionately with decreases in flow. At the time of device removal, the ACT should be approximately 225 seconds. If the patient is to be bridged to transplant and supported for >7–10 days, continuous heparin to maintain the ACT at 200 seconds is probably the safest regimen. The centrifugal pump head should also be routinely changed (every 48–72 hours).

The anticoagulant requirement for pneumatic pulsatile VADs is less than that required by centrifugal and roller pumps (Table 2). For postcardiotomy patients, pneumatic devices are inserted using systemic heparinization with ACTs >400 seconds. Once the device is inserted and operational and adequate flows have been established, the heparin is reversed with a proportional dose of protamine. The patient should be observed for approximately 12–24 hours. Once the postoperative chest tube drainage has decreased to <75 cc/hr for 3 consecutive hours, low-molecular-weight dextran is started at 25 cc/hr. As along as the flows are maintained above 4L/min, the patient is maintained on a regimen of dextran for 5–7 postoperative days or until weaning is initiated. At this time a continuous infusion of heparin is initiated to maintain the ACT between 175–200 seconds. During weaning, heparin dosage is increased in proportion with decreases in device flow. For bridge-to-transplant patients, the early postoperative anticoagulant regimen is similar to that for postcardiotomy patients (Table 3). After device placement under full systemic heparinization, the heparin is reversed with protamine. Once it is established that no significant bleeding has occurred, low-molecular-weight dextran is initiated at 25 cc/hr. The patient is maintained on dextran alone for 5–7 days or until hemostatic variables (partial thromboplastin

TABLE 3.   Anticoagulant Protocol (St. Louis University) for Bridge to Transplant

Implant using full heparinization

Dextran at 25 ml/hr
  1. Start when bleeding stops (<75 cc/hr from chest tubes for 3 consecutive hours and PTT, PT <1.6 times control)
  2. Discontinue dextran when heparin started or PT > 1.3 times control

Intravenous heparin
  1. Begin heparin (10 U/kg/hr) on the 5th–7th postoperative day unless the PT is >1.3 times control
  2. Obtain PTT 6 hours after beginning heparin and daily (maintain PTT 1.3–1.5 times control) when only on heparin

Oral anticoagulation
  1. Begin warfarin (PT 1.3–1.5 times control) once the patient is extubated and tolerating oral fluids
  2. Warfarin may be given NG for patients on a ventilator >4 days
  3. Heparin should be started (10 U/kg/hr) for a PT <1.3 times control and discontinued when the PT is ≥ 1.3 times control
  4. Begin aspirin 85 mg/day for patients with elevated PRA levels, patients with symptoms of TIAs, and patients whose duration of support is anticipated to be >30 days.

PTT = partial thromboplastin time; PT = prothrombin time; NG = nasogastric tube; TIA = transient ischemic attack; PRA = panel reactive antibody.

time [PTT], prothrombin time [PT], platelet count, and fibrinogen) have normalized. At this point a continuous infusion of heparin is started to maintain the PTT at 1.3–1.5 times control. The patient may be maintained on intravenous heparin for some period of time or switched to warfarin if able to tolerate oral medications. Once the PT reaches 1.3–1.4 times control, the intravenous heparin is discontinued. The PT is maintained at 1.4–1.5 times control with warfarin. Some investigators add dipyridamole and/or aspirin once hematocrits are stabilized. At St. Louis University we have successfully supported several patients on Thoratec or Novacor VADs with warfarin alone. However, because of the continued increase in average duration of support and several recent experiences with transient ischemic attacks in patients maintained only on warfarin, we have now added aspirin (80 mg/day) to our long-term anticoagulant regimen (Table 3).

VADs with textured surfaces, such as the Thermocardiosystems ventricular assist system (VAS), are designed to be used with little or no anticoagulation.[11] The unique feature of this VAS is a textured rather than a smooth blood contacting surface, which promotes the development of a viable biologic lining. Patients have been successfully supported with this device for up to 321 days on dipyridamole and/or aspirin.

We have developed anticoagulant protocols specific to the different devices used at our university. The anticoagulant regimen described above for pneumatic pulsatile VADs is the same protocol used for the Novacor LVAS (Table 3). For the most part, we have found warfarin to be easy to regulate, especially after 30 days of support. On occasions the PT has fallen to <1.3 times control despite close regulation of the warfarin. In these cases, we start an intravenous infusion of heparin at 10 U/kg/hr and maintain this dosage until we are able to increase the PT to >1.3 times control by increasing the warfarin. This continuous low dose of heparin has proved to be effective and requires no regulation.

Our anticoagulant protocols have evolved as the result of improved experience, better devices, and the need to support patients for longer durations. Our early patients were supported for short durations and for the most part were anticoagulated with intravenous heparin. Nonetheless, a fair number of thromboembolic events occurred, often related to device design or mechanical obstructions to flow that resulted in thrombus formation. In the mid 1980s, with use of mechanical support as a bridge to transplantation, came the necessity of supporting patients for extended periods. To reduce infectious complications, we attempted to remove all intravenous catheters, thus eliminating the possibility of using intravenous heparin as a long-term anticoagulant. In addition, we had frequent problems with regulating heparin over extended periods of time. For these reasons, we developed an oral anticoagulant protocol centered on warfarin. We have found this regimen to be extremely useful in patients with pneumatic and electrical pulsatile VADs. Patients supported with pneumatic TAHs have also been successfully maintained with similar oral regimens. Oral warfarin seemed effective in patients supported for <30 days. However, several of our patients supported >30 days have experienced transient ischemic attacks (TIAs). TIAs were initially treated with intravenous boluses of heparin followed by heparin infusion for 24 hours and the addition of aspirin (325 mg/day). Our protocol has now been modified with the addition of aspirin (80 mg/day) to warfarin in patients with stable hematocrits and no bleeding complications who have been supported for 4 weeks.

CLINICAL RESULTS AT ST. LOUIS UNIVERSITY

Postcardiotomy Shock

Since 1981, 42 patients have been supported with a Thoratec VAD at St. Louis University after cardiac procedures. All patients were maintained on intravenous regimens.[14] The anticoagulant protocol previously described for postcardiotomy patients with pneumatic VADs was followed in this group (Table 2). Seventeen patients received both dextran and heparin. Seven patients received dextran only; 3 received heparin only; and 15 patients received no antiplatelet or anticoagulant drugs. Nine of these 15 patients died in the operating room. In 5 patients thrombus was identified in the device at removal. Only 1 of these 5 patients suffered a thromboembolus. Within the VADs of 3 additional patients with thromboembolus, no thrombus was found. Thomboembolism was confirmed by computed tomography and/or postmortem examination. Of the 4 patients with thromboemboli (Table 4), 3 received both heparin and dextran during the interval of support and 1 received nothing. Two of the 4 patients had concurrent septic complications. Univariant analysis comparing 23 factors, such as age, type of support (LVAD, RVAD, BVAD), VAD flows, PT, PTT, fibrinogen, platelet count,

TABLE 4.   Patients with Thromboemboli—Postcardiotomy Shock (St. Louis University)
(n = 4)

Patient No.	Type of Support	Duration of Support (days)	Thrombi in VAD	Location of Emboli	Possible Cause	Survived
2	LVAD(T)	5.5	No	Cerebral	Unknown	No
3	BVAD(T)	3.5	No	Cerebral	Decreased flow (weaning)	Yes
4	LVAD(T)	12.0	No	Cerebral	Sepsis	No
9	BVAD(T)	12.0	No	Coronary arteries	Sepsis	No

VAD = ventricular assist device; LVAD = left ventricular assist device; BVAD = biventricular assist device; T = Thoratec.

TABLE 5.   Bridge to Transplantation—St. Louis University (n = 44)

Antithrombotic Regimen	No. of Patients	Duration of Support (days)	Thrombi in Pump	TE	TIA	Tx	Weaned	Sur
Nothing	6	2.2 (0.125–5)	1	1	0	2	0	2
Dextran only	4	3.1 (2.2–4)	0	1	0	2	0	2
Heparin only	2	14.2 (6.5–22)	1	1	0	1	0	1
Heparin + dextran	4	15.2 (2–30)	0	0	0	0	0	0
Warfarin	14	29 (6–89)	3	1	2	10	2	11
Warfarin + dipyridamole	7	49.4(12–87)	2	1	0	6	0	6
Warfarin + aspirin	4	55 (24–95)	0	0	0	2	1	3
Warfarin + dipyridamole + aspirin	3	300 (91–440)	1	0	1	3	0	2
Total	44	48 (0.2–440)	8	5	3	26	3	27

TE = thromboemboli; TIA = transient ischemic attack; TX = transplantation; Sur = survived.

number of days on dextran, and number of days on heparin, showed no significant difference between patients with thromboembolism and those without. Two of the 4 patients with thromboemboli survived. In this small group we have been unable to identify predictors for the development of thromboemboli.

Bridge to Cardiac Transplantation

Devices have been inserted in 44 patients as a bridge to cardiac transplantation at St. Louis University. The anticoagulant regimens for this population have undergone considerable evolution because of the increasing durations of support. The anticoagulant regimens and results are summarized in Table 5. Eight patients had thrombus located within the device at the time of explant, but only 2 of the 8 suffered a thromboembolus. In 3 additional patients with thromboemboli, however, no thrombus was found in the device at the time of explant (Table 6).

TABLE 6.   Patients with Thromboemboli—Bridge to Transplant (St. Louis University) (n = 5)

Pt. No.	Type of Support	Duration of Support (days)	Thrombi in VAD	Location of Emboli	Possible Cause	Survived
61	BVAD(T)	6.5	No	Cerebral, renal, pulmonary	Fungal sepsis	No
55	BVAD(T)	27	Yes	Renal, cerebral	Stopped anticoagulation due to bleeding	No
48	LVAD(T)	24	Yes	Cerebral	Mechanical failure	Yes
60	BVAD(T)	4	No	Cerebral	Embolus from LV during VAD insertion	No
11	LVAD(N)	87	No	Cerebral	Unknown	No

VAD = ventricular assist device; LVAD = left ventricular assist device; BVAD = biventricular assist device; T = Thoratec; N =Novacor.

DISCUSSION

The level of anticoagulation maintained often has a significant influence on the patient's clinical course. Antithrombotic protocols are still evolving. Thromboembolic events remain random and unpredictable, even in patients believed to be adequately anticoagulated. This may be due to alterations in hemorrheology, embolization from another source (native ventricle), or sepsis.[6,8,12] It has yet to be demonstrated if one type of device is more thrombogenic than another. For example, it is unknown whether devices with mechanical valves are more prone to thromboembolism than devices with bioprosthetic valves. The lack of uniformity among the anticoagulant protocols of individual investigators makes it difficult to evaluate the available results. Other factors, such as the type of cannulation (left atrial or left ventricular), mode of device operation, and minimal acceptable flows, have significant potential to affect the development of thrombus within a device. Some of the thrombi that form within mechanical circulatory support devices apparently result from disruption of normal flow.[18] It is also apparent that the formation of a thrombus within a device does not necessarily correlate with embolization. On the other hand, it is not unusual to find a device clean of thrombi at removal in patients who suffered thromboembolic events. These results raise several possible theories: (1) The artificial surfaces of the device are never pacified, resulting in intermittent platelet activation, accumulation, and embolization. This random blood/surface interaction would be triggered by some yet unknown factor. (2) The surface of the device is pacified, but thrombus formation and embolization result from factors such as infection and reduction or interruption of normal flow. (3) Despite passivation, embolization will occur if a certain level of anticoagulation is not maintained.

For the most part, preclinical animal studies to evaluate currently available VADs used little if any anticoagulant or platelet-deaggregating drugs. The results of animal studies usually showed little if any thrombus formation within the device and a low instance of documented thromboemboli. When clinical trials were started, most investigators felt the need to give antiplatelet or anticoagulant drugs until device safety could be demonstrated clinically. Unfortunately, as clinical trials progressed, it became apparent that the information gained from the animal studies did not directly correlate with the early clinical experience. For these reasons, most devices in clinical trials use considerably more anticoagulant and/or antiplatelet drugs than were used in the animal experiments.

Thromboembolism remains a real and constant threat to any patient undergoing mechanical circulatory support. The best results to date are from the Thermocardiosystems VAS clinical trial, probably because of the device's neobiologic surface. It remains difficult to relate the frequency of thromboembolism to the various types of devices. Thromboembolism rarely occurs within the first 3 days unless the normal flow pattern is disrupted. Data from the ASAIO-ISHLT Registry show that the risk of thromboembolism increases with the duration of support (Table 7). Clinical data clearly show that all current devices are associated with some risk of thromboembolism. Therefore, anticoagulant and/or antiplatelet therapy is advised for all patients who require assistance for more than a few days.

TABLE 7.   Duration of Support vs. Thromboembolus in Bridge to Transplant*
(VADs Only—All Types)

Duration	<30 Days		30–60 Days		>60 Days	
	Alive (n = 111)	Dead (n = 166)	Alive (n = 26)	Dead (n = 11)	Alive (n = 30)	Dead (n = 12)
Embolus	3%	10%	8%	27%	17%	50%
Total incidence	7%		13%		27%	

* ASAIO-ISHLT Registry.

REFERENCES

1. Anderson JM, Kottke-Marchant K: Platelet interactions with biomaterials and artificial devices. CRC Crit Rev Biocompatibility 1:111, 1985.
2. Bernhard WF, Poirier V, LaFarge CG, Carr JG: A new method for temporary left ventricular bypass: Preclinical appraisal. J Thorac Cardiovasc Surg 70:880, 1975.
3. Boralessa H, Shifferli JA, Zaime F, et al: Perioperative changes in complement associated with cardiopulmonary bypass. Br J Anaesth 54:1047, 1982.
4. Boretos JW, Pierce WS: Segmented polyurethane: A new elastomer for biomedical applications. Science 158:1481, 1967.
5. Chenoweth DE: Complement activation produced by biomaterials. ASAIO Trans 32:226, 1986.
6. Didisheim P, Olsen DB, Farrar DJ, et al: Infections and thromboembolism with implantable cardiovascular devices. ASAIO Trans 35:54, 1989.
7. Gibbon JH Jr: Artificial maintenance of circulation during experimental occlusion of the pulmonary artery. Arch Surg 34:1115, 1937.
8. Hung TC, Borovetz HS, Kormos RL, et al: Hemorrheology and transient ischemic attacks. ASAIO Trans 36:132, 1990.
9. Joist JH, Pennington DG: Platelet reactions with artificial surfaces. ASAIO Trans 33:341, 1987.
10. Matsuda T, Iwata H: Mechanistic aspects of in vivo antithrombogenicity of segmented polyurethane. In Akutsu T (ed): Artificial Heart 1. Berlin, Springer Verlag, 1986, pp 11–22.
11. McGee MC, Parnis SM, Nakatani T, et al: Extended clinical support with an implantable left ventricular assist device. ASAIO Trans 35:614, 1989.
12. Nakatani T, Noda H, Beppu S, et al: Thrombus in a natural left ventricle during left ventricular assist: Another thromboembolic risk. ASAIO Trans 36:711, 1990.
13. Norman JC: Intracorporeal partial artificial hearts: Initial results in ten patients. Artif Organs 1:41, 1977.
14. Pennington DG, McBride LR, Swartz MT, et al: Use of the Pierce-Donachy ventricular assist device in patients with cardiogenic shock after cardiac operations. Ann Thorac Surg 47:130, 1989.
15. Pierce WS, Brighton JA, O'Bannon W, et al: Complete left ventricular bypass with paracorporeal pump: Design and evaluation. Ann Surg 180:418, 1974.
16. Salzman EW, Merrill EW: Interaction of blood with artificial surfaces. In Colman RW, Hirsh J, Marder VJ, Salzman EW (eds): Hemostasis and Thrombosis. Philadelphia, J.B. Lippincott, 1987, p 1335.
17. Szukalski EA, Reedy JE, Pennington DG, et al: Oral anticoagulation in patients with ventricular assist devices. ASAIO Trans 36:M700, 1990.
18. Termuhlen DF, Swartz MT, Pennington DG, et al: Thromboembolic complications with the Pierce-Donachy ventricular assist device. ASAIO Trans 35:616, 1989.
19. Turitto T, Baumgartner HR: Platelet-surface interactions. In Colman RW, Hirsh J, Marder VJ, Salzman EW (eds): Hemostasis and Thrombosis. Philadelphia, J.B. Lippincott, 1987, p 555.

BILL B. DAILY, MD, PhD
WILLIAM S. PIERCE, MD

MANAGEMENT OF SECONDARY ORGAN DYSFUNCTION

Bill B. Daily, MD, PhD
Assistant Professor of Surgery
Division of Cardiothoracic Surgery
Washington University School
 of Medicine
The Jewish Hospital of St. Louis
St. Louis, Missouri

William S. Pierce, MD
Evan Pugh Professor and Chief
Division of Cardiothoracic Surgery
The Pennsylvania State University
 College of Medicine
The Milton S. Hershey Medical
 Center
Hershey, Pennsylvania

Reprint requests to:
Bill B. Daily, MD, PhD
Division of Cardiothoracic Surgery
Washington University School
 of Medicine
216 S. Kingshighway Blvd.
St. Louis, MO 63110

As our knowledge of pathophysiology grows and our technology improves, our ability to care for the critically ill improves. With each advance, we learn about new problems that limit patient survival. Initially, these problems are often poorly understood; definitions are descriptive (syndromes) rather than mechanistic (pathophysiology). Patient management is empirical, and treatments are often supportive rather than specific. These treatments are ineffective in many cases. Until scientific research yields specific solutions, we can only emphasize prevention. For this reason we emphasize prevention in the management of secondary organ dysfunction in patients who require ventricular assistance.

THE ORIGIN OF COMPLICATIONS ASSOCIATED WITH MECHANICAL VENTRICULAR ASSISTANCE

Data from the Combined Registry for the clinical use of mechanical ventricular assist devices (VADs), 1985–1990, show that 80% of patients who undergo VAD implantation suffer at least one serious complication. Table 1 lists these complications in order of decreasing frequency.

To improve patient care, we try to minimize complications by studying why they occur. The cause of a particular complication may be easily identified, or it may be entirely obscure. In the field of ventricular assistance, investigators have long recognized that some complications result directly from device flaws; e.g., thromboembolism (TE) from crevices between device components. Other complications may be due to errors in

CARDIAC SURGERY: State of the Art Reviews—Vol. 7, No. 2, 1993
Philadelphia, Hanley & Belfus, Inc.

399

TABLE 1. Complications in Ventricular Assist Patients*

Complication	Incidence (%)[†]
Bleeding	41.9
Renal failure	30.1
Biventricular failure	22.7
Respiratory failure	16.4
Infection	14.9
Inadequate cardiac output	11.7
Neurologic—not embolic	10.9
Embolus	7.9
Perioperative myocardial infarction	7.7
Hemolysis	7.3
Disseminated intravascular coagulation	7.0
Thrombus	5.6
Cannula obstruction	2.4
Mechanical failure	1.9
Cyanosis	1.5
Patent foramen ovale	1.0

* Data taken from the Combined Registry for the Clinical Use of Mechanical Ventricular Assist Devices.
[†] The number of patients is 1,195.

surgical technique, such as massive anastomotic bleeding from failure to tie a knot properly. Still other complications, such as multiorgan failure, are probably best attributed to severe antecedent cardiogenic shock and the critical nature of the patient's illness.

Often complications are caused by many contributing factors. In these cases, precise cause-and-effect relationships are difficult to specify. Nevertheless, it is important to identify and investigate all of the contributing factors. Only then can we determine which factors can be eliminated and whether such elimination will resolve the complication. For this reason we view direct and indirect device-related complications as separate categories.

Direct Device-related Complications

Direct device-related complications such as mechanical failure, hemolysis, or thromboembolism are now relatively infrequent. The blood-handling characteristics of the centrifugal pumps and pulsatile VADs available today are generally quite good. In the early postoperative period, hemolysis depends strongly on the events leading to VAD insertion. In a recent review, Richenbacher and Pierce[27] found that for a spectrum of devices, plasma hemoglobin levels were rarely more than 100 mg/dl and generally about 10 mg/dl. Hemolysis can be reduced by minimizing cardiopulmonary bypass (CPB) time and the use of cardiotomy suckers, by avoiding long-term cardiac support with a roller pump, and by limiting pump flows to 2.5 L/min/m² body surface area. When pulsatile pneumatic systems are used, hemolysis can often be decreased further by lowering the systolic air pressure and increasing the systolic duration to empty the pump. Reducing hemolysis is particularly important in patients with renal or hepatic insufficiency.

Although the incidence of major complications from systemic emboli remains low, the threat of thromboembolism looms for each device. Available data for individual devices are limited and uncontrolled with respect to several key variables, making direct comparisons difficult. These data, nonetheless, give us some sense of the relative importance of the problem. TE, usually manifested by focal, primarily transient neurologic symptoms, has been documented for 11/154 (8%) patients with the Thoratec device[6] and 7/68 (10%) patients with the Novacor device.[16] Furthermore, explanted devices have sometimes contained thrombus in the blood chamber, on the valves, or in the cannulae.[23,29] The recorded incidence of thromboembolism—2/60 (3%)—is somewhat lower for the Thermo Cardiosystems Inc. (TCI) pneumatic LVAD, but fewer patients have been studied.[5]

Current recommendations for anticoagulation vary for each device. Studies are ongoing to determine the effectiveness of these recommendations.

Indirect Device-related and Surgical Complications

By definition, the ideal VAD would be implanted in an appropriately selected patient with standard surgical technique and would itself never cause a complication. If a complication occurs that cannot be attributed directly to the device, to deviations from standard surgical technique, or to patient-related causes, then we consider it an indirect device-related complication. Such complications are often improperly classified. Although commonly attributed to surgical technique, they are frequently due as much to the incompatibility of current device design and biomaterials with human anatomy and living tissues. For this reason, many surgeons consider the devices "user unfriendly." For example, the mechanical properties of most biomaterials are quite different from those of living tissue. Cannulae are often relatively stiff, resisting both shearing and bending. Slight malposition of such a cannula can generate forces and torques that are transmitted to compliant tissue, resulting in distortion of the tissue and stresses at the suture line. Cannula obstruction and bleeding, especially with high dP/dt pulsatile flow, are then more likely.

In addition to mechanical incompatibilities, the barrier properties of biomaterials predispose to infection. Most biomaterials currently in use resist vascular ingrowth and cellular movement. Some materials even provoke activation of leukocytes.[5a] This creates a macroscopic interface between material and tissue that contains at least some fluid and does not support normal immune function. Infections are practically impossible to eradicate without removal of the foreign material.

The incompatibility of biomaterials and living tissue magnifies other problems. For instance, superficial wound infections that might easily be managed under other circumstances can lead to catastrophe. Accordingly, while we await fundamental breakthroughs in device design and biomaterials research, we must maintain a low tolerance for complications in using the current generation of assist devices.

Patient-related Complications

Notwithstanding direct and indirect device-related complications, the majority of complications in patients undergoing VAD insertion are due to preexisting conditions associated with the patient's critical illness. Patients who require a VAD after cardiotomy have often undergone a prolonged period of CPB. This period usually includes intervals of low cardiac output and high venous pressures during weaning attempts. Multiple blood transfusions, vasoconstrictive drugs, and hypothermia contribute to poor tissue perfusion, leaky capillaries, coagulopathy, and immune dysfunction. Underlying chronic disease that limits the functional reserve of individual organs exacerbates the organ dysfunction that results from the acute global insults listed above.

Patients who require VAD insertion as a bridge to transplantation frequently suffer the side effects of chronic congestive heart failure (CHF), which may include pulmonary, hepatic, and renal dysfunction from marginal cardiac output and high venous pressures. Prolonged inactivity, reduced appetite, and altered gastrointestinal function can contribute to malnutrition with poor wound healing, coagulopathy, and reduced immunocompetence. Drugs sometimes used in the management of endstage heart disease may also have deleterious side effects. The most notable examples are amiodarone, which predisposes some patients to adult respiratory distress syndrome (ARDS),[12,18] and broad-spectrum antibiotics, used to treat suspected nosocomial infections, which predispose to colonization with resistant microorganisms.

ASSESSMENT OF ORGAN DYSFUNCTION

The assessment of organ dysfunction in a VAD patient is the same as in any critically ill patient. Table 2 lists the commonly accepted parameters of organ dysfunction with associated etiologies and pathology.

The development of organ dysfunction is a key determinant of prognosis in any critical illness. In establishing prognosis, the current methods of assessing organ dysfunction are seriously deficient. Except in the extremes, single parameter values do not consistently correlate with outcome. More data and perhaps new parameters are needed before we can rely heavily on these measures to make individual clinical determinations.

Before granting an investigational device exemption (IDE), the FDA requires each VAD manufacturer to establish exclusion criteria. These criteria include indicators of secondary organ dysfunction, such as creatinine >5.0 mg/dl or bilirubin >10.0 mg/dl. These criteria, however, are means to establish protocols, not means to predict individual outcomes or to establish future practice limitations. In our opinion, the decision to implant a VAD in a patient with secondary organ dysfunction must ultimately depend on the judgment of the surgeon and the wishes of the patient.

PREVENTION OF ORGAN DYSFUNCTION

The goal of VAD implantation is to prevent irreversible secondary organ damage while the natural heart recovers or until a donor heart is located. Success depends on appropriate patient selection and early implantation of a VAD system that can provide consistent, adequate cardiac output with acceptable filling pressures (central venous pressure [CVP] and left atrial pressure [LAP] <15 mmHg). Keeping the MAP-CVP >40 mmHg helps to ensure adequate tissue perfusion. These devices can sustain the living; they cannot resurrect the dead.

Patient Selection

Because the majority of complications are patient-related, the single most important issue in preventing organ dysfunction is proper patient selection. Until recently, the need for ventricular support has been based solely on established hemodynamic criteria that define cardiogenic shock. This assumes optimal medical management and no corrective surgical options. Experience, especially with chronically ill bridge patients, has highlighted the need to expand these entrance criteria. We need to include indications based on the natural history of a particular disease process or on an estimation of the patient's physiologic reserve.

TABLE 2. Assessment of Organ Function

Organ System	Indicators of Dysfunction	Associated Etiologies	Pathology
Respiratory	↑ A-aO$_2$ gradient ↓ Pulmonary compliance (ARDS)	↓ CO, postoperative effects, CPB Sepsis,* aspiration	Alveolar epithelial and capillary endothelial damage Interstitial and alveolar exudate
Cardiac	Persistent ↓ CO	RV failure (improper device selection) Cannula obstruction Tamponade	Myocardial infarction Cardiomyopathy
Vascular	Edema (↑ capillary permeability)	↓ CO, CPB, sepsis	Capillary damage
Renal	↓ Creatinine clearance (↓ GFR) Altered fluid and electrolyte metabolism	↓ CO Altered paracrine and endocrine function	Acute tubular necrosis
Gastrointestinal			
Hepatobiliary	↑ Transaminases ↑ Bilirubin (↓ excretory function) ↑ PT ↓ Albumin (↓ synthetic function)	↑ CVP, ↓ CO, sepsis	Centrilobular congestion Hepatocellular necrosis
Intestinal	Ileus	↓ CO, sepsis, fluid and electrolyte abnormalities	
Hematologic/Immune			
Erythrocyte	Anemia (Hct 25–30%)	↓ CO, sepsis hemolysis	↓ RBC production in bone marrow Schistocytes, RBC fragments
Leukocyte	↑ or ↓ WBC Anergy ↑ Susceptibility to infection	↑ CO, sepsis	
Platelet and serum coagulation cascade	Coagulopathy (DIC)	CPB, sepsis	
Neurologic	Mental status changes, CVA	↓ CO, emboli, sepsis	Infarction (watershed or vascular distribution)

A-a = alveolar-arterial, ARDS = adult respiratory distress syndrome, CO = cardiac output, CPB = cardiopulmonary bypass, RV = right ventricle, GFR = glomerular filtration rate, PT = prothrombin time, Hct = hematocrit, RBC = red blood cell, WBC = white blood cell, DIC = disseminated intravascular coagulation, CVA = cerebrovascular accident.
* Sepsis is defined as the physiologic response of an immunocompetent host to bloodstream invasion by microorganisms; e.g., fever, hypermetabolism, leukocytosis.

For example, hemodynamic stability at the expense of high-dose inotropes or an IABP should not be a contraindication to VAD implantation. Our goal is to prevent sudden death and irreversible damage to vital organs. We need more data to determine the optimal time for VAD placement.

It is difficult to agree on exclusion criteria because exclusion means death for nearly 100% of patients. For pulsatile devices, the FDA mandates compliance with criteria established under the manufacturer's IDE. Working within the FDA's framework, investigators have tried to refine these criteria. Pae et al.[20] have analyzed the data submitted to the Combined Registry, 1985–1990. For 272 patients with postcardiotomy cardiogenic shock (PCCS) who were supported with a pulsatile VAD, the following factors were statistically associated with failure to wean from support: renal failure, biventricular failure, cyanosis secondary to shunting through a patent foramen ovale (PFO), and inlet cannula obstruction with inadequate cardiac output. For the 476 bridge patients supported with a VAD or TAH, the following univariate predictors of not receiving a transplant were identified in a group of 148 patients: bleeding, ventricular failure, renal failure, respiratory failure, infection, and multiorgan failure.[19] In both PCCS and bridge groups, older patients (>70 and >60 years, respectively) had lower hospital discharge rates. Unfortunately, many of these risk factors become identifiable only after ventricular assistance has been initiated.

Reedy et al.[26a] emphasize the importance of identifying preoperative predictors of success or failure. Based on a retrospective analysis of 26 bridge patients, they recommend that patients with progressive renal insufficiency or uncontrollable systemic infection, patients whose hemodynamic condition cannot be stabilized with conventional medical therapy within 24 hours, or patients who require intubation for more than 5 days or a high fraction of inspired oxygen (>0.7) should not be accepted for bridging to transplantation.

How to use this information to make individual clinical decisions is the real question: Which factors indicate irreversible damage, and which will respond to improvements in patient management techniques? Fifteen years ago, the mortality of pancreatitis associated with 6 positive Ranson's criteria was nearly 100%.[25] Today, many of these patients survive.[26] At this time, there are too many uncertainties to expect a consensus. The potential for organ recovery during ventricular assistance is debated (see below). These issues cannot be resolved on the basis of available data.

Intensive Care: Hemodynamic, Metabolic, and Immunologic Support

Intensive care unit (ICU) practices reflect current knowledge and assumptions about the prevention of multiorgan failure (MOF). The principles of current practice include the maintenance of tissue oxygenation, reversal of net catabolism and provision of adequate nutrition, and the prevention and aggressive treatment of infection.[15] Applied to VAD patients, these principles translate into the following recommendations:

1. Establish adequate hemodynamic support expeditiously.
   a. Select a device based on the patient's needs, device availability, and the surgeon's experience.
   b. Ensure proper device fit and function before leaving the operating room. As long as the filling pressures suggest adequate intravascular volume, low cardiac output after VAD implantation indicates cannula obstruction or biventricular failure. Neither of these conditions is likely to resolve in the ICU.[24]
   c. Evaluate the interatrial septum, either by visual inspection or palpation. To prevent interatrial shunting, close any defect identified, including a patent foramen ovale.[14]
2. Ensure hemostasis before leaving the operating room.[11]
3. Reduce pharmacologic hemodynamic support as soon as possible.
4. Optimize fluid and electrolyte balance.

5. Minimize the risk of infection. Remove indwelling tubes, lines, and catheters as soon as possible. Maintain diligent care of all wounds and percutaneous tube sites. Suspect sepsis in cases of unexplained organ dysfunction, mental status changes, or rising bilirubin. Monitor for infection and focus treatment. Avoid prolonged use of broad-spectrum antibiotics.
6. Assess nutritional status and provide adequate nutritional therapy via the least invasive route available.
7. Institute anticoagulation as recommended for a particular device to reduce the risk of thromboembolism.
8. Institute serial monitoring of organ system function to determine improvement or deterioration.

MANAGEMENT OF ORGAN DYSFUNCTION

Pulmonary Dysfunction

A wide spectrum of pulmonary dysfunction is encountered in patients undergoing VAD placement. A few bridge-to-transplant patients may develop only mild insufficiency characterized by mild transient hypoxemia (arterial $pO_2 < 60$ torr with the fraction of inspired oxygen [FiO_2] 21% in room air). This may be attributed to preexistent chronic lung disease, traditional postoperative complications such as atelectasis, the pulmonary effects of CPB and hypothermia, and the effects of volume overload and poor left ventricular function. With judicious use of diuretics, improvement in fluid and electrolyte balance is often demonstrable within 24–48 hours after VAD placement. Extubation frequently follows shortly thereafter. Improvement in the appearance of the chest x-ray may lag several days.

Many patients manifest moderate pulmonary insufficiency characterized by more severe and lasting hypoxemia ($0.21 < FiO_2 < 0.50$ with positive end-expiratory pressures [PEEP] <10 cm H_2O to keep arterial $pO_2 > 60$ torr) and a modest reduction in pulmonary compliance. In addition to the etiologies described above, pulmonary dysfunction may result from preoperative mechanical ventilation (oxygen toxicity, barotrauma, or loss of respiratory muscle strength); preoperative use of amiodarone; a period of shock, especially when associated with multiple blood transfusions; sepsis, or pulmonary infection; and aspiration of gastric contents. These patients require a longer period of mechanical ventilation. The FiO_2 and peak airway pressures should be minimized to reduce ongoing lung injury. Fluid and electrolyte balance is more difficult to achieve. Metabolic and immunologic support is required to reverse catabolism, to treat infections and malnutrition, and to permit tissue repair. If other complications can be avoided or successfully managed during this period, pulmonary function may gradually improve.

A limited number of patients undergoing VAD placement develop severe ARDS and respiratory failure, which clinically are characterized by (1) hypoxemia and hypoventilation that do not readily respond to increases in inspired oxygen concentration or minute ventilation; (2) a progressive decrease in pulmonary compliance requiring increasing mean airway pressures; and (3) a chest x-ray showing diffuse bilateral interstitial infiltrates, commonly recognized by their "ground glass" appearance. Pathologically, this severe form of ARDS is characterized by alveolar destruction with hyaline deposition and irreversible pulmonary fibrosis. Despite maximal care, oxygen requirements and pulmonary pressures may continue to rise, often in association with evolving multiorgan dysfunction. This syndrome carries a very high mortality.[8]

Extracorporeal membrane oxygenation (ECMO) has been used in a few cases to sustain LVAD patients with pulmonary insufficiency and right heart failure.[13] Although an occasional patient may survive, the overall mortality, based on the results of previous trials using ECMO to treat PCCS, ARDS, or MOF,[2] is high.

Cardiac Dysfunction

BIVENTRICULAR FAILURE

Failure of the contralateral ventricle in patients receiving univentricular support has been a frequently reported cause of morbidity and mortality in both postcardiotomy[21] and bridge-to-transplant[19] groups. Hemodynamic criteria are the most useful in determining the type of support needed. Generally, the atrium with the higher pressure indicates the ventricle with predominant failure. In practice, because severe left ventricular dysfunction is present in most VAD candidates, most surgeons establish left ventricular (LV) support and then assess right ventricular (RV) function. Prior to LVAD insertion, it is impossible to predict which patients will require biventricular support,[13] except perhaps patients with a right atrial pressure >20 mmHg.[23] Even after LVAD insertion, it may be difficult to determine the need for biventricular support. Failure of the CVP to fall significantly (e.g., to below 15 mmHg) and the need for increasing RV inotropic support may suggest the need for biventricular support.[13]

In cases of uncertainty, we believe biventricular support is preferable. All of these patients are critically ill, and many have suffered severe physiologic insults prior to ventricular assistance. Postoperative care is often complicated by bleeding, cardiac tamponade, arrhythmias, fluid shifts, multiorgan dysfunction, and occasionally inaccurate hemodynamic measurements. The need for intravenous antiarrhythmic drugs (almost all are negative inotropes) and high-dose inotropic support only worsens the situation. Device-related complications are relatively uncommon, and the additional theoretical risk of a second device is probably small.[23] Failure to recognize and treat biventricular failure early significantly lowers the survival rate in postcardiotomy[22] and bridge[5,19] patients.

ARRHYTHMIAS

Two recent reports suggest that the incidence of ventricular arrhythmias (VA) following VAD insertion ranges from 44% in bridge patients with ischemic heart disease[1] to about 30% in recovery patients.[17] In the bridge group, VAD insertion significantly reduced the incidence of VA, and in both groups it greatly simplified the management of VA. During periods of arrhythmia, including sustained ventricular tachycardia or ventricular fibrillation, only minimal hemodynamic deterioration was noted. Standard medical therapy was frequently used to reduce ectopy. The development of VA during VAD support did not increase mortality risk in either group.

Hematologic Dysfunction: Coagulopathy (Bleeding)

Bleeding is the most frequently reported complication in many series of VAD implantation.[13,16,28] The detrimental effects of massive transfusion and cardiac tamponade are important causes of morbidity and mortality in VAD patients. Despite widespread recognition and the best efforts of experienced surgeons, bleeding continues to be be a common and serious problem.

To achieve hemostatic atrial cannulation, we use two concentric pursestrings. Felt pledgets are placed at each external passage of the outer pursestring. We use deep, felted mattress sutures to secure an apical ventricular cannula. This compresses adjacent myocardium against the felt collar of the cannula. Positioning the cannula in the center of the ventricle is crucial to achieve unobstructed inflow. Dacron arterial conduits must be preclotted. Albumin curing of detachable grafts (25% albumin rinse followed by 3 minutes in the autoclave at 270° F) or treatment with cryoprecipitate, activated thrombin, and platelets is effective.[13,16]

VAD candidates with severe, chronic congestive heart failure may have limited hemostatic reserve. Baseline coagulation studies (prothrombin time, partial thromboplastin time, platelet count, bleeding time) may not accurately detect increased tissue fragility and impaired hepatic and bone-marrow function. When coupled with shock, bacteremia, anesthesia, surgery with cardiopulmonary bypass, and massive transfusion, this limited hemostatic reserve often results in coagulopathy. Thrombocytopenia, altered platelet aggregation, reduced soluble coagulation factors, fibrinolysis, and disseminated intravascular coagulation have been documented.

To reduce the severity of the coagulopathy often encountered in these patients, we attempt to minimize preoperative delays and time spent on CPB. A well-defined protocol for the management of patients in cardiogenic shock expedites decision-making and sets standards that can be evaluated and improved. On termination of CPB, heparin is fully reversed with protamine, and the activated clotting time is serially monitored for several hours. In high-risk patients, we administer fresh frozen plasma and platelets liberally. We add cryoprecipitate if fibrinogen levels are low. We often use topical agents, such as fibrin glue, Surgicel, or powdered Gelfoam, but these probably play a limited role. The use of increased PEEP may also be helpful once the chest is closed. Most important, however, is to control bleeding in the operating room.

Recently, several new approaches to reduce blood loss in patients undergoing CPB have been tested. Aprotinin, a serine protein inhibitor, reduces bleeding after coronary artery bypass grafting by approximately 50%.[3,9] Although its exact mechanism of action is not fully understood, reduction in fibrinolysis and attenuation of the normal increase in postoperative bleeding times have been demonstrated. In addition, heparin-bonded surfaces that permit CPB with greatly reduced systemic heparin are undergoing trials in Europe and the U.S.

Fluid and Electrolyte Imbalance, Renal Dysfunction

Profound hypervolemia often complicates the postoperative management of VAD patients. These patients frequently weigh more than 15 kg above their dry weight and have a CVP >15 mmHg. Their renal function is usually inadequate to permit as rapid a diuresis as desirable. Postsurgical neuroendocrine changes and low plasma oncotic pressures contribute to fluid retention. Continuous arteriovenous hemofiltration (CAVH) permits gradual fluid removal and may promote mobilization of third-space fluid without the hemodynamic instability often caused by acute hemodialysis. Ultrafiltration may be initiated intraoperatively with CPB and continued postoperatively with conventional CAVH. A simplified method of hemofiltration, incorporating extracorporeal continuous flow VADs, has also been described.[13a]

The management of renal dysfunction in VAD patients is similar to that in non-VAD patients:

1. Ensure renal perfusion. Maintain an adequate cardiac output; keep the (MAP-CVP) > 40 mmHg and the CVP < 15 mmHg. Patients with renal artery stenosis or hypertensive nephropathy may require an even greater difference. Avoid hypovolemia and minimize the use of alpha adrenergic agents.

2. Optimize fluid and electrolyte balance. Dialysis may be required in cases of severe renal failure.

3. Avoid nephrotoxins (aminoglycosides, intravenous contrast dye, products of hemolysis).

4. Provide metabolic support to enable tissue regeneration.

Conceptually, mechanical ventricular assistance is the ideal means to ensure renal perfusion during heart failure. Practically, however, recovery of renal function in VAD patients that develop renal failure has been limited at best. In 1987 Kanter et al.[11a] published a retrospective analysis of 27 patients with refractory cardiogenic shock who were successfully managed with a Pierce-Donachy VAD. The development of renal dysfunction (blood urea nitrogen [BUN] >30 mg/dl and a creatinine >2.0 mg/dl at any time during hospitalization) was highly predictive of mortality (1 of 12 survivors, 13 of 15 nonsurvivors). Because the renal pathology in these cases was variable and because many patients had evidence of multiorgan dysfunction, the authors concluded that renal failure reflected the severity of the underlying disease. More recent publications from the same institution seem to confirm these findings.[26a,28]

Recent reports describing the initial experience with the TCI pneumatic LVAD offer some promise for partial recovery of renal function in bridge patients who can be stabilized with ventricular assistance. Burnett et al.[4] analyzed the recovery of renal function in a select group of 11 bridge patients supported with pneumatic TCI LVAD for more than 30 days. They report that before transplantation urine volumes normalized in 8/9 oliguric patients and that mean (range) BUN and serum creatinine levels decreased from 59 mg/dl (17–132) to 29 mg/dl (13–90) and from 3.1 mg/dl (1.1–9.3) to 1.5 mg/dl (0.7–1.7), respectively. Two patients remained on hemodialysis. The authors demonstrate that excluding these patients from the analysis only increases the differences between the pre- and postsupport means. Four patients required hemodialysis before VAD implantation. Renal function recovered in 2 of these patients, and hemodialysis was discontinued. In 2 patients, renal failure persisted. One patient died of MOF, and the other underwent successful renal transplantation. These results suggest that in some patients renal function can improve during prolonged LVAD support if support is initiated before multiorgan damage becomes irreversible. How to select patients with reversible organ dysfunction remains the key question.

Hepatic Dysfunction

There is no specific treatment for liver dysfunction in VAD patients. The management principles—ensuring hepatic perfusion, reducing venous congestion, avoiding hepatotoxins—are the same as for other organs.

The majority of VAD candidates show some hepatic dysfunction. Many patients have evidence of hepatocellular injury (↑ transaminases) and reduced excretory function (↑ bilirubin). Some also show impaired synthetic function (↑ prothrombin time [PT], ↓ albumin). Current data are insufficient to determine the prognostic significance of these laboratory findings. Relevant reports are just now beginning to appear. Investigators at the Texas Heart Institute[4,7] have reported improvement in liver function during prolonged LVAD support. Patients with substantial preimplant hepatic dysfunction routinely underwent a transvenous liver biopsy to rule out cirrhosis, a contraindication to LVAD support and cardiac transplantation. In noncirrhotics, elevated preimplant liver function tests (LFTs) frequently normalized before transplantation. Mean values decreased from the time of implantation to explantation as follows: total bilirubin, from 4.4 to 1.6 mg/dl; serum glutamic oxaloacetic transaminase (SGOT), from 1,233 to 52.3 IU/L; serum glutamic pyruvic transaminase (SGPT), from 756 to 70.7 IU/L; and PT, from 13.3 to 12.0 seconds.[14]

Dasse et al.[5] have reported that these patients require an average of about 50 days for normalization of the total bilirubin and SGOT values. Based on their recent experience, Hershon et al.[10] suggest that an elevated PT (in patients not taking Coumadin) may be the most significant indicator of hepatic dysfunction in the evaluation of VAD candidates. They recommend extra caution before proceeding with VAD implantation in patients with even a mildly elevated PT. All of the current information regarding liver dysfunction in VAD patients must be considered preliminary. More experience and data analysis are required to resolve the issue.

Multiorgan Dysfunction and the Gastrointestinal (GI) Tract

Progressive or sequential dysfunction in multiple organ systems indicates systemic illness. Abnormalities in capillary permeability, intermediary metabolism, and immune function have been documented. The pathogenesis of MOF is of intense interest in critical care medicine. Overwhelming infection, hemodynamic instability, major surgery, burns, pancreatitis, and multiple trauma have been identified as events that may trigger the pathophysiology recognized as MOF. Traditionally, this pathophysiology is associated with an overwhelming infection caused by invading microorganisms. Despite multiple cultures, however, invading microorganisms often cannot be isolated in MOF. This has led to a distinction between the concept of infection, a microbiological phenomenon, and sepsis, a host phenomenon representing the physiologic response to exogenous and endogenous mediators of the immune system.[15]

Recently, much research has focused on the role of the immune mediators such as endotoxin, tumor necrosis factor, and interleukin-1 in perpetuating the pathophysiology of MOF. The connections between the triggering event and the release of mediators are largely unknown. Some investigators have postulated an important role for the GI tract.[15] Translocation of pathogenic intestinal flora from the lumen of the GI tract to regional lymph nodes has been seen in animal models. Animal models also suggest that changes in normal gut flora and increases in gut permeability may lead to changes in systemic physiology. Moreover, translocation is promoted by many of the same events that can trigger MOF.

Whether alterations in gut flora and gut permeability predispose critically ill patients to infections or MOF is uncertain. Investigators at the University of Pittsburgh have instituted a regimen of oral antibiotics (gentamicin, colistin, and mycostatin for 2 weeks or until transplantation) to achieve selective bowel decontamination in patients bridged with the Novacor device. Such protocols may help to answer some of these questions.

CONCLUSION

Technologic advances have substantially reduced the incidence of device-related complications, making possible prolonged mechanical ventricular assistance. Further advances should reduce indirect device-related complications by making devices easier to implant and more resistant to infection. Patient-related complications cause the majority of morbidity and mortality in VAD patients. The development of organ failure is a key determinant of prognosis. Prevention of irreversible injury is crucial for success. Prevention depends on appropriate patient selection and early VAD implantation to restore tissue perfusion. These clinical decisions are frequently difficult to make because the point at which irreversible injury occurs is poorly defined in terms of the current means of assessing organ damage. Although the FDA has important regulatory functions, we believe that the decision to implant a VAD in a patient with organ dysfunction must ultimately depend on the judgment of the surgeon and the wishes of the patient.

The assessment and management of organ dysfunction in VAD patients is not substantially different from that in any critically ill patient. The principles of management include maintenance of tissue oxygenation, reversal of net catabolism, provision of adequate nutrition, and aggressive treatment of infection. Available data suggest that prolonged mechanical ventricular assistance can reverse many forms of organ dysfunction. More data and perhaps new parameters are needed to distinguish more clearly between potential survivors and patients who will inevitably develop irreversible MOF.

REFERENCES

1. Arai H, Swartz MT, Pennington DG, et al: Importance of ventricular arrhythmias in bridge patients with ventricular assist devices. ASAIO Trans 37:M427–M428, 1991.
2. Bartlett RH: Extracorporeal life support for cardiopulmonary failure. Curr Probl Surg 27:621–705, 1990.
3. Blauhut B, Gross C, Necek S, et al: Effects of high-dose aprotinin on blood loss, platelet function, fibrinolysis, complement, and renal function after cardiopulmonary bypass. J Thorac Cardiovasc Surg 101:958–967, 1991.
4. Burnett CM, Sweeney MS, Frazier OH, et al: Improved multiorgan function in heart transplant candidates requiring prolonged univentricular support. Presented at the Southern Thoracic Surgical Association Meeting, Orlando, FL, 1991.
5. Dasse KA, Poirier VL, Frazier OH: Current clinical experience with the TCI Heartmate 1000 IP pneumatically driven LVAD. Proceedings of the Science and Technology Conference. Bethesda, MD, The Association for the Advancement of Medical Instrumentation, 1991.
5a. Didisheim P, Olsen DB, Farrar DJ, et al: Infections and thromboembolism with implantable cardiovascular devices. ASAIO Trans 35:54–70, 1989.
6. Farrar DJ: Data presented at the Thoratec Investigators' Meeting, San Francisco, CA, November 15, 1991.
7. Frazier OH, Duncan JM, Radovancevic B, et al: Successful bridge to cardiac transplantation using a new left ventricular assist device. Presented at the 11th Annual Meeting and Scientific Sessions of the International Society for Heart Transplantation, Paris, 1991.
8. Hansen-Flaschen J, Fishman AP: Adult respiratory distress syndrome: Clinical features and pathogenesis. In Fishman AP (ed): Pulmonary Diseases and Disorders, 2nd ed. New York, McGraw Hill, 1988, pp 2201–2214.
9. Havel M, Teufelsbauer H, Knöbl P, et al: Effect of intraoperative aprotinin administration on postoperative bleeding in patients undergoing cardiopulmonary bypass operations. J Thorac Cardiovasc Surg 101:968–972, 1991.
10. Hershon JJ, Hill JD: Data presented at the Second Circulatory Support Meeting, The Society of Thoracic Surgeons. San Francisco, CA, November 16–17, 1991.
11. Hill JD, Hardesty RL, Baumgartner WA, Rose DM: Intraoperative management (panel discussion). Ann Thorac Surg 47:82–87, 1989.
11a. Kanter KR, Swartz MT, Pennington DG, et al: Renal failure in patients with ventricular assist devices. ASAIO Trans 33:426–428, 1987.
12. Kay GN, Epstein AE, Kirlin JK, et al: Fatal postoperative amiodarone pulmonary toxicity. Am J Cardiol 62:490–492, 1988.

13. Kormos RL, Borovetz HS, Gasior T, et al: Experience with univentricular support in mortally ill cardiac transplant candidates. Ann Thorac Surg 49:261–272, 1990.

13a. Macris MP, Barcenas CG, Parnis SM, et al: Simplified method of hemofiltration in ventricular assist device patients. ASAIO Trans 34:708–711, 1988.

14. Magovern JA, Pae WE Jr, Richenbacher WE, et al: The importance of a patent foramen ovale in left ventricular assist pumping. ASAIO Trans 32:449–453, 1986.

15. Marshall JC, Meakins JL: Multiorgan failure. In Wilmore DW (ed): Care of the Surgical Patient, Vol. II. New York, Scientific American, 1989, pp 1–17.

16. McCarthy PM, Portner PM, Tobler HG, et al: Clinical experience with the Novacor ventricular assist system. J Thorac Cardiovasc Surg 102:578–587, 1991.

16a. Miller CA, Pae WE, Pierce WS: Combined registry for the clinical use of mechanical ventricular assist devices. ASAIO Trans 36:43–46, 1990.

17. Moroney DA, Swartz MT, Reedy JE, et al: Importance of ventricular arrhythmias in recovery patients with ventricular assist devices. ASAIO Trans 37:M516–M517, 1991.

18. Nalos PC, Kass RM, Gang ES, et al: Life-threatening postoperative pulmonary complications in patients with previous amiodarone pulmonary toxicity undergoing cardiothoracic operations. J Thorac Cardiovasc Surg 93:904–912, 1987.

19. Oaks TE, Pae WE Jr, Miller CA, et al: Combined Registry for the Clinical Use of Mechanical Ventricular Assist Pumps and the Total Artificial Heart in Conjunction with Heart Transplantation: Fifth Official Report—1990. J Heart Lung Transplant 10:621–625, 1991.

20. Pae WE Jr, Miller CA, Pierce WS: Ventricular assist devices for postcardiotomy cardiogenic shock: A Combined Registry experience. J Thorac Cardiovasc Surg [in press].

21. Pennington DG, McBridge LR, Swartz MT, et al: Use of the Pierce-Donachy ventricular assist device in patients with cardiogenic shock after cardiac operations. J Thorac Cardiovasc Surg 47:130–135, 1989.

22. Pennington DG, Merjavy JP, Swartz MT: The importance of biventricular failure in patients with postoperative cardiogenic shock. Ann Thorac Surg 39:16–26, 1985.

23. Pennington DG, Reedy JE, Swartz MT, et al: Univentricular versus biventricular assist device support. J Heart Lung Transplant 10:258–263, 1991.

24. Pierce WS, Gray LA, McBridge LR, Frazier OH: Other postoperative complications (panel discussion). Ann Thorac Surg 47:96–101, 1989.

25. Ranson JHC, Rifkind KM, Turner JW: Diagnostic signs and nonoperative peritoneal lavage in acute pancreatitis. Surg Gynecol Obstet 143:209–219, 1976.

26. Ranson JHC, Berman RS: Long peritoneal lavage decreases pancreatic sepsis in acute pancreatitis. Ann Surg 211:708–718, 1990.

26a. Reedy JE, Swartz MT, Termuhlen DF, et al: Bridge to heart transplantation: Importance of patient selection. J Heart Transplant 9:473–481, 1990.

27. Richenbacher WE, Pierce WS: Management of complications of mechanical circulatory assistance. In Waldhausen JA, Orringer MR (eds): Complications in Cardiothoracic Surgery. St. Louis, Mosby–Year Book, 1991, pp 103–113.

28. Swartz MT, Pennington DG, McBridge LR, et al: Temporary mechanical circulatory support: Clinical experience with 148 patients. In Unger F (ed): Assisted Circulation III. Berlin, Springer Verlag, pp 132–151, 1989.

29. Wagner WR, Johnson PL, Winowich BS, et al: Evaluation of LVAD inflow and outflow valves and comparison between thromboembolic event and non-event patient groups. Proceedings of the Science and Technology Conference. Bethesda, MD, The Association for the Advancement of Medical Instrumentation, 1991.

AKIHIKO KAWAI, MD
ROBERT L. KORMOS, MD
BARTLEY P. GRIFFITH, MD

MANAGEMENT OF INFECTIONS IN MECHANICAL CIRCULATORY SUPPORT DEVICES

From the University of Pittsburgh
  Medical Center Artificial Heart
  Program
Pittsburgh, Pennsylvania

Reprint requests to:
Robert L. Kormos, MD
University of Pittsburgh Medical
  Center Artificial Heart Program
Room C-700 Presbyterian–
  University Hospital
DeSoto at O'Hara Street
Pittsburgh, PA 15213

Although bleeding (42%), renal failure (31%), and respiratory failure (17%) are complications affecting the early survival of transplant candidates after implantation of a mechanical circulatory assist device, infection is the major limiting factor to the long-term use of artificial organs. A 17–80% incidence of infectious complications has been reported with the use of mechanical circulatory support devices either in the setting of postcardiotomy failure or as a bridge to cardiac transplantation.[1-5] Up to one-quarter of patients receiving such devices were precluded from transplantation as a result of infection.[6]

The incidence of infectious complications varies with the type of device and duration of support. According to the Sixth Annual Report of the Combined Registry (ASAIO-ISHLT) for the Clinical Use of Mechanical Ventricular Assist Pumps and the Total Artificial Heart, 11% of patients in whom a centrifugal ventricular assist device (VAD) was used had an infectious complication during or after the support period, whereas 33% of patients receiving an electric VAD, 20% of patients receiving a pneumatic VAD, and 32% of patients receiving a pneumatic total artificial heart (TAH) developed an infection when the devices were used as a bridge to transplant.[7] Because the duration of support with centrifugal VADs is significantly shorter (average = 5 days) than with other VADs, it seems difficult to conclude that a centrifugal VAD has a lower

CARDIAC SURGERY: State of the Art Reviews—Vol. 7, No. 2, 1993
Philadelphia, Hanley & Belfus, Inc.

413

incidence of infectious complications. Infectious complications were highest in those patients supported >60 days (Table 1). In the postcardiotomy setting, where these devices are used for much shorter durations, the incidence of infection was 13% in 157 patients.

At the University of Pittsburgh, perioperative infection complicating transplantation has been analyzed for all patients, who are grouped according to the degree of pretransport support. The incidence of infection was 29% in patients undergoing elective transplants, 31% in patients supported by inotropic agents, 46% in patients supported by an intraaortic balloon pump (IABP), and 86% in patients bridged primarily with the total artificial heart (TAH).[8]

At the University of Pittsburgh both the TAH and the Novacor left ventricular assist device (LVAD) have been used as a bridge to cardiac transplantation. Between October 1985 and September 1990, 20 patients received the Jarvik-7 TAH, and between July 1987 and April 1992, 31 patients received the Novacor LVAD. Twenty-percent of the TAH-supported patients had an infection before implant compared with 18% of patients supported with an LVAD. During the implant period, 15% of patients bridged with a TAH had an infection, and 100% of these patients died. On the other hand, 27% of the LVAD patients developed an infection during the support period, but the mortality rate was only 14%. Finally, 41% of the TAH patients had an infection after transplantation, and 85% of these patients died. The incidence of infection after transplant in the LVAD patients was 22%, with no deaths. The experience with the TAH has been less severe at other centers,[9] which report only minor infection with an incidence of 42%. However, the average period of support in these patients was only 9 days, and 42% were bridged to transplantation as a result of postcardiotomy failure. In this setting, patients were not subjected to the effects of chronic low-output syndrome in an intensive care unit.

RISK FACTORS

Factors Related to Host Defense Mechanisms

PREIMPLANT FACTORS

Candidates for transplantation who have hemodynamic deterioration to the extent that they become eligible for mechanical support are critically ill and highly susceptible to infection because of possible multisystem organ damage, nonspecific suppression of the immune system, and malnutrition. Even when acute deterioration is immediately and appropriately handled, the patient remains at high risk for

TABLE 1. Complications of Ventricular Support

Complication	Total (%) n = 1582	<30 Days (%) n = 1480	31–60 Days (%) n = 51	>60 Days (%) n = 51
Bleeding	42	42	37	51
Renal Failure	31	30	24	25
Biventricular failure	20	21	10	12
Respiratory failure	17	17	14	12
Infection	17	15	41	47
Tromboemboli	24	13	22	47

infection from pneumonia after intubation, systemic sepsis from intravascular lines and urinary catheters, and contamination of the exteriorized portion of an IABP catheter.

Sepsis syndrome is a possible confounding factor in candidates for mechanical circulatory support. Sepsis syndrome can be defined as a systemic response to infection in the form of tachycardia, fever or hypothermia, tachypnea, and evidence of inadequate organ perfusion or organ dysfunction. The sepsis syndrome does not require the presence of a positive blood culture. Sepsis syndrome accompanied by hypotension unresponsive to fluid therapy is referred to as septic shock.[10] The pathophysiologic mechanisms underlying the cardiovascular dysfunction of septic shock are extremely complex. Microorganisms release large amounts of mediators (endotoxin, exotoxin, and teichoic acid antigens) and activate host reactions (cytokines and complement). These mediators can affect the reactivity of the systemic and pulmonary vasculature, and some substances appear to affect the myocardium directly. In patients with septic shock, the left ventricle shows a depressed ejection fraction associated with left ventricular dilatation. Left ventricular dilatation compensates for the depressed ejection fraction and maintains stroke volume in patients who survive septic shock.[11] On the other hand, an endstage heart usually lacks this compensatory mechanism, and a septiclike picture results in acute deterioration. Although the only salvation for these patients may be implantation of a circulatory assist device, the diagnosis of true bacterial sepsis versus sepsis syndrome often becomes difficult in a patient with borderline end-organ perfusion who is a potential candidate for mechanical support.

IMPLANT FACTORS

Surgical procedures have been known to cause immunologic depression in humans both in vivo and in vitro. They reduce absolute numbers of T-lymphocytes and natural killer cells as well as alter the normal helper/suppressor cell ratios.[12] Furthermore, cardiopulmonary bypass may provoke activation of the complement system, generation of C3a and C5a, sequestration and degranulation of leukocytes, and activation of the fibrinolytic cascade.[13] LVAD implantation results in prolonged exposure of blood to an artificial surface, which activates blood–biomaterial interactions. Patients who underwent TAH implantation demonstrated transient complement activation, lymphopenia, and a progressive decline in the number of peripheral blood helper/inducer T cells.[14] These changes in cellular immune response may lead to decreased immunocompetence during long-term support. T-cell recovery is influenced more by the patient's clinical status than the presence or absence of a device.

Critically ill patients also have a possibility of self-contamination with endogenous bacteria. Low cardiac output may compromise mesenteric blood flow, resulting in translocation of organisms from the gastrointestinal tract to the blood stream. These complications may be enhanced by reduced splanchnic circulation during cardiopulmonary bypass.[15]

The risk of an infectious complication increases according to the severity of illness, duration of stay in an intensive care unit, and extent of preimplant support (Table 2). Analysis of the risk factors for infection in our series of TAH and LVAD patients demonstrated that the peak bilirubin during hospitalization before TAH implant and the bilirubin immediately before implant were higher in patients who ultimately developed an implant infection. In addition, the level of

TABLE 2.   Predictors of Device Infection

	Infection		
Implant	No	Yes	*p*
TAH			
Peak bilirubin (mg/dl)	2.1	6.4	<0.004
Implant bilirubin (mg/dl)	2.1	5.6	<0.02
Mental score (0 = normal, 4 = coma)	1.2	2.7	<0.05
LVAD			
Days on IABP	8	20	<0.004
Transplant			
TAH			
Hospital days	10	23	<0.003
Days on inotropes	9	21	<0.03

mental impairment was more severe in patients who developed an implant infection, thus reflecting the degree of reduced end-organ perfusion. Implant infection in the LVAD patients was related to the length of time they were supported on an IABP before LVAD implant. Patients who developed an implant infection were supported for an average of 20 days on the IABP before implant, whereas those who did not develop an infection were supported for an average of 8 days. After transplantation, infections developed more commonly in TAH patients who had been hospitalized longer and who had been supported for a longer period of time on inotropic agents.

A number of differences between patients receiving an LVAD versus a TAH in our series may influence the incidence of infection. Emergent implantation in the face of evolving multiorgan failure was quite common in the TAH group, whereas now more emphasis is placed on implantation of an LVAD under more controlled circumstances before signs of multiorgan failure have developed. The extramediastinal location of the LVAD reduces the exposure of the mediastinum to a large foreign body and allows for better healing. The dead space produced by the mediastinal location of the TAH not only results in retention of blood clot and fibrin, which provide nutrition and a medium for bacterial growth, but also increases the distance between bacteria and neutrophils. Neutrophils cannot reach the surface of the device unless the tissue bearing the neutrophil is applied directly to the surface. Finally, exposure of neutrophils to polyurethane results in a premature release of superoxide, which renders them incapable of reacting to bacteria at a later point in time.[16]

POSTTRANSPLANT FACTORS

The final risk factor is the immunosuppressive therapy required for heart transplantation. As stated above, the risk of infection in an elective transplant patient is approximately 30%. The use of azathioprine, prednisone, and antilymphocytic therapy have been associated with an increased incidence of infection

Microbial and Device-related Factors

PREIMPLANT FACTORS

Before device implantation, patients spend variable amounts of time in the hospital. With prolonged hospitalization, organisms that latently or endogenously infect or colonize the patient are the most likely agents to produce a clinical infection. In addition, the injudicious use of broad-spectrum antibiotics as prophylaxis for infection in patients with an IABP or invasive monitoring lines results in the selection of opportunistic or resistant strains of colonizing bacteria. *Candida albicans* is often cultured from skin, oral pharynx, and respiratory and urinary tracts in this population.

IMPLANT FACTORS

The infections related to biomaterials are notoriously resistant to antibiotics and host defenses and tend to persist until the biomaterial or foreign body is removed. The organisms seen most frequently in human clinical studies are *Proteus mirabilis, Pseudomonas aeruginosa, Enterobacter cloacae, Mycoplasma hominis, Candida albicans* and *Serratia marcescens.* Many of these same organisms show a predilection for producing infection in animals undergoing TAH support, and many also tend to form affinities to biomaterials.

Biomaterial-centered infections are related to preferential, adhesive, bacterial colonization of inert or inanimate substrata in which the surfaces are not integrated or protected by living cells and intact extracellular polymers.[17] Biomaterials, as well as damaged vascular endothelium, provide a receptive substratum for colonization. Bacteria-biomaterial interaction facilitates bacterial attachment, adhesion, exopolysaccharide production, and biofilm formation.[18,19] The biofilm may provide the ideal conditions for microorganisms and protect them from the effects of circulating antibodies, antibiotics, or phagocytic cells.

Certain plasma proteins affect the adhesion of bacteria on biomaterial surface. Experiments with two bacteria commonly isolated from TAHs explanted from animals demonstrate that bacteria avidly adhere to biomaterial surfaces. Moreover, this bacterial adhesion is influenced by variables of the surface environment. Fibrinogen and fibronectin are important mediators of cellular adhesion, enhancing bacterial adhesion on biomaterial surfaces.[20] On the other hand, the formation of a biologic lining within the pump may help to prevent device-related infections because this tissue lining resists bacterial adhesion and colonization.[5,21]

Prolonged operative time and reexploration due to postoperative bleeding increase the risk of bacterial inoculation and not only jeopardize hemodynamics but also increase the chance of contamination and thus the incidence of infectious complications. As noted above, infectious complications increase with prolonged periods of support. This often results from the increased incidence of percutaneous driveline complications secondary to chronic irritation associated with increased mobility and activity. Less frequent are infections of the device or its blood-contacting components due to blood-borne infections secondary to invasive lines of infections at other sites, such as the respiratory or urinary tract. Another variable influencing the incidence of infection in patients supported for extended periods of time is the presence of complications that preclude cardiac transplantation, such as renal failure requiring dialysis or severe cerebral thromboembolism. In an effort to allow recovery from one of these complications, clinicians often support patients for extended periods, during which invasive lines for monitoring, dialysis, and feeding are required.

The greatest postoperative concern centers on hematoma formation around the pump, which may facilitate bacterial colonization that leads to mediastinitis in patients with a TAH and pocket infections in patients with an implantable LVAD.

In patients with a TAH, hematoma forms directly around the device in the mediastinum, although it often extends into the left pleural space, which is violated by the effort to position the prosthetic left ventricle and to tunnel the drivelines. In patients receiving the Novacor LVAD, the inflow conduit to the pump is routed from the left ventricular apex to the device positioned behind the left rectus abdominis muscle. This pocket communicates with the pericardial and left pleural space, often acting as a repository for shed mediastinal and pleural blood. A problem associated with postoperative bleeding is the extensive use of electrocautery and hemostatic agents to control it. The pathway for bacterial colonization could be direct inoculation of microorganisms during surgery, blood from intravascular catheters, direct extension from an adjacent site, such as the lung, or ascending infection along a driveline or blood conduits.

LOCATION OF INFECTIONS

Infections in patients supported by mechanical circulatory assist devices occur either as device-related or device-unrelated. Infections that are not device-related may occur in the respiratory, urinary, or gastrointestinal tract and are seen frequently in patients undergoing major cardiothoracic surgery. This section focuses on device-related infections.

Intradevice Infections

Infections within a device are not a frequent clinical complication even in patients with recurrent bacteremic or septic episodes. However, once the patient has bacterial growth within the prosthetic device, infection is resistant to antibiotics and persists until the device is removed. The pathway for microbial colonization in the device is usually blood from intravascular catheters, but colonization can occur as a metastatic infection from a distant site, such as the urinary tract.

Another contributing factor is thrombus formation within the device. Micro-organisms may activate the coagulation cascade and facilitate thrombus formation on the inner surface of the device, especially at the prosthetic valves and its connectors. In a retrospective study of 330 animals with TAHs, 31% had microbially infected thrombi[22]; however, the cause and the specific route of infection were unclear. An infected skin lesion may be an important source of pathogens because 50% of the animals had skin lesions. Of these, 23% had blood or prosthesis cultures identical to those found in the concurrent skin lesions. Infected thrombi are also observed in clinical specimens.[23] In humans the most common organism seen within the device, especially within the vascular conduits to the pulmonary artery or aorta, is *Candida albicans*. In these cases, infected thromboemboli result in associated cerebral infarction and/or hemorrhage. At the University of Pittsburgh, only 2 patients in the total series of the combined 54 TAH and LVAD patients demonstrated intradevice infections. Infectious sites were limited to the valves and adjacent conduits in 1 patient with a TAH and 1 patient with an LVAD; *Candida albicans* was detected in each case. Pump chambers were free from infections.

Extradevice Infections

Extradevice infections may occur around the external housing of the pump, the driveline, and the wound itself. Primary wound infections, however, are relatively rare in this series of patients.

The external housing and driveline are the portions of the TAH and VAD most vulnerable to infections. Several factors may play a role in minimizing the risk of infection in the Novacor LVAD versus the TAH. Tissue ingrowth into the velour-covered driveline and development of the fibrous capsule around the pump housing contribute to the prevention of serious device-related infections. In devices such as the Thoratec paracorporeal pneumatic LVAD, the inflow and outflow conduits are also susceptible to infection because they exit the skin to connect with a pump external to the body. Drivelines provide direct access to external bacterial environments and bacterial–biomaterial interactions expedite biomaterial-centered infections. If tissue ingrowth into the driveline or along a blood conduit is delayed, liquefying hematomas may drain chronically along the tract of a conduit or driveline.

Because bacterial colonization at the skin around the external driveline commonly occurs, regardless of the type of device, the relation between driveline infection and mediastinitis is important. Early studies of the TAH demonstrated the same bacterial colonization both on the driveline and in the mediastinum, which led surgeons to conclude that infection ascending along the driveline was the cause of mediastinitis. However, meticulous postmortem microbiologic studies have demonstrated that even in patients with concurrent mediastinitis and driveline infection, a segment at the mid-third of driveline is sterile.[23] This skip region in the driveline has provoked controversy over the clinical importance of driveline infection. During the experience with the TAH at the University of Pittsburgh, the incidence of mediastinitis was high; however, microbacterial studies showed that the pathogens found in the mediastinum were more often the same as those found in cultures of the respiratory tract as opposed to the skin exit site of the drivelines.

In our series of patients, infections during the implant period occurred most frequently in the blood (10–12%), at a driveline site (12%), or simultaneously in the blood and at a driveline (4–5%). These rates were similar in both the TAH and LVAD groups. After transplantation in the TAH-supported group, infections occurred most commonly in the mediastinum (24%) or simultaneously in the blood and mediastinum (18%). In the LVAD patients, posttransplant infections were usually limited to the blood (18%), with mediastinitis in only 1 patient. Despite the prevalence of blood stream infection, no bacterial infections occurred in the pump chambers, valves, or conduits themselves. Cultures of the mediastinum in TAH patients were often negative at the time of transplant, even though mediastinitis occurred frequently after transplantation. Driveline infections in the LVAD group were usually minor, with minimal drainage and mild erythema; the most common organism was *Staphylococcus aureus* or *Candida albicans*. Because these infections tended to occur in the most mobile patients, they were felt to be related to chronic irritation. In 1 patient, a driveline infection with *Staphylococcus aureus* and *Proteus mirabilis* followed a severe dermatitis due to the laundry detergent used to wash the bed linen. After transplantation, these same organisms contaminated the Novacor pump pocket, resulting in a pocket infection that ultimately infected the mediastinum. A second, morbidly obese patient developed a pump-pocket infection with a resistant strain of *Pseudomonas* after fat necrosis in the pocket. The Novacor LVAD pump was placed in a subcutaneous position as opposed to the traditional subrectus pocket.

Other extradevice infections may occur at sites distant from the device and are related more to risk factors associated with extensive surgical procedures in morbidly ill patients. Patients with chronic congestive heart failure may be prone to develop respiratory tract infections, especially pneumonia, when intubation is prolonged. The next most common site of infection is the urinary tract, which is vulnerable to contamination from indwelling catheters. The most frequently isolated pathogen from the sputum is a gram-negative bacillus and from the urine *Serratia marescens* or *Candida albicans*. Occasionally, infected false aneurysms have been seen at the site of frequent reintroduction of an IABP in the femoral artery.

TREATMENT OF INFECTION

Preimplant

GENERAL PRINCIPLES

All patients maintained in an intensive care setting as UNOS status I transplant candidates are also potential candidates for mechanical circulatory support. Vigilance for potential contamination of indwelling catheters and daily inspection of percutaneous access sites, including the IABP, are important for prevention of sepsis. Access sites should be examined and redressed daily. All intravascular lines, including the IABP, should be changed weekly, even if the patient is asymptomatic. Activity and physiotherapy are important for general physical well-being; moreover, mobile patients appear to be less likely to acquire serious infections. This is particularly evident in patients restricted to bed because of an indwelling IABP in the femoral artery. Every effort should be made to turn these patients regularly to prevent pressure ulceration and to keep groin areas dry. Of more importance, the length of time that patients are supported on an IABP should be minimized to <7 days; preferably no more than 72 hours should expire before device implant. Other basic principles of maintaining adequate host defense mechanisms, particularly adequate nutrition, should be followed.

ANTIBIOTIC PROPHYLAXIS

Broad-spectrum intravenous antibiotic coverage should be avoided during the preimplant phase. In some centers, intravenous cefazolin, vancomycin, or cefamandole is used in patients on an IABP. Periods of low cardiac output may compromise mesenteric blood flow, resulting in an alteration of vascular permeability and translocation of bacteria, which may lead to self-contamination of the blood. To reduce the risk of gram-negative sepsis in this setting, various protocols have been developed to reduce the colony count of these bacteria in the gastrointestinal tract. For this reason, we recommend giving patients on an IABP an elixir containing polymyxin E (100 mg), gentamicin (80 mg), and Nystatin (2 million units/20 ml). If a patient is intubated, an orabase paste with 2% solutions of the above components is applied. This mixture is given every 6 hours but may be reduced to every 8 or 12 hours if patients complain of excessive diarrhea.

SPECIFIC INFECTIONS

Before device implant the most common infections are associated with indwelling lines and the IABP. In each case the primary treatment is removal and replacement of the infected line. Any febrile episode that does not appear to be related to a urinary tract or pulmonary source should be assumed to be due to line sepsis, and all lines should be changed if they have not been recently placed (within

48 hours). Positive blood cultures are treated with culture-specific antibiotics. We recommend that a support device not be inserted within 7–10 days of a positive blood culture or documented source of sepsis, such as pneumonia, or within 5 days of an unexplained fever. In some cases, we have been faced with inserting a circulatory support device in a deteriorating patient with a recent fever only to find that a positive blood culture has been reported after implant from a specimen drawn 2–4 days earlier. The risk of infection is so great and the consequences so disastrous that one needs to resist the urge to implant a device under these circumstances.

Implant Phase

General Principles and Antibiotic Prophylaxis

Certain principles are followed during the implant procedure to optimize aseptic technique and to reduce potential contamination during surgery. All intravenous lines are changed before induction of anesthesia, and if present, the urinary catheter is replaced. The potential surgical field is washed with a Betadine soap solution; the skin is dried and then rewashed. A Betadine skin preparation is then applied from chin to knees, with care to cover the area from one side of the table to the other. Broad-spectrum intravenous antibiotic coverage is given before induction of anesthesia with cefazolin, vancomycin, or cefamandole to ensure adequate staphylococcal coverage and supplemented with additional doses every 4 hours during the procedure. If the patient has not received the gut sterilization prophylaxis mentioned above, it must be started immediately upon intubation. During implant surgery saline containing a cephalosporin antibiotic is used liberally to wash the wound margins, mediastinum, pump pocket, and exposed portions of the device and its conduits and drivelines. This procedure reduces bacteria counts on the tissues in the surgical field. Although such procedures tend to draw large groups of participants and onlookers, it is important to reduce the number of transient personnel in the operating room because bacteria counts increase with the number of people. As indicated above, hematoma formation plays a role in providing a critical environment for bacterial growth. For this reason, meticulous hemostasis is essential. In addition, both pleural spaces as well as the mediastinum require chest tubes to provide adequate drainage of potential fluid and blood collections. A drain is also inserted into the abdominal pocket containing the Novacor pump. Finally, if an IABP is present, it is removed before the patient leaves the operating room.

Intravenous antibiotics are continued during the perioperative period in the intensive care unit until the chest tubes, monitoring lines, and urinary catheter are removed. The drain in the Novacor pocket is removed last because this appears to be the area in which chronic fluid collections persist the longest. In most cases it is removed within 5 days of surgery. An effort is made to remove all invasive monitoring lines and to extubate the patient as soon as possible; the patient should be transferred from the intensive care unit to an intermediate care setting as soon as practical. Continued antibiotic administration is frequently required because of prolonged intubation. Antibiotic coverage is adjusted according to the sensitivities of the cultural flora. Finally, physiotherapy and rehabilitation are stressed immediately to promote early and full mobilization. This reduces the risk of pressure ulceration, which, because of cardiac cachexia, may pose a problem in debilitated patients, and also helps to prevent pulmonary complications, such as atelectasis and pneumonia.

Surgical Management of Specific Infections

Driveline Infections. The incidence of driveline infections in LVAD (Novacor and Thoratec) patients was 13%. The pathogens were *Staphylococcus epidermidis* and *aureus, Candida albicans,* and *Proteus mirabilis.* A similar incidence was seen in the TAH patients with a similar spectrum of organisms. The treatment of driveline contamination and infection begins with meticulous attention to a rigorous protocol for dressing change, adapted from the protocol for long-term hemodialysis access catheters. A semiocclusive dressing provides a barrier against organisms and prevents skin excoriation. This same protocol is used for Novacor drivelines and has been modified for use around the blood conduits of the Thoratec VAD. In the intensive care unit dressings for the sternotomy, abdominal pocket, chest tube insertion sites, LVAD pocket drain, and percutaneous leads are changed once a day. All dressing changes are performed by a nurse using sterile technique. After the old dressing is removed, the wound and driveline near the skin are cleansed with a bacteriocidal solution. The incision and driveline sites are then washed with sterile water and dried. Using clean gloves, the wounds are redressed with an absorbent, semiocclusive dressing with an adhesive perimeter (Viasorb). The driveline itself is sandwiched between two pieces of transparent dressing material with no tract to air. Finally, methods of supporting the driveline on a sling against the leg or to the waist have been devised to reduce friction and tension on the driveline and to prevent corrosion around the skin edges. In the case of local erythema or serous drainage, the dressing changes have been increased to twice a day, with local antibiotic (cephalosporin) irrigation. If the patient complains of pain or if local tenderness or purulent drainage is seen, a 7-day course of intravenous antibiotics, appropriate for the organisms cultured at the site, is administered, followed by an additional 7 days of oral antibiotics.

In 2 patients, this method successfully controlled local infections with *Staphylococcus aureus* (day 29 of 72 days of support) and *epidermidis* (intermittently between days 40 to 115 of 140 days of support) and led to no sequelae after transplantation. In 1 patient, a mixed culture of *Candida albicans, Staphylococcus aureus,* and *Proteus mirabilis* was detected on day 34. Mediastinal drainage at the time of transplantation on day 86 also revealed *Staphylococcus* and *Proteus.* Despite antibiotics, mediastinitis due to these organisms occurred at day 21 after transplantation but was successfully treated with a skeletal muscle flap. The final case occurred in a morbidly obese patient in whom the pump was placed into a subcutaneous pocket. Subsequent to fat necrosis and dehiscence of the abdominal incision, the patient became infected with a resistant strain of *Pseudomonas,* which also drained through a tract to the driveline site. Mechanical support was discontinued on day 94 after the development of multisystem organ failure. One other patient, who was supported for 5 months, had a 12″-long, nonhealed driveline tract; however, with the above dressing method and occasional irrigation of the tract, organisms did not grow from this area.

Mediastinitis. The incidence of mediastinitis in 34 patients who underwent LVAD implantation was 3%; all cases occurred after a driveline infection and were successfully treated after transplantation, as mentioned above. This rate compares with an incidence of 30% and a mortality of 83% in the TAH group. In most cases, the sepsis from mediastinitis was so overwhelming from the gram-negative organisms that few patients survived the perioperative period, despite appropriate intravenous antibiotics, adequate drainage, and mediastinal antibiotic irrigation. Immunosuppression was modified to keep cyclosporine and prednisone dosages at approximately one-half the usual levels; immuran was avoided. Unfortunately, with this type of infection, the options are somewhat limited because patients rarely tolerate removal of the device; thus the infection is fatal. In rare circumstances an infection limited to the Novacor pocket has been successfully treated by exteriorizing the pump, letting the infection drain, and closing the defect at transplantation with a rectus muscle flap. Similar infections have been seen in the Thoratec LVAD series[4] with involvement of the inflow or outflow conduits near the skin. Again, local treatment combined with intravenous antibiotics is the main therapy.

All foreign material and parts must be removed from any device at the time of transplantation. In 1 patient, a portion of plastic conduit-reinforcing material was left in the subcostal tract between the left ventricular apex and the subrectus pump pocket. Although the patient never had a fever or elevated white blood cell count, he returned 3 months after transplantation with recurrent left subcostal and abdominal pain. Although CT scan showed a mild fluid collection, his lack of symptoms for infection resulted in no further treatment. Five months later, after recurrent bouts of pain, the area was explored, and the purulent material that was drained grew *Pseudomonas*. The retained portion of the conduit was removed at that time. Although symptoms subsided, he required further rib resection and drainage 5 months later; currently, 1½ years later, he is free of complaints.

FUTURE

The current experience with infections in mechanical circulatory support patients reveals that external drivelines remain the weak link in all systems. A totally implantable device not only will improve a patient's quality of life but also may reduce the risk of device infection. However, a totally implantable system requires implantation of additional foreign bodies, such as a controller and an internal battery system. Antibiotic-pervaded biomaterials may be effective in diminishing bacterial colonization in these circumstances.

Microthrombus formation is related to thromboembolic episodes and intradevice infection. An intradevice surface precoated with endothelial cells may reduce the incidence of bacterial adhesion and thrombogenic episodes.

Interactions between bacteria and a substratum surface depend on the surface and nearsurface atomic structure as well as the composition of implanted biomaterials. Modifications to biomaterial surfaces at an atomic level will allow the programming of cell-to-substratum events, thereby diminishing infection by enhancing tissue compatibility or integration or by directly inhibiting bacterial adhesion.[19]

Finally, the lessons learned in the TAH era emphasize the risks incurred by selection of patients in cardiogenic shock or in prolonged low output states. With proper patient selection, many series now show good infection-free survival with the TAH. Much has yet to be learned about the host-defense mechanism and susceptibility to bacterial translocation during low flow states.

REFERENCES

1. Farrar DJ, Lawson JH, Litwak P, Cederwall G: Thoratec VAD system as a bridge to heart transplantation. J Heart Transplant 9:415–423, 1990.

2. Frazier OH, Rose EA, Macmanus Q, et al: Multicenter clinical evaluation of the HeartMate 1000 IP left ventricular assist device. Ann Thorac Surg 53:1080–1090, 1992.

3. McCarthy PM, Portner PM, Tobler HG, et al: Clinical experience with the Novacor ventricular assist system bridge to transplantation and the transition to permanent application. J Thorac Cardiovasc Surg 102:578–587, 1991.

4. McBride LR, Swartz MT, Reedy JE, et al: Device related infections in patients supported with mechanical circulatory support devices for greater than 30 days. ASAIO Trans 37:M258–M259, 1991.

5. Myers TJ, McGee MG, Zeluff BJ, et al: Frequency and significance of infections in patients receiving prolonged LVAD support. ASAIO Trans 37:M283–M285, 1991.

6. Oaks TE, Pae WE, Miller CA, Pierce WS: Combined Registry for the Clinical Use of Mechanical Ventricular Assist Pumps and the Total Artificial Heart in Conjunction with Heart Transplantation: Fifth official report–1990. J Heart Lung Transplant 10:621–625, 1991.

7. Pae W, personal communication.

8. Hsu J, Griffith BP, Dowling RD, et al: Infections in mortally ill cardiac transplant recipients. J Thorac Cardiovasc Surg 98:506–509, 1989.

9. Lonchyna VA, Pifarre R, Sullivan H, et al: Successful use of the total artificial heart (TAH) as a bridge to transplantation with no mediastinitis. J Heart Lung Transplant 11:235–239, 1992.

10. Bone RC, Fisher CJ, Clemmer TP, et al: Sepsis syndrome: A valid clinical entity. Crit Care Med 17:389–393, 1989.

11. Parrillo JE, Parker MM, Natanson C, et al: Septic shock in humans: Advances in the understanding of pathogenesis, cardiovascular dysfunction, and therapy. Ann Intern Med 113:227–242, 1990.

12. Lennard TW, Shenton BK, Borzotta A, et al: The influence of surgical operations on components of the human immune system. Br J Surg 72:771–776, 1985.

13. van Oeveren W, Kazatchkine MD, Descamps-Latsha B, et al: Deleterious effects of cardiopulmonary bypass: A prospective study of bubble versus membrane oxygenator. J Thorac Cardiovasc Surg 89:888–899, 1985.

14. Stelzer GT, Ward RA, Wellhausen SR, et al: Alterations in select immunologic parameters following total artificial heart implantation. Artif Organs 11:52–62, 1987.

15. Nilsson L, Kulander L, Nström S, Eriksson Ö: Endotoxins in cardiopulmonary bypass. J Thorac Cardiovasc Surg 100:777–780, 1990.

16. Kaplan SS, Basford RE, Kormos RL, et al: Biomaterial associated impairment of local neutrophil function. ASAIO Trans 36:M172–M175, 1990.

17. Gristina AG, Dobbins JJ, Giammara B, et al: Biomaterial-centered sepsis and the total artificial heart. JAMA 259:870–874, 1988.

18. Gristina AG, Costerton JW: Bacteria-laden biofilms: A hazard to orthopedic prostheses. Infect Surg 3:655–661, 1984.

19. Gristina AG: Biomaterial-centered infection: Microbial adhesion versus tissue integration. Science 237:1588–1595, 1987.

20. Mohammad SF, Topham NS, Burns GL, Olsen DB: Enhanced bacterial adhesion on surface pretreated with fibrinogen and fibronectin. ASAIO Trans 34:573–577, 1988.

21. Graham TR, Dasse K, Salih V, et al: Neointimal development on textured biomaterial surfaces during clinical use of an implantable left ventricular assist device. Eur J Cardiothorac Surg 4:182–190, 1990.

22. Chiang BY, Burns GL, Pantalos GM, et al: Microbially infected thrombus in animals with total artificial hearts. ASAIO Trans 37:M256–M257, 1991.

23. Dobbins JJ, Johnson GS, Kunin GM, DeVries WC: Postmortem microbiological findings of two total artificial heart recipients. JAMA 259:865–869, 1988.

BRIAN L. CMOLIK, MD
STEVEN E. PARK, MD
JAMES A. MAGOVERN, MD

CARDIOMYOPLASTY AS AN ALTERNATIVE FOR CHRONIC VENTRICULAR SUPPORT

From the Department of
 Cardiothoracic Surgery
Allegheny General Hospital;
Surgical Research,
 Allegheny-Singer Research
 Institute;
 and
The Medical College of
 Pennsylvania
Pittsburgh, Pennsylvania

Reprint requests to:
James A. Magovern, MD
Department of Cardiothoracic
 Surgery
Allegheny General Hospital
320 E. North Avenue
Pittsburgh, PA 15212

End-stage congestive heart failure affects over 2 million Americans and accounts for over 400,000 deaths each year in the United States.[28] The best surgical therapy for this condition is cardiac transplantation, but the shortage of donor organs and the complications of chronic immunosuppression limit the applicability of this procedure to a small number of patients.[26] Devices for mechanical circulatory support are not yet available.

Cardiomyoplasty is a new approach that uses autogenous skeletal muscle to support the failing ventricle. Over 120 cardiomyoplasty procedures have been performed worldwide. This chapter reviews the experimental and clinical experience with cardiomyoplasty at Allegheny General Hospital (AGH) between 1985 and 1991.

CARDIOMYOPLASTY: EXPERIMENTAL STUDIES

Research on the use of conditioned skeletal muscle for cardiac assistance has been a productive research area in the past 10 years. Considerable progress has occurred in basic research on cardiomyoplasty, with subsequent important clinical application. Experimental studies have been the foundation of our clinical cardiomyoplasty program.

The first general area for investigation was chronic muscle stimulation to demonstrate the

CARDIAC SURGERY: State of the Art Reviews—Vol. 7, No. 2, 1993
Philadelphia, Hanley & Belfus, Inc.

425

feasibility of using skeletal muscle for cardiac assistance. Sheep latissimus dorsi muscle was made fatigue-resistant by chronic electrical stimulation, and the conversion was documented by histochemical, biochemical, and ultrastructural analysis. Ninety-two percent of the conditioned muscle fibers were type I fatigue-resistant fibers compared with 33% of the unconditioned muscles. In a separate experiment, the strength of the sheep latissimus dorsi muscles was tested in a fatigue test. The conditioned muscle maintained 91% of its initial strength during a 2-hour fatigue test, whereas the unconditioned muscle maintained only 47% of its initial strength. This difference was highly significant ($p = < 0.05$).[20]

The conditioned sheep latissimus dorsi muscle was able to produce up to 1.2 watts/kg of muscle power. The human heart requires an average power output of 1.05 watts. The adult male human latissimus dorsi muscle weighs 0.220–0.480 kg, which could yield a theoretical maximum of 0.55 watts. Therefore, the power output of a single latissimus dorsi muscle could effectively assist circulation, but could not support the entire circulation.[19]

Several experiments were done to determine the most effective means of stimulating skeletal muscle, and two general conclusions were reached: (1) Voltage thresholds for muscle contraction were much less when the thoracodorsal nerve was stimulated directly than when intramuscular leads were used.[15,16] (2) Burst stimulation yielded greater maximal force and hemodynamic augmentation than single-pulse stimulation.[15,18]

The influence of muscle fiber orientation on the hemodynamic response to cardiomyoplasty was then examined. Dynamic cardiomyoplasty with the conditioned left latissimus dorsi demonstrated significantly greater cardiac augmentation when the muscle fibers were perpendicular to the interventricular septum than when they were parallel to the septum. This was the first suggestion that skeletal muscle orientation was a critical factor in improving cardiac performance.[18]

These findings stimulated further interest in various types of cardiomyoplasty and different skeletal muscle orientations. The use of both latissimus dorsi muscles simultaneously was investigated to determine if biventricular hemodynamic augmentation could be achieved. Bilateral cardiomyoplasty and left posterior cardiomyoplasty were compared. The bilateral procedure resulted in significant biventricular augmentation with stimulation. The hemodynamic benefits of the left posterior wrap were significant, but less dramatic, especially with regard to right ventricular function.[23]

Next, the bilateral anterior cardiomyoplasty and its components—the left anterior cardiomyoplasty and the right anterior cardiomyoplasty—were analyzed in an acute canine experiment.[12,14] The right anterior cardiomyoplasty demonstrated cardiac performance equal to that of bilateral anterior cardiomyoplasty. The contribution of the left anterior cardiomyoplasty appeared only to augment right-heart hemodynamic variables (Fig. 1).

These hemodynamic studies of cardiomyoplasty were performed in animals with normal heart function—a simple model to use for initial studies, but not a good model of the clinical situation. Accordingly, efforts were made to develop an animal model of heart failure that could be used to analyze the effects of cardiomyoplasty.

We have recently published a model of left ventricular failure caused by intracoronary infusion of adriamycin.[22] Adriamycin (10 mg) was infused into the left main coronary artery each week for a total of 5 weeks. No systemic toxicity was noted, but the animals developed left ventricular failure. Adriamycin-induced

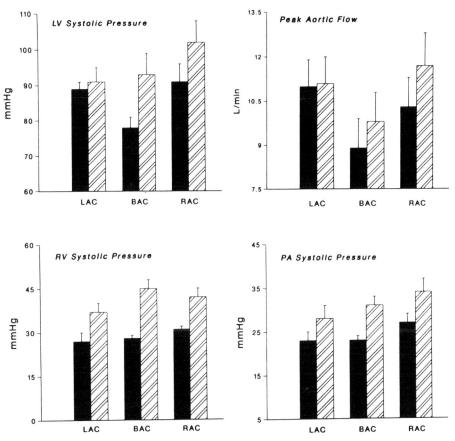

FIGURE 1. Component analysis of cardiomyoplasty on right and left ventricular function parameters. LAC = left anterior cardiomyoplasty; BAC = bilateral anterior cardiomyoplasty; RAC = right anterior cardiomyoplasty; ■ = nonstimulated; ▨ = stimulated.

changes in the left ventricle were noted histologically. Presently, we are using this model to evaluate the hemodynamic effects of cardiomyoplasty on chronic heart failure.

Future plans in the laboratory are to develop a specific muscle stimulation program for cardiomyoplasty. The focus will enlarge to encompass contractile speed, relaxation time, and strength as well as fatigue-resistance. An additional goal is to characterize further the effects of cardiomyoplasty on systolic and diastolic heart function. Initial studies using sonomicrometry and a left ventricular pressure transducer demonstrate large increases in stroke work and decreases in ventricular volume with stimulation of the muscle (Fig. 2).

CARDIOMYOPLASTY: CLINICAL APPLICATION

The first dynamic cardiomyoplasty in the U.S. was performed at AGH in September 1985. As of January 1992, 23 patients have undergone the procedure. All patients were initially considered for cardiac transplantation, but this option was excluded because of age, peripheral vascular disease, microvascular complications

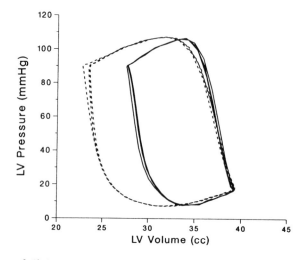

FIGURE 2. Pressure-volume loops of stimulated (dotted .lines) and unstimulated (solid lines) beats. Changes in stroke work and stroke volume with stimulation of the cardiomyoplasty are significant.

of diabetes mellitus, unsuitable psychosocial setting, or patient refusal. Patients with New York Heart Association (NYHA) functional class III and IV were considered for cardiomyoplasty. Our initial experience with the operation clearly demonstrated that the results with class III patients were better than those with class IV. Some functional reserve is necessary to withstand the operation and the 2-month postoperative muscle-conditioning program before any significant hemodynamic improvement can be expected.

Our preoperative evaluation process has evolved as our experience grows. Presently, all potential candidates have the following tests: right- and left-heart catheterization with coronary angiography, echocardiography, multiple-gated acquisition (MUGA) scan, exercise thallium scan, and measurement of maximal oxygen consumption and work capacity. Routine blood work and pulmonary function tests are obtained. Likely candidates also have a computed tomographic scan of the chest to assess cardiac size, thoracic cavity volume, and size of the latissimus dorsi muscle. Exclusion criteria are (1) age >70; (2) significant pulmonary dysfunction (FEV_1 <2 L/min); (3) renal insufficiency (creatinine clearance <30 ml/min); (4) symptomatic ventricular arrhythmias; (5) hepatic dysfunction; (6) degenerative neuromuscular disorders; and (7) previous division of the latissimus dorsi muscle on the side of the proposed procedure. Patients who are dependent on intraaortic balloon counterpulsation or intravenous inotropes are not candidates for cardiomyoplasty.

The AGH experience may be broken into 3 subsets correlating with 3 separate time periods. These subsets reflect the development and advancement of the operation. Patients' preoperative characteristics are presented in Table 1. Group 1 consisted of 5 patients (cases 1–5), on whom left latissimus dorsi muscle cardiomyoplasty was performed in conjunction with other cardiac procedures between 1985 and 1988. A left ventricular aneurysm was resected in 3 patients, and coronary bypass grafting was performed in 2. Cardiomyoplasty was accomplished in a single stage by harvesting the left latissimus dorsi muscle, placing the pacing and sensing leads, and wrapping the muscle around the heart. Orientation was left anterior cardiocostal (Fig. 3), using the standardized nomenclature.[11] Dual-chambered pacemakers were used for stimulating the latissimus dorsi. The atrial channel of the pacemaker sensed the QRS complex, and the ventricular channel stimulated the muscle.

TABLE 1. Patients' Preoperative Characteristics

	Age	LVEF	RVEF	LVEDP	CT Ratio	CI
Overall (n = 23)	55.2 ± 1.9	25.4 ± 1.5	49.6 ± 4.1	20.4 ± 1.7	0.56 ± 0.02	2.6 ± 0.2
Group 1 (n = 5)	55.0 ± 4.1	28.8 ± 3.4	46.8 ± 7.2	24.8 ± 0.9	0.60 ± 0.02	3.2 ± 0.6
Group 2 (n = 10)	56.3 ± 2.4	22.1 ± 2.4	39.8 ± 6.3	20.6 ± 3.2	0.55 ± 0.03	2.3 ± 0.3
Group 3 (n = 8)	53.9 ± 4.1	27.5 ± 1.8	63.5 ± 4.7	18.0 ± 2.3	0.54 ± 0.02	2.7 ± 0.1

Mean ± SEM.
LVEF = left ventricular ejection fraction; RVEF = right ventricular ejection fraction; LVEDP = left ventricular end-diastolic pressure; CT ratio = cardiothoracic ratio; CI = cardiac index.

Group 2 consisted of 10 patients (cases 6–15), who underwent a left latissimus dorsi cardiomyoplasty between December 1988 and January 1991. All procedures were completed in two stages in this group. The first stage consisted of harvesting the latissimus dorsi muscle and placing the pacing leads. The second stage consisted of translocation of the muscle into the thoracic cavity, performance of the cardiomyoplasty, and implantation of the cardiomyostimulator. The Medtronic SP1005 cardiomyostimulator was used in all group 2 patients. This stimulator delivers a burst stimulus to the muscle after a specified delay from the QRS complex, which results in greater tension development by the muscle. A right ventricular sensing lead and two intramuscular pacing leads were used in each case.

The final group (group 3) consisted of 8 patients (cases 16–23) whose operations took place between February 1991 and January 1992. All of these

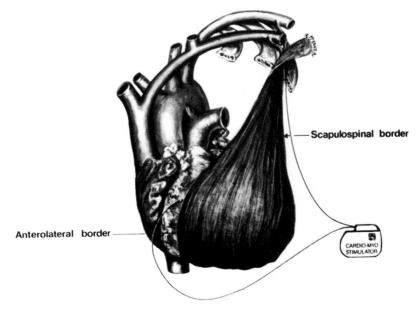

FIGURE 3. Anterior view of the left anterior cardiocostal (LACC) cardiomyoplasty.

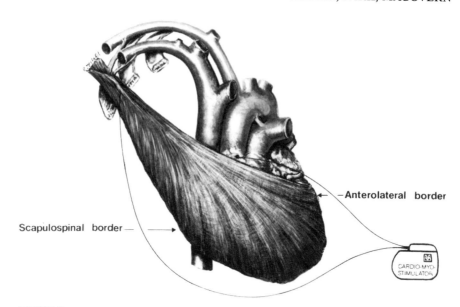

Scapulospinal border —

—Anterolateral border

CARDIO-MYO-STIMULATOR

FIGURE 4.   Anterior view of the right anterior cardiocostal (RACC) cardiomyoplasty.

patients had a right anterior latissimus dorsi cardiomyoplasty (Fig. 4). The procedure was performed in two stages in the first patient, but the other 7 have been completed in a single stage. The Medtronic SP1005 was used for muscle stimulation in each case, and the lead arrangement was the same as in the previous group.

Different muscle-conditioning protocols were used in the 3 groups. Group 1 patients received a single-pulse stimulus, beginning with 4 hr/day of stimulation at low voltage. The voltage and duration of stimulation increased gradually over 6 weeks until the muscle was stimulated 24 hr/day.[25] Group 2 patients were conditioned with a similar program in which the muscles were stimulated for increasing periods of time, voltage, and burst frequency over a 6-week period. The stimulation protocol for group 3 is specified in the phase II clinical trial of the procedure and corresponds to the conditioning program originally developed by Chachques and Carpentier (Table 2).[9]

TABLE 2.   Current Training Protocol

Time Postoperatively	Frequency (Hz)	Pulse Train (# pulses/pulse train)
Weeks 1 and 2	No pacing	—
Weeks 3 and 4	5	1
Weeks 5 and 6	10	2
Weeks 7 and 8	15	3
Week 9	20	4
Week 10	25	5
Week 11	30	6

Stimulation continues 24 hr/day once it is initiated.

RESULTS

Operative Morbidity and Mortality

Overall operative mortality was 17% (4/23). Group 1 mortality was 0% (0/5); group 2, 40% (4/10); and group 3, 0% (0/8). All operative deaths were due to cardiac factors: 2 from low cardiac output and 2 from ventricular arrhythmias.

Significant morbidity occurred in 8 patients. Four patients had prolonged endotracheal intubation (mean: 5 days), and 2 of these had adult respiratory distress syndrome. One patient suffered acute renal failure, 1 developed coagulopathic bleeding, and 1 had acute cholecystitis. Three patients had wound seromas at the muscle-flap harvest site that resolved with needle aspirations. These complications were not concentrated in any one group of patients.

Late Morbidity and Mortality

Seven deaths have occurred after discharge from 1½–30 months postoperatively. Five patients died suddenly, probably secondary to arrhythmias, and 2 others died from congestive heart failure. Two of the 5 with sudden death also had congestive heart failure as a late problem. Late complications otherwise were minor, consisting of 2 pacer-site problems, 1 with erosion and 1 with infection. The latter required replacement and translocation of the generator, but chronic infection recurred and ultimately led to removal of the second generator without replacement. One patient had a pulse generator turned off for an unknown length of time by environmental electromagnetic interference. This patient had become increasingly symptomatic with shortness of breath and weight loss. The generator was simply turned back on, and the symptoms resolved. Of the first 23 patients, 10 have been readmitted to the hospital for management of heart failure on at least one occasion. All responded rapidly to intravenous diuretics, low-dose dopamine, or retiming of the SP1005 cardiomyostimulator.

Functional Class

Preoperatively 10 patients were NYHA class IV, 11 were class III, and 1 was class II. The mean NYHA class was 3.2. All hospital survivors except 1 improved by at least one functional class. The average improvement was 1.6 classes. Patient with right cardiomyoplasty had an average pre- and postoperative functional class of 3.0 and 1.6, respectively, whereas those with left cardiomyoplasty had pre- and postoperative classes of 3.7 and 1.8, respectively.

Cardiac Function

Some changes in cardiac function were seen in many of the patients who survived the operation. Table 3 presents data obtained by radionuclide scanning approximately 8 weeks after the procedure. All patients in group 1 had concomitant cardiac procedures, consisting of 3 repairs of left ventricular aneurysm and 2 coronary bypass procedures. Pacer-off vs. pacer-on studies in these patients demonstrated changes in ejection fraction from 32.3 ± 3.6 to 34.3 ± 4.9 when the stimulator was turned on. However, the concomitant procedures could have also contributed to the overall improvement in this group, especially in patients with repair of left ventricular aneurysm.

Groups 2 and 3 each had two patients who underwent coronary bypass surgery. All patients underwent a preoperative stress thallium scan, and none had evidence of major reversible ischemia. The grafting was done because of a

TABLE 3. Pre- and Postcardiomyoplasty Results in Operative Survivors

Group	LVEF		RVEF		LVEDV	
	Pre	Post	Pre	Post	Pre	Post
I (n = 4)	31 ± 3	36 ± 4	54 ± 3	56 ± 6	*	255 ± 61
II (n = 6)	20 ± 2	25 ± 3	44 ± 7	51 ± 9	444 ± 40	433 ± 86
III (n = 7)	28 ± 2	33 ± 2	64 ± 5	69 ± 3	340 ± 19	305 ± 21

* No preoperative LVEDF.
LVEF = left ventricular ejection fraction; RVEF = right ventricular ejection fraction; LVEDP = left ventricular end-diastolic volume.

high-grade stenosis in a major vessel to prevent arrhythmia or infarction in the case of abrupt closure. Therefore, improved function on the basis of coronary bypass grafting is not likely in any of these patients.

Group 2 patients had cardiomyoplasty with the left latissimus dorsi, whereas group 3 patients had the procedure with the right latissimus dorsi. Operative mortality was significant in group 2, but no operative deaths occurred in group 3. Of note is the finding of reduced left ventricular end-diastolic volume and improved left ventricular ejection fraction (LVEF) in patients with right cardiomyoplasty (group 3). The late results of the first patient to undergo right latissimus dorsi for left ventricular failure were recently published.[24] Increases were found in stroke volume (from 78 to 96 ml), left ventricular stroke work (from 57 to 74 g/m), and LVEF (from 23% to 34%). Left ventricular end-diastolic volume decreased from 422 to 346 ml, pulmonary artery pressure fell from 40/26 to 26/11 mmHg, and the pulmonary capillary wedge pressure dropped from 24 to 15 mmHg. This type of consistent improvement in many aspects of cardiac function has not been seen in our experience with left cardiomyoplasty.

OPERATIVE TECHNIQUE

Mobilization of the Latissimus Dorsi

The latissimus dorsi muscle is harvested in the method described by Heckler.[17] The patient is placed in the lateral decubitus position, and the surgical field is widely prepared from the shoulder to the hip. The arm is positioned so that it can be easily manipulated during the procedure. A curvilinear incision is made from the axilla to the level of the iliac crest along a line immediately posterior to the free border of the latissimus dorsi. Both the anterior and posterior skin flaps are dissected with electrocautery to minimize blood loss. When the entire muscle is exposed, submuscular dissection is begun along the free border of the muscle. The vascular branch from the thoracodorsal artery to the serratus anterior muscle is identified early in the dissection. This branch runs parallel to the line of the incision and provides a landmark for locating the thoracodorsal pedicle. After identification of the thoracodorsal pedicle, the remainder of the submuscular dissection is completed. The limits of the dissection extend inferiorly to the level of the iliac crest and posteriorly to the spine. Once the submuscular dissection of the body of the muscle is completed, attention is turned to the axillary portion of the muscle. The serratus and the circumflex scapular branches are divided, and the thoracodorsal pedicle is mobilized up to the level of the axillary vessels. The tendon of the latissimus dorsi inserts onto the humerus. This tendon is divided, giving an additional 5–6 cm of length to the latissimus dorsi and minimizing arm motion during muscle stimulation.

After division of the tendinous insertion of the latissimus dorsi, the surgeon transilluminates the subcutaneous surface of the muscle. Illumination of the muscle in this way demonstrates the course of the main neurovascular pedicles. A bipolar, intramuscular electrode system is used for muscle stimulation in our current protocol. Two intramuscular electrodes are placed into the humeral portion of the muscle, with care not to injure the neurovascular pedicles. The anode is positioned near the main bifurcation of the thoracodorsal bundle. The cathode is positioned 6 cm distally and oriented perpendicular to the course of the thoracodorsal nerve branches. After placement of the electrodes, attachments of the latissimus dorsi to the iliac crest are divided.

Transposition of the latissimus dorsi into the thoracic cavity requires resection of a portion of the third rib. Five to seven centimeters of the axillary portion of the rib are resected. Because the origin and insertion of the latissimus dorsi are now completely divided, the only remaining attachment is the pedicle. The latissimus dorsi is delivered into the pleural space with care not to place undue tension on the thoracodorsal pedicle. The tendon of the latissimus dorsi is sutured into the periosteum of the resected rib with pledgeted, nonabsorbable suture. The wound is closed over two suction drainage systems. The drains are left in place until output is minimal. Early removal of the drains has resulted in seromas that required percutaneous aspiration. The patient is then repositioned in a supine position for the next stage of the operation.

Cardiomyoplasty

At our institution the muscle-wrap portion of the operation is performed through a median sternotomy. The procedure can also be performed through a left thoracotomy,[4] but we believe median sternotomy provides the advantage of better exposure, particularly when cardiopulmonary bypass is required for concomitant procedures.

Various orientations of the latissimus dorsi muscle have been used to wrap the dysfunctional myocardium. Furnary et al. developed a standard nomenclature to describe the variations of latissimus dorsi cardiomyoplasty.[11] The most common orientation has been left posterior cardiocostal (Fig. 5). In this procedure the pericardium is cut back to the level of the left phrenic nerve. The heart is lifted and the scapulospinal portion of the muscle is applied to the posterior ventricle. The anterior border of the muscle is brought around the apex of the heart to complete the wrap. The muscle can be sutured to the myocardium or to the adjacent pericardium. Suturing to the myocardium is difficult if cardiopulmonary bypass is not used because of the cardiomegaly that is always present and the hemodynamic disturbance that occurs with lifting the heart. Most frequently, we suture the muscle to the posterior pericardium at the level of the atrioventricular groove with pledgeted, nonabsorbable sutures.

A left anterior cardiomyoplasty has also been described. This technique was originally developed as a procedure to augment ventricular function after repair of left ventricular anterior aneurysm and was found to be superior to the posterior orientation in an experimental study.[18] In this procedure the muscle is first brought around the anterior surface of the heart. The scapulospinal border covers the cardiac apex. This technique has not been widely adopted in the clinical setting.

The right latissimus dorsi cardiomyoplasty differs in several respects from procedures using the left muscle. The right muscle is best used in an anterior orientation because compression of the right atrium and inferior vena cava occurs when the muscle is brought posteriorly. In addition, the right cardiomyoplasty

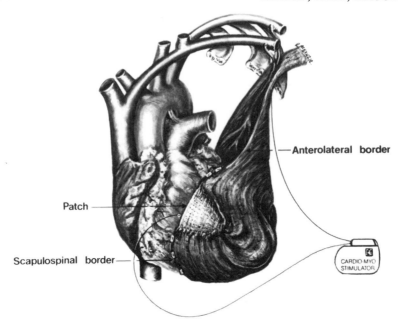

FIGURE 5.   Anterior view of the left posterior cardiocostal (LPCC) cardiomyoplasty.

does not circumferentially wrap the heart. Instead, the muscle is brought across both ventricles and sutured to the myocardium or pericardium at the level of the atrioventricular groove. The scapulospinal portion of the muscle covers the diaphragmatic surface of the right ventricle. Placement of the sensing lead and connections to the cardiomyostimulator do not differ from the techniques used for left procedures.

In general, cardiopulmonary bypass has not been used unless concomitant cardiac procedures were planned. To date, 3 patients have had repair of left ventricular aneurysm, and 10 have had coronary bypass grafting. When a concomitant procedure is performed with cardiomyoplasty, the muscle wrap is done after removal of the aortic cross-clamp, but before weaning from bypass.

The remainder of the procedure involves implantation of an epicardial screw-in electrode on the right ventricle for sensing the native QRS complex and of the cardiomyostimulator (Medtronic SP1005). The pacing and sensing leads are tunneled into the rectus sheath and connected to the stimulator. We bury the device behind the rectus muscle to reduce the risk of erosion and infection, but many investigators leave the device in a subcutaneous pocket.

Postoperative Care

This operation is performed only for patients with significant heart failure. The stress of the surgery and the repeated lifting of the heart result in some deterioration in hemodynamic function in most patients. Inotropic support or insertion of an intraaortic balloon pump was required in 74% and 39% of the patients, respectively.

Management of these patients is no different from that of other patients with compromised cardiac function. We maintain inotropic support until patients are extubated, at a mean of 2.5 days after operation. Thereafter inotropes are reduced, and the patients are started on angiotensin converting-enzyme inhibitors to reduce afterload. Digoxin and diuretics are also resumed in all patients. The average duration of stay in the intensive care unit has been 5 days. Muscle conditioning is started 2 weeks after surgery and increased as outlined in Table 2. Cardiac rehabilitation is instituted as soon as the patient can tolerate it, usually about 1 week after operation. The average hospital stay has been 28 days, but it has been decreasing as our experience and confidence with the procedure grow.

OTHER USES OF AUTOLOGOUS SKELETAL MUSCLE

The focus of this chapter has been dynamic cardiomyoplasty. However, use of autologous skeletal muscle need not be limited to cardiomyoplasty. Another approach that has been investigated extensively in the laboratory is the construction of pouches made from skeletal muscle, called skeletal muscle ventricles (SMVs).

Numerous experimental studies on SMVs have been published. They have been used to replace the right ventricle[7] and to generate diastolic aortic counter-pulsation.[1-3,5,6,10,27] Recently, left atrial-to-aortic and left ventricular-to-aortic SMVs have been reported. The major advantage of SMVs over cardiomyoplasty is the absence of geometric constraints that result from the shape of the muscle and the position of the neurovascular bundle. The muscle and pumping chamber can be conformed in such a manner to maximize pressure generation. The major disadvantage of SMVs is that they pump blood and require prosthetic valves to ensure unidirectional flow; thus blood contacts foreign surfaces, which introduce the problems of thrombosis and thromboembolism. SMVs are also less compliant than the cardiac ventricles; thus relatively high filling pressures are necessary to maintain optimal pumping characteristics.

Other investigators have used skeletal muscle to compress either the ascending or descending aorta for diastolic counterpulsation.[8,21] This approach has been successful in experimental animals but has not yet been attempted in humans. Another concern is the long-term consequence of chronic compression of an atherosclerotic aorta.

DISCUSSION

We have included dynamic cardiomyoplasty as an option in the treatment of heart failure since 1985. Clinical results with left latissimus dorsi cardiomyoplasty demonstrated improvement in the functional status of the patient. Patients who survived the operative procedure improved by an average of two NYHA classes.[13] Patients who showed the greatest improvement in objective measurements of ventricular function underwent concomitant resection of left ventricular aneurysm. Those patients who had only left latissimus dorsi cardiomyoplasty did not have objectively measurable changes in ventricular function.

Because of these clinical findings, we sought to develop a method to achieve more consistent improvement in left ventricular function. Bilateral latissimus dorsi cardiomyoplasty was investigated in the laboratory.[14,23] Component analysis of this model showed the right latissimus dorsi to be the major contributor to the resulting hemodynamic changes and provided a basis for investigation of right latissimus dorsi cardiomyoplasty. Results of acute experiments in dogs showed marked improvement in hemodynamic variables resulting from use of the right latissimus dorsi muscles. With the experimental findings as a foundation, we performed right latissimus dorsi cardiomyoplasty in the clinical setting.

The right latissimus dorsi was first used clinically in the spring of 1991. Since that time a total of 8 right latissimus dorsi cardiomyoplasties have been performed. Because of encouraging early results, this technique has been used exclusively at AGH since March 1991. We are optimistic about the clinical results obtained with the right muscle. Other centers in the U.S. and abroad are continuing studies with the left latissimus. Therefore, more clinical data on right vs. left latissimus cardio-myoplasty will be available in the near future, allowing comparison of our data with that from other centers.

Hemodynamic changes after right latissimus dorsi cardiomyoplasty can be attributed to several factors. Muscle orientation may be a critical factor in improving ventricular function after cardiomyoplasty. The right latissimus dorsi is secured posteriorly along the atrioventricular groove. Variations in the level at which the muscle is transposed into the chest allow for positioning along the long or short axis. The muscle in effect acts as a pulley; its line of force may be directed along the left ventricular outflow tract or across the short axis of the heart. The right latissimus dorsi provides biventricular coverage, as does the left latissimus dorsi. Finally, the power for the right latissimus dorsi flap is derived from the proximal portion of the muscle flap, which is thicker and has better vascularity than the distal portion, which serves only to anchor the flap.

Cardiomyoplasty is in its early stages for the treatment of heart failure. Ideas for using skeletal muscle power to assist the failing myocardium continue to grow. Cardiomyoplasty, skeletal muscle ventricles, and direct counterpulsation are developing rapidly in the laboratory. The attraction of using autologous muscle for cardiac support lies in its ability to avoid the problems associated with cardiac transplantation and mechanical circulatory support. To date, cardiomyoplasty is the only method that has been applied clinically. Early studies are encouraging but not conclusive. The use of skeletal muscle to provide circulatory support has the potential to benefit thousands of patients, but long-term improvements in ventricular function or the natural history of heart failure must be demonstrated before these methods will become commonplace.

REFERENCES

1. Acker MA, Anderson WA, Hammond RL, et al: Skeletal muscle ventricles in circulation: One to eleven weeks experience. J Thorac Cardiovasc Surg 94:163–174, 1987.
2. Acker MA, Hammond RL, Mannion JD, et al: An autologous biologic pump motor. J Thorac Cardiovasc Surg 92:733–745, 1986.
3. Acker MA, Hammond RL, Mannion JD, et al: Skeletal muscle as a potential power source for a cardiovascular pump: Assessment in vivo. Science 236:324–327, 1987.
4. Almada H, Molteni L, Ferreira R, et al: The value of the echo-doppler in cardiomyoplasty procedures. J Card Surg 6(Suppl):113–118, 1991.
5. Anderson WA, Bridges CR, Chin AJ, et al: Pneumatic aortic counterpulsation powered by a skeletal muscle. Surg Forum 39:276, 1988.
6. Bridges CR Jr, Hammond RL, Anderson DR: Skeletal muscle-powered counterpulsation: A critical overview. In Carpentier A, Chachques JC, Grandjean P (eds): Cardiomyoplasty, Mount Kisco, NY, Futura, pp 227–237, 1991.
7. Bridges CR, Hammond RL, Dimeo F, et al: Functional right heart replacement with a skeletal muscle ventricle. Circulation 80(Suppl III):183–191, 1989.
8. Chachques JC, Grandjean PA, Fischer EC, et al: Dynamic aortomyoplasty to assist left ventricular failure. Ann Thorac Surg 49:225–230, 1990.
9. Chachques JC, Grandjean PA, Schwartz K, et al: Effect of latissimus dorsi dynamic cardiomyoplasty on ventricular function. Circulation 78(Suppl III):203–216, 1988.
10. Chiu RC-J, Walsh GL, Dewar ML, et al: Implantable extra-aortic balloon assist powered by transformed fatigue resistant skeletal muscle. J Thorac Cardiovasc Surg 94:694–701, 1987.

11. Furnary AP, Christlieb IY, Magovern JA, Magovern GJ: A standardized nomenclature for latissimus dorsi cardiomyoplasty. J Card Surg 6:74–79, 1991.
12. Furnary AP, Magovern JA, Christlieb IY, Trumble DR: Improved ventricular augmentation with right latissimus dorsi cardiomyoplasty. Surg Forum 42:307–309, 1991.
13. Furnary AP, Magovern JA, Christlieb IY, et al: Clinical cardiomyoplasty: Preoperative factors associated with outcome. Ann Thorac Surg 1992 (in press).
14. Furnary AP, Magovern JA, Christlieb IY, et al: Component analysis of bilateral anterior cardiomyopathy. Ann Thorac Surg 1992 (in press).
15. Furnary AP, Trumble DR, Vu TQ, et al: Perineural leads and burst stimulation optimize contraction of skeletal muscle. ASAIO Trans 37:M164–M166, 1991.
16. Furnary AP, Vu TQ, Trumble DR, Kao RL: Muscle stimulation and force generation determined by cathode position. FASEB J 5:A1036, 1991.
17. Heckler FR, White MJ: Isolation of skeletal muscle for biomechanical circulatory assist. Semin Thorac Cardiovasc Surg 3:128–131, 1991.
18. Kao RL, Christlieb IY, Magovern GJ, et al: The importance of skeletal muscle fiber orientation for dynamic cardiomyoplasty. J Thorac Cardiovasc Surg 99:134–140, 1990.
19. Kao RL, Trumble DR, Arelt LP, Magovern GJ: Power output of fatigue resistant muscle. FASEB J 5:A1036, 1991.
20. Kao RL, Trumble DR, Magovern JA, et al: Fatigue resistant muscle with preserved force and mass for cardiac assist. J Card Surg 6:210–217, 1991.
21. Li CM, Hill A, Colson M, Desrosiers C, Chiu RC-J: Implantable rate-responsive counterpulsation assist system. Ann Thorac Surg 49:356–362, 1990.
22. Magovern JA, Christlieb IY, Badylak SF, et al: A model of left ventricular dysfunction caused by intracoronary adriamycin. Ann Thorac Surg 53:861–863, 1992.
23. Magovern JA, Furnary AP, Christlieb IY, et al: Bilateral latissimus dorsi cardiomyoplasty. Ann Thorac Surg 52:1259–1265, 1991.
24. Magovern JA, Furnary AP, Christlieb IY, et al: Right latissimus dorsi cardiomyoplasty for left ventricular failure. Ann Thorac Surg 53:1120–1122, 1992.
25. Magovern GJ, Heckler FR, Park SB, et al: Paced skeletal muscle for dynamic cardiomyoplasty. Ann Thorac Surg 45:614–619, 1988.
26. Magovern JA, Magovern GJ Jr, Magovern GJ, et al: Surgical therapy for congestive heart failure: Indications for transplantation versus cardiomyoplasty. J Heart Lung Transplant May/June:1992 (in press).
27. Rochamba G, Desrosiers C, Dewar M, et al: The muscle powered dual chamber counterpulsation: Rheologically superior implantable cardiac assist device. Ann Thorac Surg 45:620–624, 1988.
28. Smith WM: Epidemiology of congestive heart failure. Am J Cardiol 55:3A–8A, 1980.

G. RABAGO, MD, I. GANDJBAKHCH, MD
A. PAVIE, MD, V. BORS, MD
P. CORBI, MD, P. LEGER, MD
J. P. LEVASSEUR, MD, E. VAISSIER, MD
J. SZEFNER, MD, C. & A. CABROL, MD

BRIDGE TO TRANSPLANT WITH THE SYMBION TOTAL ARTIFICIAL HEART

From the Department of Thoracic
    and Cardiovascular Surgery
La Pitié Hospital
Paris, France

Reprint requests to:
G. Rabago, MD
Chirurgie Cardiovasculaire
Hôpital de la Pitié/Salpetriere
47-83, Bld de l'Hôpital
75013 Paris, France

Demikhov[1] was the first surgeon to remove a dog's heart and to replace it with a mechanical device. In 1969 Cooley attempted the first clinical use of a total artificial heart (TAH) as a bridge to transplantation.[2] Technical development of the TAH continued for another 14 years before DeVries implanted the first Jarvik-7 TAH (Symbion Inc., Salt Lake City, UT) in a patient who was mechanically supported for 112 days. Three years later the first successful use of the Jarvik-7 TAH as a bridge to transplantation took place.[3] Since then, the use of the Jarvik-7 TAH has become a clinical reality, and data from clinical trials have identified infection,[4] major organ dysfunction,[5] and misfit of the device[6] as the major causes of support failure.

Our clinical TAH program at Hospital la Pitié began in April 1986. Our current indications for implantation of the TAH include three conditions: (1) patients in chronic endstage cardiac failure who have already been selected for transplantation and are waiting for a donor heart; (2) patients who develop acute heart failure without a potential organ donor; and (3) patients who cannot be weaned from cardiopulmonary bypass (CPB).

SYMBION TAH SYSTEM

Symbion Ventricle

The Symbion ventricle consists of a housing that contains an air-driven intracorporeal diaphragm coated with polyurethane urea. Two

CARDIAC SURGERY: State of the Art Reviews—Vol. 7, No. 2, 1993
Philadelphia, Hanley & Belfus, Inc.

439

Medtronic valves are positioned in the outflow and inflow orifices. Two sizes are available: the Jarvik-7-70, with a stroke volume of 70 cc, and the Jarvik-7-100, with a stroke volume of 100 cc.

Symbion Controller

The Symbion Utah-drive heart controller operates with an internal fixed rate. Three parameters should be assessed before initiating support: heart rate (0–99 beats per minute [BPM]), drive pressure (0–300 mmHg), and percent systole (0–99%). Each console is equipped with two controllers: a primary active controller and a backup. The console also provides for vacuum (0 to –20 mmHg), which is used in case of poor ventricular filling.

A Cardiac Output Monitoring and Diagnostic Unit (COMDU) (Symbion Inc., Salt Lake City, UT) is attached to the Utah-drive system. The COMDU provides continuous estimates of cardiac output for each ventricle based on the airflow returning to the console during diastole. The COMDU displays waveforms for device filling rate as well as driveline pressure.

PATIENT POPULATION AND METHODS

From April 1986 to June 1992 60 patients underwent mechanical circulatory support with the Jarvik-7 TAH as a bridge to cardiac transplantation. Patient age ranged from 18–56 years (average: 39 ± 11 years); only 9 of the patients were women. The main indications for implantation were (1) acute decompensation while waiting for transplantation (n = 21); (2) ischemic disease (n = 20); (3) allograft rejection (n = 5); (4) acute graft failure (n = 4); (5) postoperative failure or patients unable to be weaned from CPB (n = 3); (6) postpartum cardiomyopathy (n = 4); and (7) miscellaneous (n = 3). Criteria for selection of patients are outlined in Table 1.

Patients were divided into two groups based on the type of decompensation. The acute group included patients who presented with sudden decompensation during the 2 weeks before TAH implantation. The chronic group included patients with decompensation of known etiology in whom deterioration occurred over a long period of time.

Because of the urgent conditions under which implantation often occurs, a computed tomogram may not be available; thus selection of the Jarvik-7-70 or the Jarvik-7-100 is based on the patient's size and thoracic dimensions. Since 1988 the Jarvik-7-70 has been selected for the majority of patients; only exceptionally large patients received the Jarvik-7-100. The Jarvik-7 100 was implanted in patients (n = 22) with a body surface area (BSA) >1.8 m² (average: 1.84 ± 0.12 m²), whereas the Jarvik-7 70 was implanted in patients (n = 38) with a smaller BSA (average: 1.78 ± 0.14 m²). In all patients the TAH was implanted in the medial position,[7] which avoids opening the left pleura and does not require excision of the left pericardium.

TABLE 1.   Selection Criteria for Implantation of TAH Jarvik-7

No major contraindication for transplantation
Age <60 years
Cardiac index <2 L/m/m²
Systolic blood pressure <80 mmHg
Pulmonary capillary pressure >20 mmHg
Urine output < 20 ml/h
In spite of optimal drug therapy

SURGICAL TECHNIQUE

Through a median sternotomy[8] the pericardium is opened from the ascending aorta to the diaphragm. First the ventricle drivelines are placed through two separate skin incisions in the left upper quadrant of the abdomen, and a tunnel is formed from the skin incisions to the pericardial cavity. Once the drivelines are perfectly placed, both ventricles are carefully checked. CPB is initiated with two right-angled caval cannulae that are inserted anteriorly and an arterial cannula that is placed into the ascending aorta.

The native heart should be carefully excised to permit subsequent cardiac transplantation. The pulmonary artery and the aorta are transected just above their respective valves. The right and left native ventricles are transected 2-3 cm in length distally to the atrioventricular groove. The coronary sinus ostium and the venous coronary sinus are closed to avoid bleeding.

The anastomosis between the atrial cuffs and the atrioventricular remnants is begun at the cephalic portion of the septum. A double anastomosis is performed, with a simple running suture joining the two cuffs to the remnant septum. Then each cuff is sutured to its respective right and left free ventricular wall. The aortic and pulmonary grafts (7 cm long) are sutured end-to-end to their respective vessels. Before testing the suture line, all anastomoses are supplemented with gelatin resorcin formol (GRF) adhesive. The artificial ventricles are then attached to their corresponding cuffs. After deairing, support is initiated by starting first the left artificial ventricle, then the right artificial ventricle. When the hemodynamics are satisfactory, CPB is stopped.

POSTOPERATIVE CARE

All patients with a TAH are placed in private rooms in the intensive care unit; maximal asepsia is maintained. Cap, mask, boots, and sterile gown are required. Management of patients involves three major aspects: (1) coagulation control, (2) major organ function, and (3) hemodynamic and device control.

Coagulation Control

The complex interaction between blood and the TAH (i.e., the presence of 4 mechanical valves, the large exposure between foreign materials and blood, and the localized turbulent blood flow) requires a systematic and personalized approach to avoid thromboembolic complications.[9] All of our patients are assessed for platelet function, thrombin formation pathways, and fibrinolytic status at least daily (Table 2). Dipyridamole is used to stabilize platelet activity, and aspirin (ASA) is used to lower aggregation. If a pathologic fibrinolytic state is found, aprotinin is given until laboratory data and clinical status are normalized. All mechanisms involved in hemostasis are controlled according to individual need (Table 3).

Major Organ Function

Hepatic and renal function are evaluated with daily determination of biochemical indices. Urine output is calculated every 6 hours from the immediate preoperative period through the first 72 hours after implantation. Daily urine output is monitored thereafter. Renal function is also evaluated by daily determination of serum creatinine and urea. Significant renal dysfunction is defined as urea or creatinine levels over twice the upper normal limit (UNL), oliguria (<240 ml/day), or dialysis.

TABLE 2.   Coagulation Monitoring Checklist

Platelet functions
    Platelet aggregation to ADP, epinephrine, collagen, and arachidonic acid by Born method
    Platelet count, hematocrit
    Platelet aggregate evaluation by Wu-Hoak method
    Ivry-Borchgrevink bleeding time
    Platelet factor 4 (PF-4)
    Beta-thromboglobulin (BTG)

Thrombin Formation and Its Regulatory Pathways
    Prothrombin time
    Activated partial thromboplastin time (APTT)
    Fibrinogen titration
    Thromboelastography recalcified whole blood (TEG)
    Plasma and serum antithrombin III titration
    Calculation of antithrombinic potential (API) as API = plasma ATIII–serum ATIII
    Raby's transfer test on plasma by thromboelastography
    Protein C–protein S–heparin cofactor II

Fibrinolytic system
    Reptilase time
    Fibrinogen degradation products (FDP)
    Alpha-2-antiplasmin (A-2-AP)
    Plasminogen

Hepatic function is assessed by serum levels of total bilirubin, conjugated bilirubin, glutamic oxaloacetic transaminase (GOT), and glutamic pyruvic transaminase (GPT). Significant liver dysfunction is defined as bilirubin levels over twice UNL or levels of alanine aminotransferase (ALT) or aspartate aminotransferase (AST) exceeding 5 times UNL.

Respiratory function is evaluated by blood gas analysis every 3 hours. Intubation and mechanical ventilation are maintained until pulmonary function is satisfactory.

Hemodynamic and Device Control

The Jarvik-7 is driven at a rate of 100 BPM and 55% systole, without diastolic vacuum during weaning from CPB. Left and right drive pressures are adjusted to ensure complete ejection from each ventricle. Changes are made at bedside to stabilize device output and hemodynamics. Hemodynamic performance of the TAH is evaluated by right and left stroke volume, device output, and waveforms recorded in the COMDU. Minute averages of these variables are reviewed every 10 minutes during the first 6 hours after implantation, every 20 minutes during the next 18 hours, and hourly thereafter up to 72 hours. Ventricular driving pressures, percent systole, and diastolic vacuum are reviewed. The average diastolic duration is calculated and used to estimate the average diastolic filling rate. Waveforms of actual ventricular filling are reviewed in each patient for signs

TABLE 3.   Anticoagulation Regimen

Heparin 1000–5000 IU/day IV	*Only when indicated*
Dipyridamole 150–300 mg/6 hr IV	Ticlopidine 250 mg/ 2–3 days
Aspirin 50 mg/day	Fresh frozen plasma
Aprotinin 12,500 KIU/bolus IV, then	Antithrombin III concentrates
500 KIU/min in continuous drip	Blood cell concentrates
Pentoxyphylline 400 mg/day	Fibrogen concentrates

of inflow obstruction. Central venous pressure (CVP) is monitored in the superior vena cava or right atrium, and left atrial pressure (LAP) is measured with a catheter placed during surgery.

TRANSPLANTATION

The mean support period for the entire patient population was 26 ± 81 days. Five patients had <2 days of TAH support (2 received transplants; 3 died of various causes). The remaining patients were supported >6 days (range: 6–602 days).

When the patient with the TAH becomes stable and a suitable donor heart is obtained, orthotopic heart transplantation is performed. The patient is again placed on CPB, and the Jarvik is stopped. The artificial ventricles are disconnected from their atrial and arterial cuffs. The pulmonary artery and aorta are transected distally to the suture lines, and the right and left atrial walls are transected proximal to the suture lines and atrial appendages. Then heart transplantation is performed in the usual fashion.

STATISTICAL ANALYSIS

Student's t-test was used to establish the differences between parameters in the different groups. Discriminating variables were compared with the chi-square test with Yates's correction and Fischer's exact test. A probability (p) <0.05 is considered to be statistically significant. All reported values are expressed as a mean $\pm$ standard deviation.

RESULTS

TAH support was assessed primarily by whether a given patient could restore and maintain adequate end-organ function to be considered for transplantation. Hence, results were analyzed for two groups. Group 1 consisted of patients who could not undergo transplantation and died during TAH support, whereas group 2 consisted of patients who experienced functional recovery and underwent successful transplantation.

Group 1

Thirty-six patients (60%), including 5 women, were unable to undergo transplantation and died during mechanical support. The mean age of group 1 is 41 ± 11 years. Fifty-eight percent (21 patients) were in chronic decompensation before implantation. Twelve patients presented with a primary etiology of coronary artery disease, including 2 with postoperative cardiac failure. Thirteen patients presented with dilated cardiomyopathy (2 postpartum), and 8 needed TAH after transplantation (3 for graft failure, 5 after cardiac rejection).

The BSA of group 1 was 1.78 ± 0.13 m^2; 64% (23 patients) were supported with a Jarvik-7-70. Mean support time for the entire group was 30 ± 102 days; 5 patients were supported > 30 days (Table 4). Mean time for extubation in these patients was 7.3 ± 5.4 days.

Analysis of group 1 shows three main causes of death: (1) progressive deterioration of hemodynamic function associated with multiorgan failure and inability to maintain stable blood pressure in spite of vasoactive drugs (11 patients); (2) untreatable sepsis (9 patients); and (3) pulmonary complications (5 patients) (Table 5).

TABLE 4.   Support Time in Group 1 and Group 2

Time	Group 1	Group 2
1–5 days	5 (14%)	5 (21%)
5–15 days	21 (58%)	12 (50%)
15–30 days	5 (14%)	5 (21%)
>30 days	5 (14%)	2 (8%)

Group 2

Transplantation after TAH support was performed only when the patient's underlying conditions were corrected and stable (24 patients). Four patients (16%) were women. The mean age for group 2 is 36 ± 11 years (range: 19–45 years). Fifteen patients (62%) were in acute decompensation before TAH implantation. The underlying disease was ischemic cardiomyopathy in 10 patients (1 with low cardiac output syndrome after surgery); dilated cardiomyopathy in 12 patients (2 postpartum); graft failure after transplantation in 1 patient; and hypertrophic cardiomyopathy in 1 patient.

BSA was 1.86 ± 0.16 m^2; 16 patients (67%) had a Jarvik-7-70 TAH. The mean period of support was 20 ± 28 days; 50% of patients were supported for 1–2 weeks (Table 4). The mean time for extubation during TAH support was 2.7 ± 1.8 days.

Fourteen patients (58%) in group 2 were discharged from the hospital. Ten patients (42%) died in the hospital after transplantation. The main causes of death were sepsis (3 patients) and multiorgan failure (2 patients).

Comparison Between the Two Groups

Data show that nontransplanted patients were older than transplanted patients, but the difference is not statistically significant. In group 2, 62% of patients presented with acute decompensation compared with 41% in group 1; this difference is statistically significant. The distribution of Jarvik size is the same for both groups. Two parameters are clearly different for groups 1 and 2: (1) BSA is larger in group 2 ($p = 0.001$), and (2) the time for extubation is shorter in group 2 ($p = 0.05$). The support time (excluding patients supported over 31 days) is longer in group 1 than in group 2 (12.3 ± 8 days compared with 9.8 ± 5.4 days) ($p = 0.05$).

Other data were also analyzed. Patients younger than 40 years (n = 30) had a 56% chance of transplantation compared with a 23% chance ($p = 0.001$) for patients older than 40 years. From the entire population, 50% of patients presented with an acute decompensation, of whom 50% (15 patients) underwent

TABLE 5.   Causes of Death During Support

Multiple organ failure	10
Sepsis	9
Pulmonary problems	5
Pneumonia	2
Hemorrhage	1
Emboli	1
Insufficiency	1
Bleeding	3
Device-related	2
Mismatch	1
Others	5

successful transplantation compared with only 23% of patients with chronic decompensation. When the patient population was divided according to BSA, 75% of transplant patients had a BSA <1.8 m^2. The Jarvik-7-70 was used in 67% of patients with BSA <1.8 m^2. Sixty percent of patients had a BSA >1.8 m^2.

Preoperative liver or kidney function or both were considerably impaired in our TAH population. Twenty-two percent had a kidney disorder; 15% had liver failure; and 41% had failure of both organs. Fifty-three percent of patients regained hepatic and renal function during the immediate preoperative period; of these, 75% underwent successful transplantation.

DISCUSSION

Criteria for patient selection to improve transplantation in patients with a TAH remain poorly defined. We compared two groups of patients with a TAH and tried to identify critical parameters for indicating TAH implantation as a bridge to transplantation in patients with endstage cardiac disease. Age, type of decompensation, primary etiology, and BSA have been identified as predictors of successful outcome among patients supported with a TAH.[10,11]

Younger patients were more likely to undergo transplantation than to die during TAH support; however, the difference was not statistically significant. The data also show that patients under the age of 40 years have a higher chance of undergoing transplantation.

The type of decompensation could be considered a risk factor. Patients with chronic decompensation are likely to have more end-organ dysfunction because of the chronicity of their disease. In this respect, however, no difference was found when we compared transplanted with nontransplanted patients. A small but statistically insignificant difference was found when the entire population was classified according to type of decompensation (acute patients had a transplantation rate of 50% vs. 30% in chronic patients).

BSA was the only preoperative variable associated with a significant difference between patients with and without subsequent transplantation. Patients with a large BSA should have a better match between thorax and device, but the rate of successful transplantation in patients with a large BSA did not vary between the 70-ml and the 100-ml TAH (22% vs. 22%). Conversely, patients with a small BSA had poorer results after implantation. These data seem to implicate a poor fit between the TAH and the patient's thorax as a cause of obstruction in systemic or pulmonary venous return. This observation has been noted by some authors as a theoretical explanation of end-organ dysfunction, secondary to an increased pressure in the inferior vena cava.[5]

Preoperative organ disorder appears to be associated with a smaller chance of recovery. Nonetheless, as a result of mechanical support, 53% of patients recovered from hepatic or renal dysfunction after TAH implantation and thus had a higher possibility of transplantation. As other authors have shown, the earliest variable to distinguish patients with subsequent recovery is increased initial postoperative urine output, which correlated directly with renal function recovery.

Nontransplanted patients required longer periods of intubation, which generally indicate primary pulmonary failure or pulmonary failure secondary to multiorgan failure or sepsis, although the Jarvik-7 TAH provides potent respiratory support through the cardiogenic oscillations it generates.[12]

Favorable outcome for patients with TAH support was associated with rapid extubation (3 days) and marked improvement of renal and hepatic function, which provided more favorable conditions for transplantation.

The primary cause of death during TAH support was multiorgan failure (lungs, kidney, and liver).[13] Abnormal flow to the kidney and liver may be the underlying reason. In experiments with the TAH or VADs, high portal vein pressures and pathologic changes in tissues surrounding the hepatic artery were noted.[14] Alterations in abdominal circulation influence passage through the intestinal membrane and permit toxins and bacteria to enter the portal venous system, thus increasing the risks of dysfunction and infection. Lesions found in the necropsic study of these patients showed centrolobular hepatic necrosis with a tubulonephritis syndrome, [15] which is clear evidence of early organ failure.

CONCLUSION

The Jarvik-7 TAH is a powerful device for bridging to transplantation, but patient selection is important to ensure good recovery of end-organ function and successful transplantation. The best indications for a successful TAH bridge are younger age, acute cardiac decompensation, large BSA, and good preoperative end-organ function.

REFERENCES

1. Demikhov VP: Experimental Transplantation of Vital Organs (translated by Basil Haig). New York, Consultant Bureau, 1947, p 212.
2. Cooley DA, Liotta D, Hallman GL, et al: Heart transplantation after use of a total artificial heart. Am J Cardiol 24:723–730, 1969.
3. Copeland JG, Emery RW, Levinson MM, et al: The role of mechanical support and transplantation in treatment of patients with end-stage cardiomyopathy. Circulation 72(Suppl II):7–12, 1985.
4. Griffith BP, Kormos RL, Hardesty RL, et al: The artificial heart: Infection-related morbidity and its effect on transplantation. Ann Thorac Surg 45:409–414, 1988.
5. Kawaguchi AT, Muneretto C, Pavie A, et al: Hemodynamics characteristics of the Jarvik-7 total artificial heart. Circulation (Suppl III):152–157, 1989.
6. Jarvik RK, DeVries WC, Sem B, et al: Surgical positioning of Jarvik-7 artificial heart. J Heart Transplant 5:184–195, 1986.
7. Cabrol C, Solis E, Muneretto C, et al: Orthotopic transplantation after implantation of a Jarvik total artificial heart. J Thorac Cardiovasc Surg 97:342–350, 1989.
8. Solis E, Muneretto C, Cabrol C: Total artificial heart. In Cooper DK, Novitzky D (eds): The Transplantation and Replacement of Thoracic Organs. Dordrecht, Kluwer Academic Publishers, 1990, pp 144–182.
9. Szefner J, Bellon JL, Cabrol C: Coagulation et coeur artificiel. Paris, Masson Ed., 1988.
10. Kawaguchi AT, Cabrol C, Gandjbakhch I, et al: Preoperative risk analysis in patients receiving Jarvik-7 artificial heart as bridge to transplantation. Eur J Cardiothorac Surg 5:509–514, 1991.
11. Kawaguchi AT, Gandjbakhch I, Pavie A, et al: Factors affecting survival in total artificial heart recipients before transplantation. Circulation 82(Suppl IV):322–327, 1990.
12. Rouby JJ, Leger PH, Arthaud M, et al: Respiratory effects of the Jarvik-7 artificial heart. J Appl Physiol 66:1984–1989, 1989.
13. Charbonneau P, Suisse A: Le syndrome de défaillance multiviscérale. Rev Prat Réanimation 40:2329–2336, 1990.
14. Sukehiro, Flameng W: Effects of left ventricular assist for cardiogenic shock on cardiac function and organ blood flow distribution. Ann Thorac Surg 50:374–384, 1990.
15. Chomette G, Auriol M, Louahlia S, et al: Coeur artificiel (Jarvik-7): Conséquences anatomiques. Arch Anat Cytol Pathol 5-6:273–277, 1987.

ROQUE PIFARRÉ, MD; HENRY J. SULLIVAN, MD;
ALVARO MONTOYA, MD; BRADFORD BLAKEMAN, MD;
DAVID B. CALANDRA, MD; MARIA ROSA
COSTANZO-NORDIN, MD; VASSYL LONCHYNA, MD;
THOMAS HINKAMP, MD; JEANINE M. WALENGA, PhD

BRIDGE TO TRANSPLANTATION WITH THE TOTAL ARTIFICIAL HEART: THE LOYOLA EXPERIENCE

From the Department of Thoracic
and Cardiovascular Surgery and
Section of Cardiology
Loyola University Medical Center
Maywood, Illinois

Reprint requests to:
Roque Pifarré, MD
Professor and Chairman
Department of Thoracic and
Cardiovascular Surgery
Loyola University Medical Center
2160 South First Avenue
Maywood, IL 60153

The number of candidates for cardiac transplantation has increased steadily, but the number of donors has not kept pace. The longer the patient remains on the waiting list, the further the condition deteriorates—until eventually the patient fails to respond to the usual medications for treatment of congestive heart failure and cardiac arrhythmias and reaches the point that without some kind of mechanical support, life cannot be prolonged any longer. Intraaortic balloon pumping (IABP) has been the most commonly used method of mechanical support. In many cases IABP is successful in sustaining life until a donor heart becomes available. However, in some cases, despite maximal medical therapy and IABP, the heart continues to fail, and the only possible hope is use of the total artificial heart (TAH) as a bridge. The purpose of the TAH is to stabilize and improve the patient's condition until a donor heart becomes available.

HISTORICAL BACKGROUND

Several methods of mechanical support have been used. In 1978 Reemtsma[14] reported the first successful case of mechanical support as a bridge to transplantation with the IABP. Its ease of insertion and excellent mechanical support have made the IABP the most commonly used method of support. For some patients, however, the

CARDIAC SURGERY: State of the Art Reviews—Vol. 7, No. 2, 1993
Philadelphia, Hanley & Belfus, Inc.

447

support provided by the IABP may not be sufficient; a device that provides greater circulatory support may be necessary for survival. In 1984 Pennington et al.[10] reported the use of extracorporeal membrane oxygenation (ECMO) as a bridge.

In 1969 Cooley et al.[3] reported the first use of an artificial heart as a bridge to transplantation. Although transplantation was successful, the patient died after suffering complications. Cooley reported 3 cases of staged cardiac transplantation in 1982.[2] In 1985 Copeland et al.[4] reported long-term survival of patients who underwent a transplant after implantation of a TAH as a bridge. In 1986 Joyce et al.[8] reported the world experience with clinical use of the TAH. The permanent use of the TAH was reported by DeVries in 1988.[5] The Pittsburgh group[6] reported their experience with the Jarvik-7 in 1987. Cabrol et al. reported their extensive experience in 1989.[1] Encouraged by these reports, the first TAH was implanted at the Loyola University Medical Center in 1988.[11]

THE JARVIK-7 TOTAL ARTIFICIAL HEART

Our experience is based on use of the Jarvik-7-70 and Jarvik-7-100. This TAH consists of two separate prosthetic ventricles connected to an external drive unit by percutaneous tubes. It is pneumatically powered. The ventricles are spherical in shape and made of polyurethane. Pulses of compressed air displace a flexible diaphragm made of Biomer. The prosthetic ventricles are emptied by the motion of the flexible diaphragm. The TAH has four prosthetic valves made by Medtronic to control the direction of the blood flow. The control of cardiac output is based on a variable stroke volume as well as heart rate.

The TAH is a passive filling device that depends on atrial filling pressure to open the inflow valve and collapse the flexible diaphragm. Increases in the atrial filling pressure reduce the diastolic time necessary to fill completely each ventricle. The heart rate, left ventricular drive pressure, and percentage systolic duration are regulated to maintain cardiac output and systemic arterial pressure at levels only slightly greater than the preoperative levels. After the first 24 hours of support, the heart rate and left and right drive-pressure settings require little adjustment.

INDICATIONS

From February 16, 1988 until December 30, 1990, 19 patients underwent placement of the Jarvik-7 TAH as a bridge to transplantation at the Loyola University Medical Center (LUMC) (Table 1). Seventeen (89%) underwent transplantation.

The indications for placement of the TAH were failure to wean from cardiopulmonary bypass in 8 patients (42%) and cardiogenic shock in 11 patients (58%). Sixteen patients (84.2%) had a previous insertion of IABP before the TAH was implanted. One patient (5.2%) had been supported with a left ventricular assist device (Biomedicus, Medtronics, Inc., Minneapolis, MN) before transfer to the LUMC (Table 2). The ages of the patients ranged from 16–64 years (mean: 44 years). Seventeen (89%) were men. Weights ranged from 51–109 kg (mean: 76.7 kg). The Jarvik-7-70 model (70 cc capacity) was used in 18 patients; in the other patient a Jarvik-7-100 (100 cc capacity) was implanted (Table 3).

The diagnosis was ischemic cardiomyopathy in 12 patients (63.3%), dilated cardiomyopathy in 5 (26.3%), myocarditis in 1 (5.2%), and failure of a previously transplanted heart in 1 (5.2%) (Table 1).

The 19 patients were considered candidates for support with the TAH if they could not be weaned from cardiopulmonary bypass despite use of vasopressors and the IABP or if they met the following hemodynamic parameters:

TABLE 1. Jarvik TAH Implantation at LUMC

Patient No.	Age/ Sex	Weight (kg)	Diagnosis	Implanta- tion Date	Implant Duration (days)	Trans- plantation Date	Outcome
1	56/M	72	Ischemic CM	02/16/88	2	02/18/88	Alive
2	52/M	68	Ischemic CM	02/23/88	2	02/25/88	Alive
3	42/M	81	Ischemic CM	02/24/88	8	03/03/88	Died 3/21/88 (acute rejection)
4	62/M	85	Ischemic CM	03/30/88	2	NA	Died 4/1/88 (brain death)
5	58/M	89	Ischemic CM	04/17/88	1	04/18/88	Alive
6	55/M	109	Ischemic CM	04/28/88	34	06/01/88	Died 10/3/88 (CMV and pneumocystis pneumonia)
7	26/M	82	Ischemic CM	06/16/88	10	06/26/88	Died 8/25/89 (chronic rejection)
8	25/F	67	Dilated CM	06/20/88	3	06/23/88	Alive
9	17/M	84	Myocarditis	07/07/88	6	07/13/88	Alive
10	52/M	65	Failure tx heart	08/01/88	17	08/18/88	Alive
11	44/M	84	Ischemic CM	08/03/88	33	09/05/88	Died 9/19/88 (multiple cerebral infarcts)
12	60/F	51	Ischemic CM	08/15/88	5	08/20/88	Died 5/7/89 (sepsis, broncho- pneumonia, multi- organ failure)
13	16/M	61	Dilated CM	10/12/88	2	10/14/88	Alive
14	64/M	56	Dilated CM	11/08/88	14	11/22/88	Alive
15	62/M	81	Ischemic CM	12/14/88	23	01/06/89	Alive
16	25/M	80	Dilated CM	01/05/90	2	01/07/90	Alive
17	19/M	80	Dilated CM	04/03/90	2	04/05/90	Alive
18	43/M	89	Ischemic CM	07/09/90	1	NA	Died 7/10/90 (coagulopathy)
19	59/M	74	Ischemic CM	08/14/90	3	08/17/90	Alive

All patients received Jarvik-7-70, except patient 3, who received Jarvik-7-100. M = male; CM = cardiomyopathy; NA = not applicable; CMV = cytomegalovirus; F = female; tx = transplanted.

TABLE 2. Jarvik TAH: Indications

Indication	No. Patients
Failure to wean from cardiopulmonary bypass	8
Coronary artery bypass grafting (patients 1, 3)	
Coronary artery bypass grafting + valve (patients 7, 12)	
Valve (patient 4)	
Coronary artery bypass grafting, ventricular aneurysm, mapping (patient 11*)	
Ventricular septal defect (patient 19)	
Failed heart transplant (patient 10)	
Cardiogenic shock	11
Ischemic (patients 2, 5, 6*, 18†)	
Dilated cardiomyopathy (patients 8†, 13, 14, 16, 17)	
Myocarditis (patient 9)	
Total	19

* Malignant ventricular arrhythmias.
† Cardiac arrest.

TABLE 3. Jarvik TAH: Characteristics

Size	
Jarvik-7-70	18 patients
Jarvik-7-100	1 patient
Transplants	17 (89.5 %)
Duration of implantation (days)	1–34 (mean: 9.8)

1. Cardiac index <1.8 L/min/m^2
2. Right and/or left atrial pressure >20 mmHg
3. Pulmonary wedge pressure >25 mmHg
5. Systolic arterial pressure <88 mmHg despite maximal medical management with positive inotropic drugs and IABP
5. Oliguria
6. Elevated systemic vascular resistance (SVR)
7. Evidence of decreasing peripheral perfusion

Other factors should also be considered, including the amount of drug support needed to maintain the blood pressure and urinary output as well as the general clinical impression of patient deterioration.

TECHNIQUE OF IMPLANTATION

The chest was entered through a median sternotomy, and the pericardium was opened longitudinally. The patient was placed on cardiopulmonary bypass with bicaval cannulation. The aorta was cross-clamped, and the cardiectomy was performed. Care should be taken to transect the aorta and pulmonary artery just distal to their respective valves to maintain long stumps of native artery for suture of grafts. The atria are transected close to the atrioventricular junction.

The technique of implantation is similar to that described by Jarvik and DeVries,[7] with the following modifications: (1) The cuffs of the TAH are sewn to the native atrial wall, using Teflon felt strips in the atrial side of the suture line as reinforcement, to facilitate hemostasis and to prevent bleeding (Fig. 1). The vascular grafts are sewn to the great vessels. Teflon felt strips are used to reinforce the side of the anastomosis and to prevent bleeding (Fig. 2). (2) After connecting the ventricles to the atrial cuffs, the drivelines are brought out subcostally and connected to the driving unit. The cuffs designed to fit around the tubes connected to the driving unit are eliminated to expedite the passage of the tubes through the chest wall.[13] These cuffs were designed for permanent use of the TAH and not as a bridge. The purpose was to prevent infection with the ingrowth of tissue into the cuffs. In our judgment the driving tubes are no different from the chest tubes inserted for drainage of the mediastinum and chest cavities.

All patients supported with the TAH received broad-spectrum antibiotics for the duration of support. In most cases vancomycin and cefazolin sodium were used. The antibiotics were changed only in response to isolation of organisms in routine cultures.

ANTICOAGULATION

Anticoagulation of the patients began 8–24 hours after the operation was completed and surgical bleeding came under adequate control. Heparin was given intravenously at a rate of 500–1200 U/hr to maintain the activated clotting time (ACT) between 170–200 seconds. The longer the support with the TAH, the higher

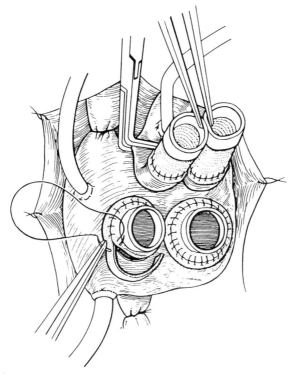

FIGURE 1.   Suturing of the atrial cuffs. Note the use of a strip of Teflon felt on the atrial site to reinforce the suture line.

the required dose of heparin, indicating that the patient was developing some degree of heparin resistance. The heparin was supplemented with 100 mg of dipyridamole every 6 hours.

Our patients and those of other institutions have experienced varying degrees of hemorrhagic complications and occasional thrombotic episodes. To understand further the effect of the TAH on the hemostatic system of this population, we undertook a study to investigate the hemostatic profile of TAH recipients.[15] We evaluated specific plasma and cellular markers of thrombotic, fibrinolytic, platelet, and endothelial function (Tables 4 and 5). Alterations in these variables indicate the initial changes that occur at specific biochemical sites associated with activation of the hemostatic system. These variables appear to demonstrate alternatives in coagulation prior to changes in standard prothrombin time (PT), activated partial thromboplastin time (APTT), and fibrinogen assays. It is now possible to detect not only a hypocoagulable state leading to hemorrhage, but also a hypercoagulable state leading to thrombosis. Clinical use of these hemostatic markers makes possible a more defined diagnosis and thus a more targeted treatment of thrombotic and hemorrhagic disorders of TAH recipients.

In this study of the TAH patient, possible abnormalities that can occur in the components of the hemostatic system were investigated: the platelets, the fibrinolytic system, the coagulation system, and the endothelium. A hypercoagulable state was determined by the increased level of the thrombin-antithrombin (TAT)

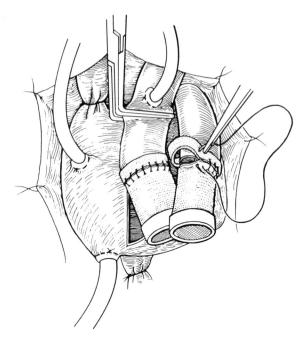

FIGURE 2. Suturing of the graft to the pulmonary artery. The aorta site is reinforced with a strip of Teflon felt.

TABLE 4. Blood Variables Measured

Coagulation System Variables	Fibrinolytic System Variables
Prothrombin time (PT)*	D-dimer
Activated partial thromboplastin time (APTT)*	Fibrinogen degradation products
Fibrinogen*	Fibrin degradation products
Fibrin/fibrinogen split products*	Total degradation products
Factor assays*	Tissue plasminogen activator (TPA)
Thrombin time*	Plasminogen activator inhibitor (PAI)
Bleeding time*	Plasminogen
Antithrombin III (ATIII)	α-2-antiplasmin
Protein C	
Protein S	
Thrombin–antithrombin (TAT) complex	

* Routine clinical order.

TABLE 5. Blood Variables Measured

Platelet Variables	Endothelium Variables	Other Variables
Platelet count*	Tissue plasminogen activator (TPA)	Complete blood count*
Platelet factor 4	Plasminogen activator inhibitor (PAI)	Plasma free hemoglobin*
Thromboxane B_2 (TxB$_2$)	PGF$_{1\alpha}$	
6-keto prostaglandin $F_{1\alpha}$ (PGF$_{1\alpha}$)		

* Routine clinical order.

complex in most patients. The TAT complex forms when thrombin is generated by activation of coagulation. With heparin treatment this interaction is modified. In 2 patients, a lower than average level of TAT complex was observed for several days. One patient sustained a stroke and the other a transient ischemic attack (TIA) after transplantation. Evaluation of the inhibitors of the coagulation cascade revealed low levels of protein C, low levels of antithrombin III (ATIII), and normal levels of protein S in the TAH-supported patients. The low levels of protein C and ATIII should contribute to the development of a hypercoagulable state.

Analysis of the fibrinolytic system with the routine fibrin/fibrinogen split products assay indicated activation of fibrinolysis in all patients at all times. Elevated levels of D-dimer are a clear indication that an organized thrombus has formed and undergone lysis (thrombolysis). Levels of plasminogen and α-2-antiplasmin were decreased only during the early days on the TAH but were normal thereafter. On the other hand, levels of tissue plasminogen activator (TPA) were significantly increased throughout all days on the TAH and levels of plasminogen activator inhibitor (PAI) were slightly elevated.

In several patients, enhanced fibrinolysis was associated with mediastinal bleeding that was treated with reexploration, fresh frozen plasma, and/or cryoprecipitate.

To assess platelet activation, thromboxane B_2 (TxB_2) and platelet factor 4 (PFA) were quantitated. All patients had a high level of TxB_2, a potent platelet-aggregating substance, and extremely high levels of PFA, which may have caused the heparin resistance.

The endothelium of TAH patients was greatly stimulated, as suggested by the higher than normal levels of prostaglandin $F_1\alpha$ ($PGF_1\alpha$), TPA, and PAI, all of which are derived from the vascular endothelium.

All aspects of the hemostatic system appeared to be greatly activated in the TAH-supported patient. The alterations in PT, APTT, ACT, and thrombin time assays were useful to monitor heparin therapy. The factor assays and platelet count were useful to evaluate patients for severe deficiencies that could be treated with blood component therapy. Patients with a TAH should be evaluated not only with the routine coagulation assays but also by more sensitive plasma markers specific for activation of coagulation, fibrinolysis, and platelets. In particular, assays of fibrinogen, TAT, protein C, TPA, PAI, D-dimer, and TxB_2 revealed diagnostically useful information.

CLINICAL RESULTS

The TAH was implanted in 19 patients, but only 17 underwent cardiac transplantation (Table 6). Patient 4, who was transferred to LUMC by airplane, suffered repeated bouts of ventricular fibrillation during transport and was comatose on arrival. Although it was suspected that he may have suffered an irreversible neurologic injury, nevertheless he underwent implantation of the TAH. Two days later he was declared brain dead, and the support was discontinued. Patient 18 deteriorated while awaiting transplantation. He was resuscitated after suffering a cardiac arrest, and the TAH was implanted. After the operation he developed a coagulopathy. He was given platelets, fresh frozen plasma, and cryoprecipitate. He received 66 units of packed red blood cells and was reexplored 3 times. He developed adult respiratory distress syndrome (ARDS) and multiorgan failure, then died 36 hours after implantation.

TABLE 6.   Jarvik TAH: Survival and Mortality

	No. of Patients (%)
Died on TAH	2 (10.5)
Transplantation	17 (89.5)
Early mortality	2 (11.7)
Late mortality	3 (17.6)
1-year survival of patients who underwent transplantation	13/17 (76.5)
Actuarial survival of patients who underwent transplantation	12/17 (70.5)

Two (11.8%) of the 17 patients who underwent cardiac transplantation died within 30 days. Patient 3 died of acute rejection 14 days after transplantation. Patient 11 suffered multiple cerebral infarcts 10 days after transplantation. He became comatose and was declared brain dead. It was suspected that clots formed in the atrial suture line and became loose, resulting in multiple brain embolism.

Three (17.6%) late deaths occurred. Patient 6 died from *Pneumocystis carinii* pneumonia 3 months after transplantation. Patient 7 died from chronic rejection 14 months after transplantation. Patient 12 died 9 months later from bronchopneumonia, sepsis, and multiple organ failure.

At present 12 patients (63%) are alive, with survivals ranging from 2–4½ years after transplantation. Six patients have shown some coronary artery disease on routine angiography. One patient has undergone an angioplasty. All 12 patients are active and rehabilitated (Table 6).

The infectious complications that occurred during the TAH implantation and after transplantation were recently reported.[9] No case of mediastinitis occurred either while the TAH was implanted or after transplantation.

Our results after heart transplantation, comparing mechanically supported versus nonsupported patients, have been previously reported.[12] No significant difference was found between the mechanically supported and nonsupported group in length of stay, 30-day survival rate, or 1-year survival rate.

CONCLUSION

After reviewing our experience with the TAH as a bridge to transplantation and the reports from other centers, we conclude that the purpose of mechanical support is to stabilize and improve the patient's condition until a suitable donor becomes available.

The Loyola experience is based on the implantation of the Jarvik-7 TAH in 19 patients. Seventeen patients were transplanted (89.5%). The 1-year survival has been 76.5% (13 of 17). At present, 12 patients have been alive from 2–4½ years. All 12 patients are active and rehabilitated.

The use of the TAH as a bridge provides excellent support and no longer should be considered experimental. It should be accepted as therapeutic mechanical support for the endstage cardiac patient on the waiting list for a donor.

REFERENCES

1. Cabrol C, Solis E, Muneretto C, et al: Orthotopic transplantation after implantation of a Jarvik total artificial heart. J Thorac Cardiovasc Surg 97:342–350, 1989.
2. Cooley DA: Staged cardiac transplantation: Report of three cases. J Heart Transplant 5:229–235, 1982.

3. Cooley DA, Liolta D, Hallman GL, et al: Orthotopic cardiac prosthesis for two-staged cardiac replacement. Am J Cardiol 24:723–733, 1969.

4. Copeland JG, Emery RW, Levenson MM, et al: The role of mechanical support and transplantation in the treatment of patients with end-stage cardiomyopathy. Circulation 72(Suppl II):7–12, 1985.

5. DeVries WC: The permanent artificial heart: Four case reports. JAMA 25:848–859, 1988.

6. Griffith BP, Hardesty RI, Vormous RL, et al: Temporary use of the Jarvik-7 total artificial heart before transplantation. N Engl J Med 316:130–134, 1987.

7. Jarvik RK, DeVries WC, Bjarre KH, et al: Surgical positioning of the Jarvik-7 artificial heart. J Heart Transplant 5:184–195, 1986.

8. Joyce LD, Johnson EK, Pierco WS, et al: Summary of the world experience with the clinical use of of total artificial hearts as heart support devices. J Heart Transplant 5:229–235, 1986.

9. Lonchyna VA, Pifarré R, Sullivan H, et al: Successful use of the total artificial heart as a bridge to transplantation with no mediastinitis. J Heart Lung Transplant 11:803–811, 1992.

10. Pennington DG, Merjary JP, Codd JE, et al: Extracorporeal membrane oxygenation for patients with cardiogenic shock. Circulation 70:130–137, 1984.

11. Pifarré R, Sullivan H, Montoya A, et al: Cardiac transplantation. Cardiol Clin 1:183–194, 1989.

12. Pifarré R, Sullivan H, Montoya A, et al: Comparison of results after heart transplantation: Mechanically supported versus nonsupported patients. J Heart Lung Transplant 11:235–239, 1992.

13. Pifarré R, Sullivan H, Montoya A, et al: The use of the Jarvik-7 total artificial heart and Symbion ventricular assist device as a bridge to transplantation. Surgery 108:681–685, 1990.

14. Reemtsma K, Kreisin R, Edie R, et al: Cardiac transplantation in patients requiring mechanical circulatory support. N Engl J Med 298:670–671, 1978.

15. Walenga JM, Hoppensteadt D, Fareed J, Pifarré R: Hemostatic abnormalities in total artificial heart patients as detected by specific blood markers. Ann Thorac Surg 53:844–850, 1992.

PRATAP S. KHANWILKAR, MS, MBA
DON B. OLSEN, DVM

FUTURE PROSPECTS FOR A TOTALLY IMPLANTABLE ARTIFICIAL HEART

From the Artificial Heart Research
  Laboratory
Institute for Biomedical
  Engineering
University of Utah
Salt Lake City, Utah

Reprint requests to:
Pratap S. Khanwilkar, MS, MBA
Artificial Heart Research
  Laboratory
Institute for Biomedical
  Engineering
University of Utah
803 North 300 West
Salt Lake City, UT 84103-1414

Totally implantable artificial hearts (TIAHs) will be commercially available for implantation in humans by the first decade of the next century. These devices will save lives until viable alternatives are fully developed by the middle of the next century. Compared with pneumatically powered devices, TIAHs will reduce infection as well as improve patient comfort, mobility, and quality of life because of reduced tethering.

The implantable portion of a TIAH must meet four basic requirements: (1) the blood pump must fit in the space made available by removal of the natural heart; (2) it must provide extremely reliable operation, from an engineering as well as from a surgical perspective; (3) it must be responsive to changing physiologic needs; and (4) it must be energy-efficient so that its total weight and volume as well as its heat dissipation are minimized. If these conditions are not met, the risks of an implantable system far outweigh the advantages. Fulfilling these requirements is the ultimate goal of a TIAH system.

Precisely when we will reach the goal of implanting a TIAH in a human and what types of devices will be widely used are unknown. Predicting the future in any field is risky at best. Predicting the future prospects for the TIAH is even more so, because environmental (legal and regulatory, financial, technologic, and societal) factors will have as much, if not more, impact on eventual use as will supply and demand.

CARDIAC SURGERY: State of the Art Reviews—Vol. 7, No. 2, 1993
  Philadelphia, Hanley & Belfus, Inc.

457

This chapter focuses on the need for, and supply of, TIAHs, and discusses the effects of environmental factors on the future prospects of the TIAH.

THE NEED FOR LONG-TERM MECHANICAL CIRCULATORY ASSISTANCE

Cardiovascular disease, the leading cause of death in the U.S. and other developed countries, has also become the major cause of adult death in developing countries.[7] The widespread use of long-term mechanical circulatory support systems (MCSSs) can alleviate this problem and prolong life. Although the precise need for MCSSs cannot be determined, the potential annual need for such devices in the U.S. has been estimated by three studies[1,14,40] (Table 1).

Estimate of the National Institutes of Health

The estimate of the National Institutes of Health (NIH)[40] was derived from a population-based study of Olmsted County, Minnesota, where the complete medical records of all residents were available. The study cautions that the data derived from several thousand deaths (from all causes) cannot be extrapolated to the national level because of the low confidence level and doubt about the representativeness of the sample. Nevertheless, the NIH review of death certificates for Olmsted County for the period 1979–1983 identified residents who died between the ages of 15 and 69 years. A review panel decided whether each patient would have been a candidate for a totally implantable MCSS.

The results for Olmsted County were compared with similar average figures obtained for the U.S. population during the same 5-year period. If one assumes that 14% of U.S. citizens who die of heart disease between the ages of 15 and 69 are potential MCSS candidates, then the annual market for MCSSs in the U.S. is 35,000.

This study underestimates need in at least three ways: (1) Because not all critically ill heart patients die suddenly, a MCSS may also be used in patients who would survive without the device. (2) Because full information on contraindications might not be available in acutely ill patients, the tendency will be to err in the direction of implanting a device. (3) The extrapolation of 14% of persons dying from heart disease as potential MCSS candidates from Olmsted County to the entire U.S. probably lowers the estimate. However, the estimate also errs in the opposite direction by presupposing general availability, access, and acceptance of MCSSs.

The Kidder-Peabody Estimate

The Kidder-Peabody analysis[1] estimates that 236,000 people who die annually from cardiac disease in the hospital are potential MCSS candidates. Their estimate is based on the breakdown of deaths due to cardiovascular disease in 1986 and on whether or not the patient was able to reach a hospital. Unlike the

TABLE 1. Annual Estimated Need for MCSSs

Study/Author	Year Published	Annual Need in the U.S.
National Institutes of Health	1985	35,000–75,000
Kidder-Peabody Equity Research	1988	236,000
Institute of Medicine	1991	35,000–70,000 (up to 200,000)

NIH estimate, this analysis includes no demographic data. The potential market is identified as patients with acute myocardial infarction (AMI) who reached the hospital but died. Including *all* patients with AMI in this category overestimates the demand. On the other hand, the Kidder-Peabody estimate ignores people who suffer from congestive heart failure.

Estimate of the Institute of Medicine

The estimate of the Institute of Medicine (IOM)[14] coincides with the earlier NIH estimate for MCSS candidates for the primary patient group, i.e., those with the greatest need. However, if the TIAH is at least as efficacious as a transplanted heart, the IOM estimates that a secondary group of about 200,000 patients annually will become potential recipients by the year 2020.

One can conclude that the IOM and NIH analyses give a conservative estimate of MCSS demand ($\sim$35,000/year), whereas the Kidder-Peabody estimate sets an upper bound on the annual demand ($\sim$236,000/year).

TRENDS

We estimate that factors increasing the number of potential recipients of MCSSs (increasing population, an increasing proportion of adults, and the epidemiologic transition of developing countries from infectious and parasitic diseases to cardiovascular diseases and cancer[36]) will slightly edge out factors tending to decrease the number. These factors, including prevention of heart disease through proper diet, exercise, and reduction of smoking, also may postpone the onset of heart disease, thus increasing the mean age of the target population. The onset of other diseases at an advanced age would diminish the positive effect of an MCSS.

On the other hand, demographic trends will increase the number of potential recipients as the population of the U.S. (and the world) increases and ages.[42] The world's population is projected to increase from the present 5.5 billion people to about 8 billion before 2005. Current estimates place the number of people aged 60 years or more at about 490 million. This number is expected to be 612 million by the year 2000.

The baby-boom generation in the U.S. will be between 35 and 55 years of age when TIAHs are predicted to hit the market between the years 2001 and 2010. People in this age group with cardiac disease will be prime candidates for MCSSs. Although attention has been focused on the U.S. market, Canada, England and Wales, Germany, and other European countries "have high enough mortality rates from coronary heart disease, as well as large enough populations, to produce a group of potential MCSS users of sufficient magnitude to warrant consideration"[10] in estimating the need for devices.

ALTERNATIVES TO THE TIAH

The alternatives to the TIAH are discussed according to the time-frame in which they are projected to be available. A category of alternatives exists now, another category is still under development, and a third will be provided by different kinds of MCSSs.

Present Alternatives

Present alternatives for the MCSS fall into three major categories: (1) heart transplants, (2) xenografts, and (3) drug therapy.

Heart Transplants. The number of transplants has remained relatively stable because of the lack of acceptable donor hearts: 3054 transplants were performed worldwide in 1990 and 2764 in 1991.[17,22] The number of heart transplants is not expected to grow significantly because of the severe lack of supply.

Xenografts. This procedure uses the hearts of related primates such as baboons as donors for heart transplantation. A xenograft may serve as a bridge to transplant, as a temporary ventricular assist device, or as a permanent heart replacement in infants and neonates.[3] Potential advantages include availability, low cost, and ease of application; risks include host immunosuppression, anticoagulation, and rejection. Only four such procedures have been performed to date.[17] This procedure has been extremely controversial[5] because it crosses the interspecies boundary and because animal rights activists have taken a stand against it.[9] Thus we expect that the procedure will never be widely accepted and will not become a viable alternative to long-term MCSSs.

Drug Therapy. Positive inotropic drugs, especially phosphodiesterase-III (PDE-III) inhibitors such as amrinomone, milrinone, and enoximone, are proving to be increasingly effective in treating heart failure.[11,35] These drugs need to be administered intravenously for a limited period of time (about 2 weeks), after which the natural heart recovers some of its function. Moreover, ACE inhibitors such as captopril and enalapril, which previously have been used to treat hypertension and heart failure, have recently proved to be effective as preventive therapy in patients with mild heart problems.[37]

Thus new uses will continue to be found for already known drugs. Conversely, new drugs will continue to be discovered to reduce the effects of heart attack and heart failure. We expect that the use of drug therapy will continue to grow in the future. This technology has proved to be effective in the short term, but long-term effectiveness in treatment of heart failure is uncertain.

Alternatives Currently Under Development

In addition to available procedures, two other potential categories of alternatives are still in the embryonic stages of development or conceptualization: (1) cardiomyoplasty and (2) genetically engineered devices and techniques.

Cardiomyoplasty. This novel technique, still in the exploratory research stage, involves supporting a damaged heart with skeletal muscle tissue from the patient's body.[6] Through appropriate training by electrical stimulation, the muscle adapts itself to contract at a higher rate and with a greater force than skeletal muscle and acquires many of the characteristics of myocardial tissue.

In a successful procedure, the latissimus dorsi is used after its origin is surgically removed. The muscle is wrapped around either the native ventricle, an artificial ventricle, or a section of the aorta replaced with elastic material. The muscle is then electrically stimulated, probably with a pacemaker, to contract in synchrony with the native heart. This technique provides partial assistance to the heart on a permanent basis.

Because it requires a pacemaker or a similar device as well as additional surgical intervention to access and train the muscle, cardiomyoplasty will be comparable in cost with implanting an MCSS. Long-term usefulness is currently limited. However, extensive development of the concept is presently pursued by at least five companies: Eli Lilly, Cordis, Medtronic, Siemens A.G., and Abiomed. We expect that cardiomyoplasty will be validated by the end of this decade, but widespread clinical use is not likely before 2010.

Genetically Engineered Devices and Techniques. Genetic engineering, using a technique called "antisense," has provided a way to stop the clogging of arteries in animals.[4] This technology reportedly will be used to prevent or reduce the reclogging of arteries in patients who have previously undergone coronary bypass surgery or angioplasty.

Continuing advances such as these make us believe that the future of artificial circulatory support lies in this technology. Whether genetically engineered TIAHs will be obtained by growing replacement hearts or by using fetal tissues to repair failing hearts, we do not know yet; no specific work has started. We expect such work to begin in another 10 years, after which it will take at least 20 years before the concept can be demonstrated and tested extensively. Because of bioethical and social considerations, a genetically engineered method to replace or augment the failing heart's long-term function is not likely to be available commercially until after the year 2025.

Permanently Implantable MCSSs

The restrictions and limitations of present technology and the extended time frames for the development of other technology leave a window of opportunity for permanently implantable MCSSs from now until about 2025, after which their use will diminish with advances in the above technologies and therapies. We expect that by 2050 viable alternatives to a TIAH will have been found and that their use will be discontinued thereafter.

Permanently implantable MCSSs can be classified into two major categories: (1) ventricular assist devices (VADs) and (2) TIAHs. A perennial source of debate is the proportion of potential MCSS recipients who will need VADs as compared to TIAHs. Cited proportions of potential MCSS recipients needing TIAHs range from 15–25% up to 78%.[12]

Ventricular Assist Devices. VADs supplement the function of the natural heart, typically only the left ventricle, instead of replacing it. Therefore they must occupy additional space within the body. VADs are further along in their development than TIAHs because of earlier and more extensive NIH funding. Currently, only Thermo-Cardio Systems Inc. (TCI, Woburn, MA) is conducting clinical trials of totally implantable VADs; Novacor (Novacor Division, Baxter HealthCare, Oakland, CA) has voluntarily withdrawn its device from NIH-sponsored clinical trials. In 1995 NIH plans to sponsor the development of next-generation VADs, which will incorporate the latest technology into their designs and presumably will be developed at a similar rate as the TIAHs.

Totally Implantable Artificial Hearts. A TIAH replaces the natural ventricles. Therefore it fits better within the human chest and reduces the compression of surrounding tissue, particularly the lungs, as compared with a VAD. A TIAH can have hard failures (i.e., its inability to pump leads to the death of a patient), whereas failure of a VAD can be soft (i.e., failure does not necessarily result in death). However, if a device, be it a TIAH or a VAD, stops for more than a few minutes, activation of the coagulation cascade would render moot this apparent advantage of a VAD over a TIAH.

SUPPLY

Development of artificial hearts has been ongoing since 1957. Since 1964 the effort has been financed primarily by the federal government through the Devices and Technology Branch of the National Heart, Lung, and Blood Institute.

TABLE 2. Key Features of NIH-funded TIAHs

Developer	Drive Mechanism	Number of Stages and Methods of Energy Conversion	Longest Animal Survivor
Penn State University/Sarns3M	Roller-screw pusher plate	2 (electromagnetic, mechanical)	350 days
Abiomed Inc./Texas Heart Institute	Electrohydraulic centrifugal flow pump with rotary valve	2 (electromagnetic, hydraulic)	5 days
Cleveland Clinic Foundation/ Nimbus Inc.	Electrohydraulic gear pump with magnetically-coupled pusher plate	4 (electromagnetic, hydraulic, magnetic, mechanical)	45 days
University of Utah	Electrohydraulic reversing axial flow pump	2 (electromagnetic, hydraulic)	102 days+

Currently, four major efforts for development of a TIAH are funded by contracts from the NIH until September 1993. The major features of these four devices are listed in Table 2.

Overall progress in these 6-year efforts has been good.[19,20,23,39] The Penn State team has recently demonstrated the long-term in vivo viability of a totally implantable system with a 118-day animal survivor. The other three groups are also progressing toward integrating their systems; in vivo results range from good to poor. All four systems aim to satisfy the same functional requirements. Key differences are primarily related to valves used to control the direction of blood flow in the artificial ventricle, which are either mechanical (Penn State, Cleveland Clinic, University of Utah) or bio-prosthetic (Abiomed) and to blood-contacting materials (Biomer, Angioflex, Biolon, Biolyzed surface), which are either polyurethanes or polyurethanes coated with a gel surface.

The choice of drive mechanism and its control primarily dictates the number of moving parts, the anatomic fit of the device, reliability, and power efficiency. Pusher-plate systems (Penn State, Cleveland Clinic Foundation) need to be oriented in a fixed way to the blood sacs. This restriction does not apply to the electrohydraulically driven systems (University of Utah, Abiomed), which take advantage of hydraulic fluid conduits to improve their anatomic fit by positioning drive mechanisms in a convenient location. However, the electrohydraulically driven systems, especially the axial flow pump used by the University of Utah, consume more power as the reversing, high-speed (15,000 rpm) axial flow pump is nonlinear over its range of operation. To function reliably, the motor bearings need to be well designed. Abiomed uses a unidirectional centrifugal pump, with a rotary valve to switch the direction of fluid flow. In addition, ventricular filling during diastole is either passive—i.e., without any driving force on the blood sac (Penn State, Cleveland Clinic Foundation)—or active—i.e., the drive mechanism pulls on the blood sac during diastole (Utah, Abiomed). Therefore, the choice of drive mechanism affects not only the engineering performance of the system, but also available methods of physiologic control. This choice implicitly defines trade-offs between key performance parameters such as fit, reliability, and efficiency.

Different physiologic control methods and philosophies also cause significant differences in device design and performance. Cardiac output is varied either by changing both stroke volume and heart rate (Penn State, Cleveland Clinic) or by changing heart rate alone (Abiomed, University of Utah) while operating each ventricle in a full-fill, full-eject mode. Philosophies of physiologic control range from relative sensitivity to preload and insensitivity to afterload[6] to the opposite scenario, with sensitivity reversed.[38]

Fluid imbalance between the systemic and pulmonary sides of the circulation is caused by the left-to-left shunt (especially in the bronchial circulation), by the greater losses of stroke volume (from valve leakage and ventricular compliance in an MCSS) in the left ventricle, and by the inertial passthrough of fluid in the right ventricle.[36] Unless corrected, this problem can quickly lead to pulmonary edema and death. Fluid imbalance is peculiar to the TIAH because in VADs, even when used for biventricular assistance, each ventricle can be driven independently to provide different cardiac outputs.

Significantly different methods are followed by each group to solve the problem of fluid imbalance. The basic tenet is to reduce the stroke volume of the artificial right ventricle as compared with the left ventricle. The most common approach is use of volume-displacement chambers (Penn State, Cleveland Clinic Foundation, Abiomed), which allow partial volume decoupling of the left and right ventricles and thus result in slightly different stroke volumes. Both Penn State and the Cleveland Clinic use a large volume-displacement chamber that is slightly larger than the device stroke volume (about 65–70 cc) to allow completely passive filling of one ventricle while the other is being pumped. Abiomed's volume-displacement chamber is small (about 20 cc) and shunts a small amount of hydraulic fluid away from the right ventricle during every stroke, thus reducing its effective stroke volume in comparison with the left ventricle. In addition to the volume-displacement chamber, Penn State uses a pulmonic valve with greater leakage than the aortic valve. The University of Utah device uses an interatrial shunt (IAS) designed as an orifice between the two artificial atrial cuffs to achieve fluid balance.[18,29] The IAS acts as an atrial septal defect, and more blood flows from the left atrium to the right atrium (~8–10 cc/stroke) than in the reverse direction (~3–5 cc/stroke).

Many features and components are common to all four devices, including pulsatile pumping of blood, like the natural heart. Unlike the natural heart, however, they pump blood in a counterpulsatile manner. The natural heart is in left and right systole (diastole) at approximately the same time; when these devices are in left (right) systole, they are also in right (left) diastole.

Device developers strive to incorporate the latest or the most reliable technology into their designs. All flexing membranes used to pump the blood are made of polyurethanes. The internal electronics are miniaturized with hybrid circuit and surface-mount technology. All four devices use a 3-phase, brushless, direct current motor, which is the most reliable and the most commonly available. To eliminate wires passing through the skin, electrical energy is transmitted transcutaneously with radio frequency waves. Implantable packaging technology is borrowed from the pacemaker and defibrillator industries. Implantable rechargeable batteries presently use the widely-available nickel–cadmium chemistry. Although they do not provide the required 45 minutes of daily operation for the lifetime of the TIAH, this limitation of battery technology does not curb TIAH development.

In addition to the NIH-funded TIAH developers, other entities, both in the U.S. and abroad, are developing artificial hearts (Table 3). Some of these researchers are also developing continuous-flow TIAHs and VADs. Continuous-flow pumps appear promising and may have significant advantages over traditional pulsatile pumps.[30]

TABLE 3. Other Major Centers Worldwide Developing TIAHs/VADs

Research Center	Industrial Partner/Sponsor	MCSS Being Developed
In-house	Jarvik Research Institute, NY	TIAH, VAD
Milwaukee Heart Institute, Milwaukee, WI	Bradley Foundation, Milwaukee, WI	TIAH
Texas Heart Institute, Houston, TX	Aerospatiale and Sagem, Paris, France	TIAH
Baylor College of Medicine, Houston, TX	Nikkiso Co. Ltd. & American Biomed, Tokyo, Japan and the Woodlands, TX	TIAH
Free University of Berlin, Berlin, Germany	Mercedes-Benz Inc., Stuttgart, Germany	TIAH
Seoul National University, South Korea	Government of South Korea	TIAH
University of Tokyo, Tokyo, Japan	Unknown	TIAH
National Cardiovascular Research Center, Osaka, Japan	Government of Japan	TIAH, VAD
University of Kyoto, Kyoto, Japan	Unknown	TIAH
Institute for Transplantation and Artificial Organs, Moscow, USSR	Government of USSR	TIAH
University of Vienna, Vienna, Austria	Unknown	TIAH
University of Bologna, Bologna, Italy	Sorin Biomedica, Saluggia (Vercelli), Italy	TIAH, VAD
University of Utah/Ottawa Heart Institute	None	VAD

In our opinion, the TIAH developers funded by NIH are currently at least 5 years ahead of other developers. The complexity of the TIAH and of its related testing requirements (in animals and later in human clinical trials, with intense regulatory scrutiny) ensures a long period of development before the devices can be marketed. Developers who have been in the field for a longer period of time are at a distinct advantage because they are further ahead on the steep learning curve of development than those who have recently entered the field.

In a recently completed review of NIH's TIAH program, IOM recommended continued support for an interim period of 3 years.[14] Recent plans announced by the NIH[28] suggest that four TIAHs will be funded for phase 1 development for 3 years after 1993; two designs will be selected for phase 2 funding in 1996 with an eye toward testing of device readiness. This testing phase will last until 2000, after which clinical trials will begin. The challenges to be tackled in phase 1 (October 1993–September 1996) will cover improvements in device design, system integration, further in vitro and in vivo testing, reliability, cost, and production issues. Phase 2 (October 1996–September 2000) will focus on in vivo testing, rigorous and statistically valid bench testing of system reliability, and preparation for approval by the Food and Drug Administration (FDA). After phase 2, NIH probably will end its role as a funder of TIAH development. It will expect the private sector to fund the marketing and commercialization of such devices.

A major challenge posed by the long periods of time required to take such complex devices from concept to market is the obsolescence of components. The TIAH designs need to be flexible and modular to accommodate advances in technology.

ENVIRONMENTAL EFFECTS

Factors such as the legal and regulatory environment, the finances and costs of TIAH technology, advances in technology, and societal solutions to ethical and moral dilemmas posed by the use of TIAHs will influence the eventual availability of a TIAH more so than the supply of and the need for such devices.

Regulatory and Legal Effects

Regulatory. Medical devices have been regulated since the Medical Devices Amendments of 1976. The passage of the Safe Medical Devices Act of 1990 increased the regulatory burden by requiring of device manufacturers the following: user reports, distributor reports, device tracking, reports of removal and correction of defects, and market surveillance.[16] In addition, the FDA was granted substantial authority for device recall and marketing suspension. Violators are now liable for civil penalties. Since the passage of this act, and with the hiring of Dr. David Kessler as its head, the FDA has shifted its role toward more enforcement. This attitude, coupled with limited FDA budgets, has slowed down the approval for new devices considerably over the last 2 years.[15]

In FDA parlance, a TIAH is a class III device, i.e., a life-sustaining device the failure of which would cause death. A class III device is the most heavily regulated and has to meet substantially higher standards of testing and documentation than devices in the two lower classes. The requirements of this regulatory classification system are taxing and will slow entry into the marketplace.

If TIAHs had existed before 1976 or if their design and usage were substantially equivalent to devices made before then, it would be much easier to obtain FDA approval for clinical trials and marketing. Unfortunately, because TIAHs are new and innovative, the FDA requires detailed and extensive applications for investigational device exemption (IDE) to allow clinical trials and for pre-market approval (PMA) to allow marketing. Thus the present regulatory environment prolongs the time-to-market and increases the developmental costs of TIAHs. These regulations pose an additional hurdle, but they will not stop the eventual widespread clinical use of TIAHs.

Legal. Companies that supply TIAH developers with key polymers (Dow Corning, Johnson & Johnson, and DuPont) are not only withdrawing materials from clinical settings, but have also stopped their supply at the prototype stage of TIAH development.[8,25,27] The primary reason is the legal exposure that the companies face for such a small segment of their business; i.e., dollar sales of their materials to TIAH developers will be low even when TIAHs are commercialized. Sales levels do not justify risking bankruptcy by exposure to lawsuits and juries that award huge payments to prosecutors.

The withdrawal of materials from use in medical devices is a systemic trend. Unless U.S. liability laws are changed by Congress, it is unlikely that any TIAH will be available for commercial use in the U.S. U.S. developers may be able to find foreign suppliers for key materials, to persuade U.S. manufacturers to let them use their materials for sale overseas, or to establish manufacturing and marketing relationships with non-U.S. firms for worldwide sales and distribution of TIAHs.

The two trends of increased regulation and withdrawal of key materials, primarily for legal reasons, constitute a major barrier to the introduction of TIAHs into the U.S. marketplace.

Financial Effects

Containment of health-care costs is on the national agenda. The forecast of lackluster growth for U.S. economy, ranging from a low of 1.5% to a high of 2.9% in gross national product (GNP) throughout the rest of this century,[34] will lead to even greater emphasis on cost-containment, especially in health care. The TIAH is a curative therapy, not a preventive one; pressure on TIAH developers to cut the life-cycle costs of such devices will be enormous. Prioritization of health-care expenses, as demonstrated by the Oregon experiment[21] but rejected by the federal government, will reduce the access of prospective patients to this technology.

The NIH estimated that the total cost of the device, its implantation, and an average of 4.5 years of follow-up is $150,000 (in 1983 dollars).[41] This estimate calculates to an annual societal expense ranging from 5.25 to 15 billion dollars. Costs are comparable to those for a number of already-established life-saving medical procedures (dialysis, cardiac transplantation, liver transplantation, bone marrow transplant, psychotic disorders, burn treatments) that represent the current state of medical and surgical technology.[41]

The IOM recently analyzed the cost-effectiveness of TIAHs.[13] This analysis normalized estimated life-cycle costs with quality-adjusted life years (QALY) to derive a figure of merit for comparing various cardiac assist and replacement technologies. The IOM estimated that TIAH technology was more expensive than cardiac transplantation. However, the analysis of cardiac transplantation assumed adequate availability of donor organs to meet the projected need. Moreover, the analysis apparently neglected the fact that TIAHs are further behind in their development cycle than both VADs and cardiac transplants. A valid comparison would use a figure of merit for all three technologies at the same stage of development. The IOM study does note that if the quality of the developed TIAH increases, so will its use and the recipient's quality of life.

Nevertheless, pressure on TIAH developers to reduce cost is enormous. Advances in design and manufacturing materials and techniques should enable us to meet the challenge of making an affordable TIAH. At the behest of the IOM, NIH will again evaluate TIAH technology in 1996 to determine if it will continue to fund development.

Technologic Effects

Technologic trends are accelerating the pace of development of TIAHs. Advances in TIAH development are mostly driven by successful incorporation of advances in different and varied technologies. Enabling technologies include:[32]

Materials

1. Lighter and stronger plastics, polymers, and composite materials with better biocompatibility, manufacturability, and reliability
2. Surface engineering (modifications of existing materials to improve biocompatibility by bonding or by changing surface topology and texture) and surface coatings (using chemical vapor deposition, thermally sprayed coatings, plasma coating, or ion implantation)
3. Metallic alloys, ceramics, and composites
4. Magnetic materials with increased energy densities that will lead to smaller and lighter motors as well as improve the anatomic fit of the device.

Electronics

Trends in electronics will provide greater functionality in a smaller physical circuit size, improved accuracy and reliability of components, and development of reliable real-time and miniaturized sensors for pressure, position, and blood gas analysis.

1. Power electronics, with advances to improve device efficiency and reduce generated heat

2. Microprocessors/microcontrollers with higher processing speeds to facilitate functionality and flexibility in design and performance

3. Microelectromechanical systems with smaller and more reliable sensors and actuators as well as more precise processing of materials and manufacturing techniques.

Imaging

Imaging technologies help designers to visualize and to measure with increased accuracy the dynamics of the TIAH during both in vitro and in vivo tests, including blood flow and real-time TIAH dynamics. Technologies such as positron emission tomography; magnetic resonance imaging; lasers; high-speed, high-resolution cameras; and infrared thermometry will drive advances in this area.

Manufacturing and Process Technologies

Manufacturing will be a focus of economic growth for the rest of the decade. It has been targeted as an area of national attention to enable the U.S. to keep its position as the world's preeminent economic power. The Omnibus Trade and Competitiveness Act of 1988 changed the mission of the National Institute of Standards and Technology, giving it the additional task of helping industry move products into the marketplace more rapidly. This act included the establishment of regional centers for the transfer of manufacturing technologies. Most high-technology industries in the U.S. now realize the importance of world-class manufacturing in delivering value-added goods to customers.

Improved manufacturing processes (including technologies for rapid product development) will enhance greatly the reliability and reduce the cost of TIAHs. Technologies and processes such as flexible manufacturing and rapid prototyping (including stereolithography) will either reduce the total investment needed to manufacture TIAHs or increase the speed at which desired changes can be incorporated into TIAH designs. Increasing computerization of the entire produce life-cycle—from idea generation, product definition, and product design stages to product prototyping stage and even during the manufacturing stage—will further increase the rate at which better TIAH designs can be developed.

Faster and easier-to-use computers will make a variety of simulation technologies available to improve TIAH design. Simulation software now makes use of advances in graphic user interfaces and menu-driven point-and-click computers to allow greater access to this technology. Simulation decreases the short-term efficiency of making a particular TIAH design, but it makes the design more effective by allowing experimentation with alternative designs and algorithms before actually building and testing a prototype.

Communication, People, and Management

The rate of TIAH development depends greatly on the ability of professionals with widely different fields of expertise to communicate effectively. The growing availability of generalists with expertise in the two areas of medicine and engineering greatly facilitates this process. In addition, the increasing attention paid to assurance of quality and reliability, along with availability of individuals trained in these areas, enhances development of the TIAH.

Societal and Ethical Effects

Social acceptance of the TIAH will greatly influence its use. The device will experience reduced use if the public perceives the technology to be risk-free and expects it to work perfectly all the time. For its own best interests, the medical device industry should educate the public on the potential risks and realities of using its products. Informed consent and advance directives are two processes that have been refined to improve communication with patients and their families.

Some potential patients may view death as an acceptable alternative to any kind of device intervention. However, survivors who have been on temporary MCSSs, as well as their spouses, have been found to be in good psychological condition after MCSS implantation.[24,33]

Ethical issues related to regular TIAH use include access, nondiscriminatory criteria for patient selection, and reduction of overall costs to society. The previous use of permanent as well as temporary MCSSs has generated extensive debate and criticism in various quarters.[2,24] Issues center on cost and affordability, patient selection, and use of the artificial heart experiments as a publicity tool.[2] However, we raise these issues only as points for debate. Device developers and manufacturers, ethicists, sponsors, clinicians, nurses, potential patients and their families, legislators and regulators, health insurers, and lay people must exchange ideas and share and solve the concerns of everyone involved in MCSS implantations.

As a result of continued dialogue, general guidelines will be developed to select and to educate potential patients and to pay for MCSS implantations.

CONCLUSIONS

Cardiac support and replacement devices will clearly satisfy an identified need worldwide. Some, if not most, patients with cardiac failure will need TIAHs for long-term survival (≥ 5 years). Excellent progress has been made by TIAH developers. Technologic trends will improve the quality of the TIAHs currently under development and lead to innovative and yet unknown methods of reliably pumping blood.

However, regulatory and legal burdens imposed on the development of TIAHs may slow the availability of such devices in the U.S. Probably TIAHs that eventually will be in clinical use worldwide will originate and be developed in the U.S. but will be manufactured and marketed by companies based elsewhere.

REFERENCES

1. Alon R: Cardiac assist devices: An emerging life-saving technology. Kidder Peabody Equity Research Industry Report, October 18, 1988.
2. Annas GJ: Made in the U.S.A.: Legal and ethical issues in artificial heart experimentation. Law Med Health Care 14:164–171, 1988.
3. Bailey LF: Biologic versus bionic heart substitutes: Will xenotransplantation play a role? ASAIO Trans 33:51–53, 1987.
4. Bishop JE: Genetic technique antisense is shown to bar clogging of arteries in animals. Wall Street J Sept 3:B2, 1992.
5. Bailey LF: Another look at cardiac xenotransplantation. J Cardiac Surg 5:210–218, 1990.
6. Chiu RCJ (ed): Biomechanical Cardiac Assist: Cardiomyoplasty and Muscle-powered Devices. Mount Kisco, NY, Futura Publishing, 1986.

7. Division of Epidemiological Surveillance and Health Situation and Trend Assessment: Global Estimates for Health Situation Assessment and Projections—1990. Geneva, World Health Organization, 1990, pp 14–15, 34–35.
8. Fancher JA: Personal communication to Dr. Don Olsen, Market Manager, Dow Plastics, March 13, 1992.
9. Francione GL: Xenografts and animal rights. Transplant Proc 22:1044–1046, 1990.
10. Funk M: Epidemiology of End-Stage Heart Disease. Appendix D. The Artificial Heart: Prototypes, Policies, and Patients. The Institute of Medicine, 1991, pp 258–259.
11. Haustein KO: Review: Therapeutic concepts of congestive heart failure. Inter J Clin Pharmacol Ther Toxicol 28:273–281, 1990.
12. Hogness JR, VanAntwerp M (eds): The Artificial Heart: Prototypes, Policies, and Paitents. Washington, DC, The Institute of Medicine, National Academy Press, 1991, pp 78–79.
13. Hogness JR, VanAntwerp M (eds): The Artificial Heart: Prototypes, Policies, and Patients. Washington, DC, The Institute of Medicine, National Academy Press, 1991, pp 107–120, 262–283.
14. Hogness JR, VanAntwerp M (eds): The Artificial Heart: Prototypes, Policies, and Patients. Washington, DC, The Institute of Medicine, National Academy Press, 1991, pp 4–5.
15. Ingersoll B: FDA attacked for holding up medical devices. Wall Street J Sept 8:B1, B4, 1992.
16. Kahan JS: The Safe Medical Devices Act of 1990. Med Device Diag Ind January 1991, pp 66–71, 154.
17. Kaye MP: The Registry of the International Society for Heart and Lung Transplantation: 9th Official Report—1992. J Heart Lung Transplant 1992, 11(Part 1):599–601, 1992.
18. Khanwilkar PS, Kinoshita M, Hansen AC, et al: An inter-atrial shunt used to balance the output of an electrohydraulic total artificial heart: Chronic in vivo results. Proc 13th Ann Inter Conf IEEE Eng Med Biol Soc 13:2085–2086, 1991.
19. Khanwilkar P, Olsen DB, Hoeppner DW, et al: Progress made in the 4th year of development of a totally implantable electrohydraulic total artificial heart. Proc Cardiovasc Sci Technol Conf 1991, p 175.
20. Kiraly R, Butler K, Masseillo A, et al: Development progress on the E4T completely implantable total artificial heart. Proc Cardiovasc Sci Technol Conf 1991, p 176.
21. Kitzhaber J: A healthier approach to health care. Issues Sci Technol Winter:59–65, 1990–1991.
22. Kriett JM, Kaye MP: The Registry of the International Society for Heart and Lung Transplantation: 8th Official Report—1991. J Heart Lung Transplant 10:491–495, 1991.
23. Kung RV, Yu LS, Ochs B, et al: Development of an electrohydraulic total artificial heart. Proc Cardiovasc Sci Technol Conf 1991, p 177.
24. Levine RJ: Mechanical circulatory support systems: Ethical considerations. Transplant Proc 22:969–970, 1990.
25. Lilenfeld R: Letter to Ethicon customers, Director, Suture Technologies, Ethicon Inc., May 29, 1992.
26. Lioi AP, Orth JL, Crump KR, et al: In-vitro development of automatic control for the actively filled electrohydraulic heart. Artif Organs 12:152–162, 1988.
27. Miller BT Jr: Personal communication to Dr. Don Olsen, Business Strategy Manager, DuPont Fibers, Inc., July 1, 1992.
28. National Heart, Lung, and Blood Institute: Decade of artificial heart research planned. HLB Newsletter 28 May 1992, pp 76–77.
29. Olsen DB, Long JW: Simplified right-left balance for the implanted artificial heart. In Akutsu T, Koyanagi H (eds): Artificial Heart 3: Heart Replacement. Tokyo, Springer Verlag, 1991, pp 235–243.
30. Olsen DB, Wampler RK: Continuous blood-flow pumps with internal and external motors. Proceedings of the International Workshop on Rotary Blood Pumps, 1988, pp 8–17.
31. Phillips DR: Health and Health Care in the Third World. Hong Kong, Longman Developmental Studies, Longman Group UK Limited, 1990, pp 31–58.
32. Rosenberg G: Technological opportunities and barriers in the development of mechanical circulatory support systems, Appendix C. In Hogness JR, VanAntwerp M (eds): The Artificial Heart: Prototypes, Policies, and Patients. Washington, DC, National Academy Press, 1991, pp 211–250.
33. Ruzevich SA, Swartz MT, Reedy JE, et al: Retrospective analysis of the psychologic effects of mechanical circulatory support. J Heart Transplant 9:209–211, 1990.
34. Saunders NC: The U.S. economy into the 21st century. Month Labor Rev 114:13–31, 1991.
35. Schlepper M, Thormann J, Kremer P, et al: Present use of positive inotropic drugs in heart failure. J Cardiovasc Pharmacol 14(Suppl 1):S9–S19, 1989.
36. Tanaka T, Takatani S, Umezu M, et al: Factors affecting left-right output differences in artificial heart implanted animals. ASAIO Trans 31:211–215, 1985.

37. Tanouye E: ACE-inhibitors found to cut coronary risks. Wall Street J Sept 3:B1–B2, 1992.
38. Weiss WJ, Rosenberg G, Snyder AJ, et al: Permanent circulatory support systems at the Pennsylvania State University. IEEE Trans Biomed Eng 37:138–145, 1990.
39. Weiss WJ, Rosenberg G, Snyder A, et al: Progress made in the development of the Penn State implantable total artificial heart. Proc Cardiovasc Sci Technol Conf 1991, p 178.
40. Working Group on Mechanical Circulatory Support of the National Heart, Lung, and Blood Institute: Artificial Heart and Assist Devices: Directions, Needs, Costs, Societal and Ethical Issues. U.S. Department of Health and Human Services, Public Health Service, National Institutes of Health, NIH Publ No. 85-2723, May 1985, pp 15–17.
41. Working Group on Mechanical Circulatory Support: Artificial Heart and Assist Devices: Directions, Needs, Costs, Societal and Ethical Issues. National Heart, Lung, and Blood Institute, May 1985, pp 19–20.
42. World Health Organization: Global Estimates for Health Situation Assessment and Projections—1990. World Health Organization Report, 1990, pp 1–3.

INDEX

Entries in **boldface type** indicate complete chapters.